W9-BSV-098

Pulmonary Physiology

Seventh Edition

Michael G. Levitzky, PhD
Professor of Physiology, Anesthesiology, and Cardiopulmonary Science
Louisiana State University Health Sciences Center
New Orleans, Louisiana

Adjunct Professor of Pediatrics and Physiology
Tulane University Medical Center
New Orleans, Louisiana

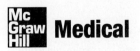 **Medical**

New York   Chicago   San Francisco   Lisbon   London   Madrid   Mexico City
Milan   New Delhi   San Juan   Seoul   Singapore   Sydney   Toronto

Pulmonary Physiology, Seventh Edition

2 3 4 5 6 7 8 9 0 DOC/DOC 0 9 8 7

Previous editions copyright © 2003, 1999, 1995, 1991, 1986, 1982 by The McGraw-Hill Companies, Inc.

ISBN-13: 978-0-07-143775-2
ISBN-10: 0-07-143775-4
ISSN: 1540-7764

Notice

Medicine is an ever-changing science. As new research and clinical experience broaden our knowledge, changes in treatment and drug therapy are required. The author and the publisher of this work have checked with sources believed to be reliable in their efforts to provide information that is complete and generally in accord with the standards accepted at the time of publication. However, in view of the possibility of human error or changes in medical sciences, neither the author nor the publisher nor any other party who has been involved in the preparation or publication of this work warrants that the information contained herein is in every respect accurate or complete, and they disclaim all responsibility for any errors or omissions or for the results obtained from use of the information contained in this work. Readers are encouraged to confirm the information contained herein with other sources. For example and in particular, readers are advised to check the product information sheet included in the package of each drug they plan to administer to be certain that the information contained in this work is accurate and that changes have not been made in the recommended dose or in the contraindications for administration. This recommendation is of particular importance in connection with new or infrequently used drugs.

This book was set in Adobe Garamond by International Typesetting and Composition.
The editors were Jason Malley and Karen G. Edmonson.
The production supervisor was Sherri Souffrance.
The cover designer was Mary McKeon.
The text was designed by Eve Siegel.
Printed by RR Donnelley.

This book is printed on acid-free paper.

International Edition: ISBN-13: 978-0-07-110468-5; ISBN-10: 0-07-110468-2
Copyright © 2007. Exclusive rights by The McGraw-Hill Companies, Inc., for manufacture and export. This book cannot be re-exported from the country to which it is assigned by McGraw-Hill. The International Edition is not available in North America.

Contents

Preface

The seventh edition of *Pulmonary Physiology* has been thoroughly updated. New figures have been added to help students visualize concepts more clearly and learn the material more effectively. New references have been added to the end of each chapter. It has been more than 25 years since *Pulmonary Physiology* was first published. The book is now older than many of the students reading it!

Perhaps the greatest pleasure associated with the first six editions has been receiving the many favorable comments and suggestions made by students, readers, and colleagues, and I have used many of these suggestions in the preparation of this new edition.

This book is intended to be used both as an introductory text for beginning students and as a review for residents and fellows in such fields as internal medicine, anesthesiology, pediatrics, and pulmonary medicine. Students who have studied the text should be able to review for licensure and certification examinations by concentrating on the figures, key concepts, tables, and appendices, which summarize nearly all of the material in the book.

My goal in writing this book is to provide first-year medical students (as well as respiratory therapy, nursing, nurse-anesthesia, and other students) with a solid background in the aspects of pulmonary physiology essential for an understanding of clinical medicine. My approach is to encourage self-sufficiency not only in studying pulmonary physiology for the first time but also in understanding the basic concepts of pulmonary physiology well enough to apply them with confidence to future patients.

I believe that the ways to accomplish this are to inform the reader of the goals of each chapter with clearly stated learning objectives, to give detailed and complete explanations of physiologic mechanisms and demonstrate how they apply to pathologic states, and to give the reader a means of self-testing by providing clinical problems and pulmonary function test data to interpret.

The challenge is to write a book that students can read without difficulty in the limited amount of time allocated to pulmonary physiology in the typical curriculum. The material must be presented in a way that discourages memorization without real comprehension, because only those students who understand the basic mechanisms are able to apply them to new situations. The result of this approach should be a book that covers the essentials of the respiratory system as concisely as possible yet raises no questions in students' minds without answering them. I hope that I have achieved these goals in writing this book.

I would like to thank the many people whose comments have helped me revise the various editions of the book including my colleagues in respiratory physiology and pulmonary medicine, my colleagues at LSU Health Sciences Center and Tulane University School of Medicine, as well as my students and readers. For this edition I give special thanks to Drs. Andy Pellett of Louisiana State University

Health Sciences Center and C. William Davis of the University of North Carolina at Chapel Hill School of Medicine. I would also like to thank everyone who has helped me prepare the manuscripts, illustrations, and proofs including my many editors at McGraw-Hill. For this edition, I would especially like to thank Betsy Giaimo, and my wife Elizabeth. Finally, very special thanks to Gail and Jim Miller of Baton Rouge, Louisiana for taking us in after Hurricane Katrina and making us feel at home for eight months.

This book is dedicated to Robert S. Alexander.

Michael G. Levitzky

Function & Structure of the Respiratory System

Most of the tissues of the body require oxygen to produce energy, so a continuous supply of oxygen must be available for their normal functioning. Carbon dioxide is a by-product of this aerobic metabolism, and it must be removed from the vicinity of the metabolizing cells. The main functions of the respiratory system are to obtain oxygen from the external environment and supply it to the cells and to remove from the body the carbon dioxide produced by cellular metabolism.

The respiratory system is composed of the lungs, the conducting airways, the parts of the central nervous system concerned with the control of the muscles of respiration, and the chest wall. The chest wall consists of the muscles of respiration—such as the diaphragm, the intercostal muscles, and the abdominal muscles—and the rib cage.

FUNCTIONS OF THE RESPIRATORY SYSTEM

 The functions of the respiratory system include gas exchange, acid-base balance, phonation, pulmonary defense and metabolism, and the handling of bioactive materials.

Gas Exchange

The exchange of carbon dioxide for oxygen takes place in the lungs. Fresh air, containing oxygen, is inspired into the lungs through the conducting airways. The forces needed to cause the air to flow are generated by the respiratory muscles, acting on commands initiated by the central nervous system. At the same time, venous blood returning from the various body tissues is pumped into the lungs by the right ventricle of the heart. This mixed venous blood has a high carbon dioxide content and a low oxygen content. In the pulmonary capillaries, carbon dioxide is exchanged for oxygen. The blood leaving the lungs, which now has a high oxygen content and a relatively low carbon dioxide content, is distributed to the tissues of the body by the left side of the heart. During expiration, gas with a high concentration of carbon dioxide is expelled from the body. A schematic diagram of the gas exchange function of the respiratory system is shown in Figure 1–1.

Other Functions

ACID-BASE BALANCE

In the body, increases in carbon dioxide lead to increases in hydrogen ion concentration (and vice versa) because of the following reaction:

$$CO_2 + H_2O \rightleftharpoons H_2CO_3 \rightleftharpoons H^+ + HCO_3^-$$

The respiratory system can therefore participate in acid-base balance by removing CO_2 from the body. The central nervous system has sensors for the CO_2 and the hydrogen ion levels in the arterial blood and in the cerebrospinal fluid that send information to the controllers of breathing. Acid-base balance is discussed in greater detail in Chapter 8; the control of breathing is discussed in Chapter 9.

PHONATION

Phonation is the production of sounds by the movement of air through the vocal cords. Speech, singing, and other sounds are produced by the actions of the central nervous system controllers on the muscles of respiration, causing air to flow through the vocal cords and the mouth. Phonation will not be discussed in detail in this book.

PULMONARY DEFENSE MECHANISMS

Each breath brings into the lungs a small sample of the local atmospheric environment. This may include microorganisms such as bacteria, dust, particles of silica or asbestos, toxic gases, smoke (cigarette and other types), and other pollutants. In addition, the temperature and humidity of the local atmosphere vary tremendously.

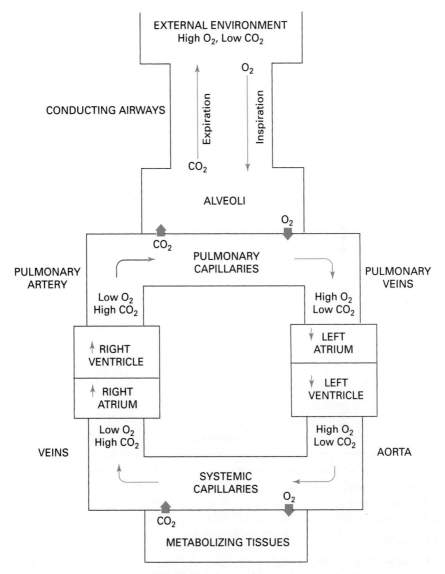

Figure 1–1. Schematic representation of gas exchange between the tissues of the body and the environment.

The mechanisms by which the lungs are protected from these environmental assaults are discussed in Chapter 10.

PULMONARY METABOLISM AND THE HANDLING OF BIOACTIVE MATERIALS

The cells of the lung must metabolize substrates to supply energy and nutrients for their own maintenance. Some specialized pulmonary cells also produce substances necessary for normal pulmonary function. In addition, the pulmonary capillary endothelium contains a great number of enzymes that can produce, metabolize, or modify naturally occurring vasoactive substances. These metabolic functions of the respiratory system are discussed in Chapter 10.

STRUCTURE OF THE RESPIRATORY SYSTEM

Air enters the respiratory system through the nose or mouth. Air entering through the nose is filtered, heated to body temperature, and humidified as it passes through the nose and nasal turbinates. These protective mechanisms are discussed in Chapter 10. The upper airways are shown in Figure 10–1. Air breathed through the nose enters the airways via the nasopharynx and through the mouth via the oropharynx. It then passes through the glottis and the larynx and enters the tracheobronchial tree. After passing through the conducting airways, the inspired air enters the alveoli, where it comes into contact with the mixed venous blood in the pulmonary capillaries.

The Alveolar-Capillary Unit

The *alveolar-capillary* unit is the site of gas exchange in the lung. The alveoli, traditionally estimated to number about 300 million in the adult (a recent study calculated the mean number of alveoli to be 480 million), are almost completely enveloped in pulmonary capillaries. There may be as many as 280 billion pulmonary capillaries, or approximately 500 to 1000 pulmonary capillaries per alveolus. The result of these staggering numbers of alveoli and pulmonary capillaries is a vast area of contact between alveoli and pulmonary capillaries—probably 50 to 100 m^2 of surface area available for gas exchange by diffusion. The alveoli are about 200 to 250 μm in diameter.

Figure 1–2 is a scanning electron micrograph of the alveolar-capillary surface. Figure 1–3 shows an even greater magnification of the site of gas exchange.

The alveolar septum appears to be almost entirely composed of pulmonary capillaries. Red blood cells (erythrocytes) can be seen inside the capillaries at the point of section. Elastic and connective tissue fibers, not visible in the figure, are found between the capillaries in the alveolar septa. Also shown in these figures are the pores of Kohn or interalveolar communications.

THE ALVEOLAR SURFACE

The alveolar surface is mainly composed of a single thin layer of squamous epithelial cells, the type I alveolar cells. Interspersed among these are the larger cuboidal type II alveolar cells, which produce the fluid layer that lines the alveoli. Although there are about twice as many type II cells as there are type I cells in the human lung, type I cells cover 90% to 95% of the alveolar surface, because the average type I cell has a much larger surface area than the average type II cell does. The alveolar surface fluid layer is discussed in detail in Chapter 2. A third cell type, the free-ranging phagocytic alveolar macrophage, is found in varying numbers in the extracellular lining of the alveolar surface. These cells patrol the alveolar surface and phagocytize inspired particles such as bacteria. Their function is discussed in Chapter 10.

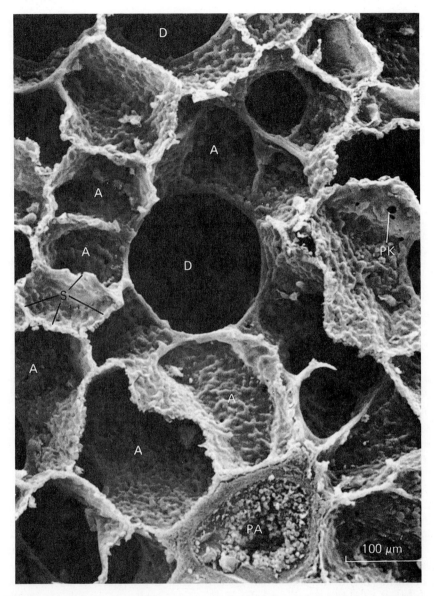

Figure 1–2. Scanning electron micrograph of human lung parenchyma. A = alveolus; S = alveolar septa; D = alveolar duct; PK = pore of Kohn; PA = small branch of the pulmonary artery. (Reproduced, with permission, From Weibel, 1998.)

THE CAPILLARY ENDOTHELIUM

A cross section of a pulmonary capillary is shown in the transmission electron micrograph in Figure 1–4. An erythrocyte is seen in cross section in the lumen of the capillary. Capillaries are formed by a single layer of squamous epithelial cells

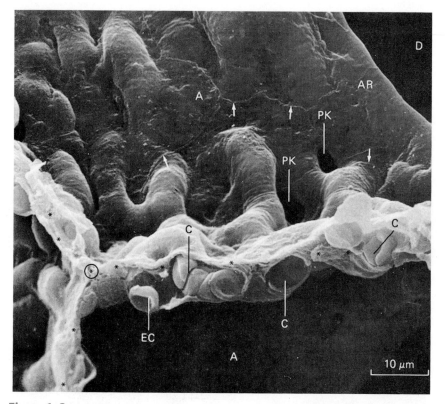

Figure 1–3. Scanning electron micrograph of the surface and cross section of an alveolar septum. Capillaries (C) are seen sectioned in the foreground, with erythrocytes (EC) within them. A = alveolus; D = alveolar duct; PK = pore of Kohn; AR = alveolar entrance to duct; * = connective tissue fibers. The encircled asterisk is at a junction of three septa. (Reproduced with permission from Weibel, 1998.)

that are aligned to form tubes. The nucleus of one of the capillary endothelial cells can be seen in the micrograph.

The barrier to gas exchange between the alveoli and pulmonary capillaries can also be seen in Figure 1–4. It consists of the alveolar epithelium, the capillary endothelium, and the interstitial space between them. Gases must also pass through the fluid lining the alveolar surface (not visible in Figure 1–4) and the plasma in the capillary. The barrier to diffusion is normally 0.2 to 0.5 μm thick. Gas exchange by diffusion is discussed in Chapter 6.

The Airways

After passing through the nose or mouth, the pharynx, and the larynx (*the upper airways*), air enters the tracheobronchial tree. Starting with the trachea, the air may pass through as few as 10 or as many as 23 *generations,* or branchings, on its

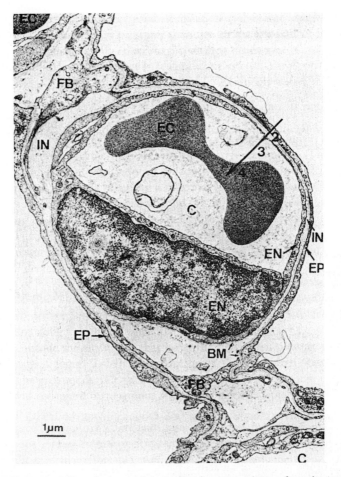

Figure 1–4. Transmission electron micrograph of a cross section of a pulmonary capillary. An erythrocyte (EC) is seen within the capillary. C = capillary; EN = capillary endothelial cell (note its large nucleus); EP = alveolar epithelial cell; IN = interstitial space; BM = basement membrane; FB = fibroblast processes; 2,3,4 = diffusion pathway through the alveolar-capillary barrier, the plasma, and the erythrocyte, respectively. (Reproduced with permission from Weibel, 1970.)

way to the alveoli. The branchings of the tracheobronchial tree and its nomenclature are shown in Figure 1–5. Alveolar gas exchange units are denoted by the U-shaped sacs.

The first 16 generations of airways, the *conducting zone,* contain no alveoli and thus are anatomically incapable of gas exchange with the venous blood. They constitute the *anatomic dead space,* which is discussed in Chapter 3. Alveoli start to appear at the 17th through the 19th generations, in the respiratory bronchioles, which constitute the *transitional zone.* The 20th to 22nd generations are lined with

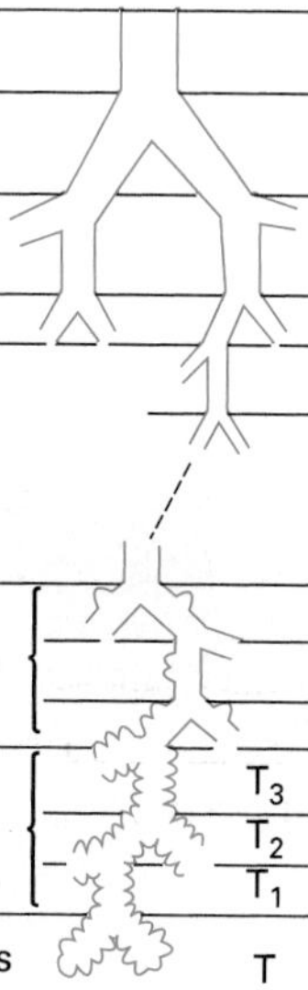

Generation			Diameter, cm	Length, cm	Number	Total cross-sectional area, cm²
trachea		0	1.80	12.0	1	2.54
bronchi		1	1.22	4.8	2	2.33
		2	0.83	1.9	4	2.13
		3	0.56	0.8	8	2.00
bronchioles		4	0.45	1.3	16	2.48
		5	0.35	1.07	32	3.11
terminal bronchioles		16	0.06	0.17	6 × 10⁴	180.0
respiratory bronchioles		17				
		18				
		19	0.05	0.10	5 × 10⁵	10³
alveolar ducts	T₃	20				
	T₂	21				
	T₁	22				
alveolar sacs	T	23	0.04	0.05	8 × 10⁶	10⁴

Left margin labels: Conducting zone; Transitional and Respiratory zones

Figure 1–5. Schematic representation of airway branching in the human lung with approximate dimensions. (Figure after Weibel, 1963. Data from Bouhuys, 1977. Reproduced with permission.)

alveoli. These *alveolar ducts* and the *alveolar sacs,* which terminate the tracheo-bronchial tree, are referred to as the *respiratory zone.*

The portion of lung supplied by a primary respiratory bronchiole is called an *acinus.* All of the airways of an acinus participate in gas exchange. The numerous branchings of the airways result in a tremendous total cross-sectional area of the distal portions of the tracheobronchial tree, even though the diameters of the individual airways are quite small. This can be seen in the table within Figure 1–5.

STRUCTURE OF THE AIRWAYS

The structure of the airways varies considerably, depending on their location in the tracheobronchial tree. The trachea is a fibromuscular tube supported ventrolaterally by C-shaped cartilage and completed dorsally by smooth muscle. The cartilage of the large bronchi is semicircular, like that of the trachea, but as the bronchi enter the lungs, the cartilage rings disappear and are replaced by irregularly shaped cartilage plates. They completely surround the bronchi and give the intrapulmonary bronchi their cylindrical shape. These plates, which help support the larger airways, diminish progressively in the distal airways and disappear in airways about 1 mm in diameter. By definition, airways with no cartilage are termed *bronchioles.* Because the bronchioles and alveolar ducts contain no cartilage support, they are subject to collapse when compressed. This tendency is partly opposed by the attachment of the alveolar septa, containing elastic tissue, to their walls, as seen in Figure 1–2 and shown schematically in Figure 2–18. As the cartilage plates become irregularly distributed around distal airways, the muscular layer completely surrounds these airways. The muscular layer is intermingled with elastic fibers. As the bronchioles proceed toward the alveoli, the muscle layer becomes thinner, although smooth muscle can even be found in the walls of the alveolar ducts. The outermost layer of the bronchiolar wall is surrounded by dense connective tissue with many elastic fibers.

THE LINING OF THE AIRWAYS

The entire respiratory tract, except for part of the pharynx, the anterior third of the nose, and the respiratory units distal to the terminal bronchioles, is lined with ciliated cells interspersed with mucus-secreting goblet cells and other secretory cells. The ciliated cells are pseudostratified columnar cells in the larger airways and become cuboidal in the bronchioles. In the bronchioles, the goblet cells become less frequent and are replaced by another type of secretory cell, the Clara cell. The ciliated epithelium, along with mucus secreted by glands along the airways and the goblet cells and the secretory products of the Clara cells, constitutes an important mechanism for the protection of the lung. This mechanism is discussed in detail in Chapter 10.

The Muscles of Respiration & the Chest Wall

The muscles of respiration and the chest wall are essential components of the respiratory system. The lungs are not capable of inflating themselves—the force for this inflation must be supplied by the muscles of respiration. The chest wall must be intact and able to expand if air is to enter the alveoli normally. The interactions among the muscles of respiration and the chest wall and the lungs are discussed in detail in the next chapter.

The primary components of the chest wall are shown schematically in Figure 1–6. These include the rib cage; the external and internal intercostal muscles and the diaphragm, which are the main muscles of respiration; and the lining of the chest wall, the visceral and parietal pleura. Other muscles of respiration include the abdominal muscles, including the rectus abdominis; the parasternal intercartilaginous muscles; and the sternocleidomastoid and scalenus muscles.

The Central Nervous System & the Neural Pathways

Another important component of the respiratory system is the central nervous system. Unlike cardiac muscle, the muscles of respiration do not contract spontaneously. Each breath is initiated in the brain, and this message is carried to the respiratory muscles via the spinal cord and the nerves innervating the respiratory muscles.

Spontaneous automatic breathing is generated by groups of neurons located in the medulla. This medullary respiratory center is also the final integration point for influences from higher brain centers; for information from chemoreceptors in the blood and cerebrospinal fluid; and for afferent information from neural receptors in the airways, joints, muscles, skin, and elsewhere in the body. The control of breathing is discussed in Chapter 9.

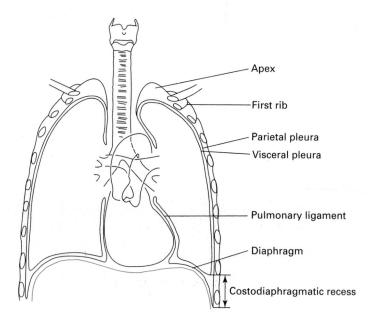

Figure 1–6. The primary components of the chest wall. (Reproduced with permission from Weibel, 1998.)

KEY CONCEPTS

1 The main function of the respiratory system is the exchange of oxygen from the atmosphere for carbon dioxide produced by the cells of the body.

2 Other functions of the respiratory system include participation in the acid-base balance of the body, phonation, pulmonary defense, and metabolism.

SUGGESTED READINGS

Bouhuys A. *The Physiology of Breathing.* New York, NY: Grune & Stratton; 1977:26–42.

Dormans JAMA. Morphology, function and response of pulmonary type I cells: a review. *Inhal Toxicol.* 1996;8:521–536.

Netter FH. The Ciba Collection of Medical Illustrations, vol 7: *Respiratory System.* Summit, NJ: Ciba; 1979:3–43.

Ochs M, Nyengaard JR, Jung A, Knudsen L, Voight M, Wahlers T, Richter J, Gundersen HJG. The number of alveoli in the human lung. *Am J Respir Crit Care Med.* 2004;169:120–124.

Weibel ER. *Morphometry of the Human Lung.* Berlin, Germany: Springer-Verlag; 1963.

Weibel ER. Morphometric estimation of pulmonary diffusion capacity, I. Model and method. *Respir Physiol.* 1970;11:54–75.

Weibel ER, Taylor CR. Functional design of the human lung for gas exchange. In Fishman AP et al, eds. *Pulmonary Diseases and Disorders.* 3rd ed. New York, NY: McGraw-Hill; 1998:21–61.

Mechanics of Breathing

OBJECTIVES

The reader understands the mechanical properties of the lung and the chest wall during breathing.

▶ *Describes the generation of a pressure gradient between the atmosphere and the alveoli.*

▶ *Describes the passive expansion and recoil of the alveoli.*

▶ *Defines the mechanical interaction of the lung and the chest wall, and relates this concept to the negative intrapleural pressure.*

▶ *Describes the pressure-volume characteristics of the lung and the chest wall, and predicts changes in the compliance of the lung and the chest wall in different physiologic and pathologic conditions.*

▶ *States the roles of pulmonary surfactant and alveolar interdependence in the recoil and expansion of the lung.*

▶ *Defines the functional residual capacity (FRC), and uses his or her understanding of lung–chest wall interactions to predict changes in FRC in different physiologic and pathologic conditions.*

▶ *Defines airways resistance and lists the factors that contribute to or alter the resistance to airflow.*

▶ *Describes the dynamic compression of airways during a forced expiration.*

▶ *Relates changes in the dynamic compliance of the lung to alterations in airways resistance.*

▶ *Lists the factors that contribute to the work of breathing.*

▶ *Predicts alterations in the work of breathing in different physiologic and pathologic states.*

Air, like other fluids, moves from a region of higher pressure to one of lower pressure. Therefore, for air to be moved into or out of the lungs, a pressure difference between the atmosphere and the alveoli must be established. If there is no pressure gradient, no airflow will occur.

Under normal circumstances, inspiration is accomplished by causing alveolar pressure to fall below atmospheric pressure. When the mechanics of breathing are being discussed, atmospheric pressure is conventionally referred to as 0 cm H_2O, so lowering alveolar pressure below atmospheric pressure is known as *negative-pressure breathing*. As soon as a pressure gradient sufficient to overcome the resistance to airflow offered by the conducting airways is established between the atmosphere and the alveoli, air flows into the lungs. It is also possible to cause air to flow into the lungs by raising the pressure at the nose and mouth above alveolar pressure. This *positive-pressure ventilation* is generally used on patients unable to generate a sufficient pressure gradient between the atmosphere and the alveoli by normal negative-pressure breathing. Air flows out of the lungs when alveolar pressure is sufficiently greater than atmospheric pressure to overcome the resistance to airflow offered by the conducting airways.

GENERATION OF A PRESSURE GRADIENT BETWEEN ATMOSPHERE & ALVEOLI

During normal negative-pressure breathing, alveolar pressure is made lower than atmospheric pressure. This is accomplished by causing the muscles of inspiration to contract, which increases the volume of the alveoli, thus lowering the alveolar pressure according to Boyle's law. (See Appendix II: The Laws Governing the Behavior of Gases.)

$$P_1 V_1 = P_2 V_2$$

Passive Expansion of Alveoli

 The alveoli are not capable of expanding themselves. They only expand passively in response to an increased distending pressure across the alveolar wall. This increased *transmural pressure gradient,* generated by the muscles of inspiration, further opens the highly distensible alveoli and thus lowers the alveolar pressure. The transmural pressure gradient is conventionally calculated by subtracting the outside pressure (in this case, the intrapleural pressure) from the inside pressure (in this case, the alveolar pressure).

Negative Intrapleural Pressure

The pressure in the thin space between the visceral and parietal pleura is normally slightly subatmospheric, even when no inspiratory muscles are contracting. This *negative intrapleural pressure* (sometimes also referred to as *negative intrathoracic pressure*) of −3 to −5 cm H_2O is mainly caused by the mechanical interaction between the lung and the chest wall. At the end of expiration, when all the respiratory muscles are relaxed, the lung and the chest wall are acting on each other in opposite directions.

 The lung is tending to *decrease* its volume because of the *inward* elastic recoil of the distended alveolar walls; the chest wall is tending to *increase* its volume because of its *outward* elastic recoil. Thus the chest wall is acting to hold the alveoli open in opposition to their elastic recoil. Similarly, the lung is acting by its elastic recoil to hold the chest wall in. Because of this interaction, the pressure is

 negative at the surface of the very thin (about 10 to 30 μm in thickness at normal lung volumes), fluid-filled pleural space, as seen on the left in Figure 2–1. There is normally no gas in the intrapleural space, and the lung is held against the chest wall by the thin layer of serous intrapleural liquid, estimated to have a total volume of about 15 to 25 mL in the average adult.

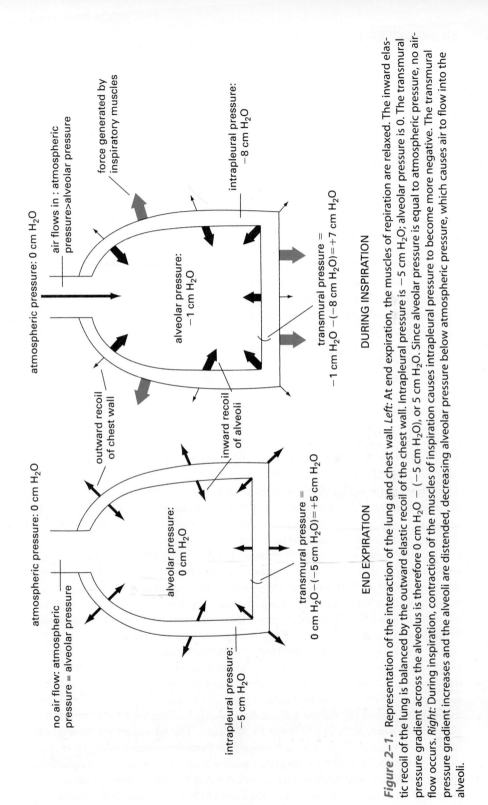

Figure 2–1. Representation of the interaction of the lung and chest wall. *Left:* At end expiration, the muscles of repiration are relaxed. The inward elastic recoil of the lung is balanced by the outward elastic recoil of the chest wall. Intrapleural pressure is −5 cm H_2O; alveolar pressure is 0. The transmural pressure gradient across the alveolus is therefore 0 cm H_2O − (−5 cm H_2O), or 5 cm H_2O. Since alveolar pressure is equal to atmospheric pressure, no air-flow occurs. *Right:* During inspiration, contraction of the muscles of inspiration causes intrapleural pressure to become more negative. The transmural pressure gradient increases and the alveoli are distended, decreasing alveolar pressure below atmospheric pressure, which causes air to flow into the alveoli.

13

Initially, before any airflow occurs, the pressure inside the alveoli is the same as atmospheric pressure—by convention 0 cm H_2O. Alveolar pressure is greater than intrapleural pressure because it represents the sum of the intrapleural pressure plus the alveolar elastic recoil pressure:

Alveolar pressure = intrapleural pressure + alveolar elastic recoil pressure

The muscles of inspiration act to increase the volume of the thoracic cavity. As the inspiratory muscles contract, expanding the thoracic volume and increasing the outward stress on the lung, the intrapleural pressure becomes *more negative.* Therefore, the transmural pressure gradient tending to distend the alveolar wall (sometimes called the *transpulmonary pressure*) increases as shown in Figure 2–1, and the alveoli enlarge passively. Increasing alveolar volume lowers alveolar pressure and establishes the pressure gradient for airflow into the lung. In reality, only a small percentage of the total number of alveoli are directly exposed to the intrapleural surface pressure, and at first thought, it is difficult to see how alveoli located centrally in the lung could be expanded by a more negative intrapleural pressure. However, careful analysis has shown *that the pressure at the pleural surface is transmitted through the alveolar walls to more centrally located alveoli and small airways.* This structural *interdependence* of alveolar units is depicted in Figure 2–2.

The Muscles of Respiration

INSPIRATORY MUSCLES

The muscles of inspiration include the diaphragm, the external intercostals, and the accessory muscles of inspiration.

The Diaphragm—The diaphragm is a large (about 250 cm^2 in surface area) dome-shaped muscle that separates the thorax from the abdominal cavity. As mentioned in Chapter 1, the diaphragm is considered to be an integral part of the chest wall and must always be considered in the analysis of chest wall mechanics.

The diaphragm is the primary muscle of inspiration. When a person is in the supine position, the diaphragm is responsible for about two thirds of the air that enters the lungs during normal quiet breathing (which is called *eupnea*). (When a person is standing or seated in an upright posture, the diaphragm is responsible for only about one third to one half of the tidal volume.) It is innervated by the two phrenic nerves, which leave the spinal cord at the third through the fifth cervical segments.

The muscle fibers of the diaphragm are inserted into the sternum and the six lower ribs and into the vertebral column by the two *crura.* The other ends of these muscle fibers converge to attach to the fibrous *central tendon,* which is also attached to the pericardium on its upper surface (Figure 2–3). During normal quiet breathing, contraction of the diaphragm causes its dome to descend 1 to 2 cm into the abdominal cavity, with little change in its shape. This elongates the thorax and increases its volume. These small downward movements of the diaphragm are possible because the abdominal viscera can push out against the relatively compliant abdominal wall. During a deep inspiration, the diaphragm can descend as much as 10 cm. With such a deep inspiration, the limit of the compliance of the abdominal

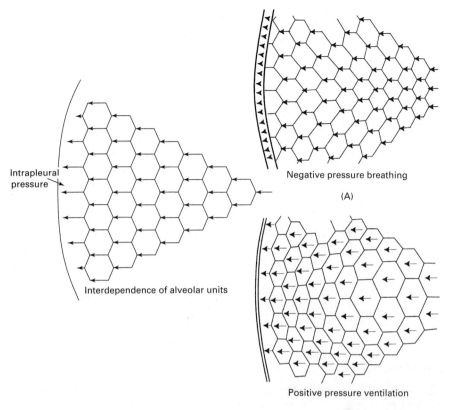

Figure 2–2. Structural interdependence of alveolar units. The pressure gradient across the outermost alveoli is transmitted mechanically through the lung via the alveolar septa. The insets show the author's idea of what might happen in negative pressure breathing and positive pressure ventilation. In negative pressure breathing (Inset A) the mechanical stress would likely be transmitted from the more exterior alveoli (those closest to the chest wall) to more interior alveoli, so the exterior alveoli might be more distended. In positive pressure ventilation (Inset B) the lungs must push against the diaphragm and rib cage to move them. The outermost alveoli might be more compressed than those located more interiorly.

wall is reached, abdominal pressure increases, and the indistensible central tendon becomes fixed against the abdominal contents. After this point, contraction of the diaphragm against the fixed central tendon elevates the lower ribs (Figure 2–3).

If one of the leaflets of the diaphragm is paralyzed (for example, because of transection of one of the phrenic nerves), it will "paradoxically" move up into the thorax as intrapleural pressure becomes more negative during a rapid inspiratory effort.

The External Intercostals—When they are stimulated to contract, the external intercostal, parasternal intercostal, and scalene muscles raise and enlarge the rib cage. The parasternal muscles, which are usually considered part of the internal intercostals, are inspiratory muscles and may be partly responsible for raising the lower ribs.

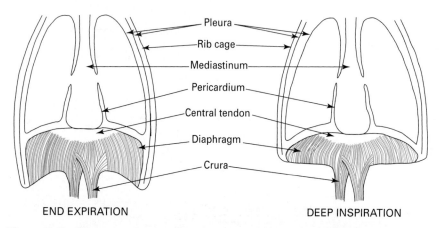

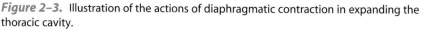

END EXPIRATION   DEEP INSPIRATION

Figure 2–3. Illustration of the actions of diaphragmatic contraction in expanding the thoracic cavity.

The scalene muscles appear to contract in normal quiet breathing and are therefore not accessory muscles. Figure 2–4 demonstrates how contraction of these muscles increases the anteroposterior dimension of the chest as the ribs rotate upward about their axes and also increases the transverse dimension of the lower portion of the chest. These muscles are innervated by nerves leaving the spinal cord at the first through the eleventh thoracic segments. During inspiration, the diaphragm and inspiratory rib cage muscles contract simultaneously. If the diaphragm contracted alone, the rib cage muscles would be pulled inward (this is called *retraction*). If the inspiratory muscles of the rib cage contracted alone, the diaphragm would be pulled upward into the thorax.

The Accessory Muscles of Inspiration—The accessory muscles of inspiration are not involved during normal quiet breathing but may be called into play during exercise; during the inspiratory phase of coughing or sneezing; or in a pathologic state, such as asthma. For example, the *sternocleidomastoid* elevates the sternum and helps increase the anteroposterior and transverse dimensions of the chest. *Dyspnea,* the feeling that breathing is difficult, is probably often related to fatigue of the inspiratory muscles. Other potential causes of dyspnea will be discussed in Chapter 9.

EXPIRATORY MUSCLES

Expiration is *passive* during normal quiet breathing, and no respiratory muscles contract. As the inspiratory muscles relax, the increased elastic recoil of the distended alveoli is sufficient to decrease the alveolar volume and raise alveolar pressure above atmospheric pressure. Now the pressure gradient for airflow out of the lung has been established.

Although the diaphragm is usually considered to be completely relaxed during expiration, it is likely that some diaphragmatic muscle tone is maintained, especially when one is in the horizontal position. The inspiratory muscles may also continue to contract actively during the early part of expiration, especially in obese people. This so-called braking action may help maintain a smooth transition between inspiration and expiration. It may also be important during speech production.

INSPIRATION   ACTIVE EXPIRATION

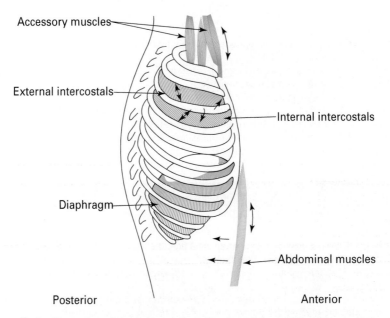

Figure 2–4. Illustration of the actions of contraction of the intercostal muscles, abdominal muscles, and accessory muscles. (Reprinted by permission of the publisher from *The Pathway for Oxygen* by Ewald R. Weibel, p. 304, Cambridge, Mass: Harvard University Press. Copyright © 1984 by the President and Fellows of Harvard College.)

Active expiration occurs during exercise, speech, singing, the expiratory phase of coughing or sneezing, and in pathologic states such as chronic bronchitis. The main muscles of expiration are *the muscles of the abdominal wall*, including the rectus abdominis, the external and internal oblique muscles, the transversus abdominis, and the *internal intercostal muscles*.

The Abdominal Muscles—When the abdominal muscles contract, they increase abdominal pressure and push the abdominal contents against the relaxed diaphragm, forcing it upward into the thoracic cavity. They also help depress the lower ribs and pull down the anterior part of the lower chest.

The Internal Intercostal Muscles—Contraction of the internal intercostal muscles depresses the rib cage downward in a manner opposite to the actions of the external intercostals.

Summary of the Events Occurring During the Course of a Breath

The events occurring during the course of an idealized normal quiet breath, which are summarized in Table 2–1, are shown in Figure 2–5. For the purpose of clarity, inspiration and expiration are considered to be of equal duration, although during normal quiet breathing, the expiratory phase is longer than the inspiratory phase.

Table 2-1. Events Involved in a Normal Tidal Breath.

Inspiration

1. Brain initiates inspiratory effort.
2. Nerves carry the inspiratory command to the inspiratory muscles.
3. Diaphragm (and/or external intercostal muscles) contracts.
4. Thoracic volume increases as the chest wall expands.[1]
5. Intrapleural pressure becomes more negative.
6. Alveolar transmural pressure gradient increases.
7. Alveoli expand (according to their individual compliance curves) in response to the increased transmural pressure gradient. This increases alveolar elastic recoil.
8. Alveolar pressure falls below atmospheric pressure as the alveolar volume increases, thus establishing a pressure gradient for airflow.
9. Air flows into the alveoli until alveolar pressure equilibrates with atmospheric pressure.

Expiration (Passive)

1. Brain ceases inspiratory command.
2. Inspiratory muscles relax.
3. Thoracic volume decreases, causing intrapleural pressure to become less negative and decreasing the alveolar transmural pressure gradient.[2]
4. Decreased alveolar transmural pressure gradient allows the increased alveolar elastic recoil to return the alveoli to their preinspiratory volumes.
5. Decreased alveolar volume increases alveolar pressure above atmospheric pressure, thus establishing a pressure gradient for airflow.
6. Air flows out of the alveoli until alveolar pressure equilibrates with atmospheric pressure.

[1]Note that Nos. 4 to 8 occur simultaneously.
[2]Note that Nos. 3 to 5 occur simultaneously.

Reproduced with permission from Levitzky MG, Cairo JM, Hall SM: *Introduction to Respiratory Care, Philadelphia*, WB Saunders and Company, 1990.

The *volume* of air entering or leaving the lungs can be measured with a spirometer, as will be described in Chapter 3 (Figure 3–4). *Airflow* can be measured by breathing through a pneumotachograph, which measures the pressure differential across a fixed resistance. The *intrapleural pressure* can be estimated by having a subject swallow a balloon into the intrathoracic portion of the esophagus. The pressure then measured in the balloon is nearly equal to intrapleural pressure. *Alveolar pressures* are not directly measurable and must be calculated.

Initially, alveolar pressure equals atmospheric pressure, and so no air flows into the lung. Intrapleural pressure is -5 cm H_2O. Contraction of the inspiratory muscles causes intrapleural pressure to become more negative as the lungs are pulled open and the alveoli are distended. Note the two different courses for changes in intrapleural pressure. The *dashed line* (which would not really be straight for reasons discussed in the next section) predicts the changes in intrapleural pressure necessary to overcome the elastic recoil of the alveoli. The *solid line* is a more accurate representation of intrapleural pressure because it also includes the additional pressure work that must be done to overcome the resistance to airflow and tissue

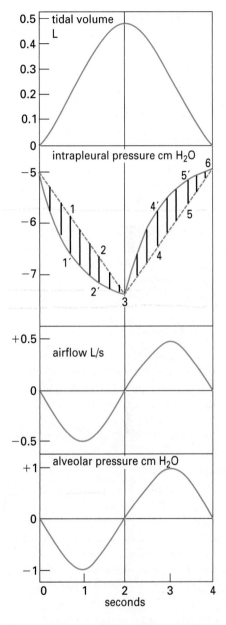

Figure 2–5. Volume, pressure, and airflow changes during a single idealized respiratory cycle. Described in text.
(Reproduced with permission from Comroe, 1974: *Physiology of Respiration,* 2d ed., Chicago, Year Book Medical Publishers.)

resistance discussed later in this chapter. As the alveoli are distended, the pressure inside them falls below atmospheric pressure and air flows into the alveoli, as seen in the tidal volume panel. As the air flows into the alveoli, alveolar pressure returns to 0 cm H_2O and airflow into the lung ceases. At the vertical line (at 2 seconds), the inspiratory effort ceases and the inspiratory muscles relax. Intrapleural pressure becomes less negative, and the elastic recoil of the alveolar walls (which is increased at the higher lung volume) is allowed to compress the alveolar gas. This raises alveolar pressure above atmospheric pressure so that air flows out of the lung until an alveolar pressure of 0 cm H_2O is restored. At this point, airflow ceases until the next inspiratory effort.

PRESSURE-VOLUME RELATIONSHIPS IN THE RESPIRATORY SYSTEM

The relationship between changes in the pressure distending the alveoli and changes in lung volume is important to understand because it dictates how the lung inflates with each breath. As mentioned before, the alveolar-distending pressure is often referred to as the *transpulmonary pressure*. Strictly speaking, the transpulmonary pressure is equal to the pressure in the trachea minus the intrapleural pressure. Thus, it is the pressure difference across the *whole lung*. However, the pressure in the alveoli is the same as the pressure in the airways—including the trachea—at the beginning or end of each normal breath; that is, end-expiratory or end-inspiratory alveolar pressure is 0 cm H_2O (Figure 2–5). Therefore, at the beginning or end of each lung inflation, alveolar-distending pressure can be referred to as the *transpulmonary pressure*.

Compliance of the Lung & the Chest Wall

The pressure-volume characteristics of the lung can be inspected in several ways. One of the simplest is to remove the lungs from an animal or a cadaver and then graph the changes in volume that occur for each change in transpulmonary pressure the lungs are subjected to (Figure 2–6).

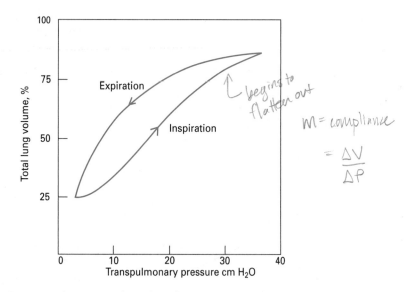

Figure 2–6. Pressure-volume curve for isolated lungs.

Figure 2–6 shows that as the transpulmonary pressure increases, the lung volume increases. Of course, this relationship is not a straight line: The lung is composed of living tissue, and although the lung distends easily at low lung volumes, at high lung volumes the distensible components of alveolar walls have already been stretched, and large increases in transpulmonary pressure yield only small increases in volume.

The slope between two points on a pressure-volume curve is known as the *compliance*. Compliance is defined as the change in volume divided by the change in pressure. Lungs with high compliance have a steep slope on their pressure-volume curves. That is, a small change in distending pressure will cause a large change in volume. It is important to remember that compliance is the *inverse* of elasticity, or elastic recoil. Compliance denotes the ease with which something can be stretched or distorted; elasticity refers to the tendency for something to oppose stretch or distortion, as well as to its ability to return to its original configuration after the distorting force is removed.

There are several other interesting things to note about an experiment like that illustrated in Figure 2–6. The curve obtained is the same whether the lungs are inflated with positive pressure (by forcing air into the trachea) or with negative pressure (by suspending the lung, except for the trachea, in a closed chamber and pumping out the air around the lung). So when the lung alone is considered, only the transpulmonary pressure is important, not how the transpulmonary pressure is generated. A second feature of the curve in Figure 2–6 is that there is a difference between the pressure-volume curve for inflation and the curve for deflation, as shown by the arrows. Such a difference is called *hysteresis*. One possible explanation for this hysteresis is the stretching on inspiration and the compression on expiration of the surfactant that lines the air-liquid interface in the alveoli (discussed later in this chapter). Another is that some alveoli or small airways may open on inspiration ("recruitment") and close on expiration ("derecruitment"). Finally, it is helpful to think of each alveolus as having its own pressure-volume curve like that shown in Figure 2–6, although some researchers believe that lung volume changes primarily by recruitment and derecruitment of alveoli rather than by volume changes of individual alveoli.

CLINICAL EVALUATION OF THE COMPLIANCE OF THE LUNG AND THE CHEST WALL

The compliance of the lung and the chest wall provides very useful data for the clinical evaluation of a patient's respiratory system because many diseases or pathologic states affect the compliance of the lung, of the chest wall, or both. The lung and the chest wall are physically in series with each other, and therefore their compliances add as reciprocals:

$$\frac{1}{\text{Total compliance}} = \frac{1}{\substack{\text{compliance} \\ \text{of the lung}}} + \frac{1}{\substack{\text{compliance of} \\ \text{the chest wall}}}$$

Compliances in parallel add directly. Therefore, both lungs together are more compliant than either one alone.

To make clinical determinations of pulmonary compliance, one must be able to measure changes in pressure and in volume. Volume changes can be measured with a spirometer, but measuring pressure changes is more difficult because changes in the *transmural pressure gradient* must be taken into account. For the lungs, the transmural pressure gradient is transpulmonary pressure (alveolar minus intrapleural); for the chest wall, the transmural pressure gradient is intrapleural pressure minus atmospheric pressure. As described previously, intrapleural pressure can be measured by having the patient swallow an esophageal balloon. The compliance curve for the lung can then be generated by having the patient take a very deep breath and exhale in stages, stopping periodically for pressure and volume determinations. During these determinations, no airflow is occurring; alveolar pressure therefore equals atmospheric pressure, 0 cm H_2O. Similar measurements can be made as the patient inhales in stages from a low lung volume to a high lung volume. Such curves are called *static compliance* curves because all measurements are made when no airflow is occurring. The compliance of the chest wall is normally obtained by determining the compliance of the total system and the compliance of the lungs alone and then calculating the compliance of the chest wall according to the above formula. *Dynamic compliance,* in which pressure-volume characteristics during the breath are considered, will be discussed later in this chapter.

Representative static compliance curves for the lungs are shown in Figure 2–7. Note that these curves correspond to the expiratory curve in Figure 2–6. Many pathologic states shift the curve to the right (i.e., for any increase in transpulmonary pressure there is less of an increase in lung volume). A proliferation of connective

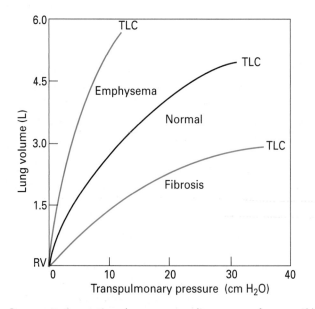

Figure 2–7. Representative static pulmonary compliance curve for normal lungs, fibrotic lungs, and emphysematous lungs. (Reproduced with permission from Murray, 1972, 1986.)

tissue called *fibrosis* may be seen in sarcoidosis or after chemical or thermal injury to the lungs. Such changes will make the lungs less compliant, or "stiffer," and increase alveolar elastic recoil. Similarly, pulmonary vascular engorgement or areas of collapsed alveoli (atelectasis) also make the lung less compliant. Other conditions that interfere with the lung's ability to expand (such as the presence of air, excess fluid, or blood in the intrapleural space) will effectively decrease the compliance of the lungs. Emphysema *increases* the compliance of the lungs because it destroys the alveolar septal tissue that normally opposes lung expansion.

The compliance of the chest wall is decreased in obese people, for whom moving the diaphragm downward and the rib cage up and out is much more difficult. People suffering from a musculoskeletal disorder that leads to decreased mobility of the rib cage, such as kyphoscoliosis, also have decreased chest wall compliance.

Because they must generate greater transpulmonary pressures to breathe in the same volume of air, people with decreased compliance of the lungs must do more work to inspire than those with normal pulmonary compliance. Similarly, more muscular work must be done by someone with decreased chest wall compliance than by a person with normal chest wall compliance.

As noted in the beginning of this section, lung compliance is volume-dependent. It is greater at low lung volumes and lower at high lung volumes. For this reason, the term *specific compliance* is often used to denote compliance with reference to the original lung volume.

The total compliance of a normal person near the normal end-expiratory lung volume (the *functional residual capacity [FRC]*) is about 0.1 L/cm H_2O. The compliance of the lungs is about 0.2 L/cm H_2O; that of the chest wall is also about 0.2 L/cm H_2O.

Elastic Recoil of the Lung

So far the elastic recoil of the lungs has been discussed as though it were only due to the elastic properties of the pulmonary parenchyma itself. However, there is another component of the elastic recoil of the lung besides the elastin, collagen, and other constituents of the lung tissue. That other component is the surface tension at the air-liquid interface in the alveoli.

Surface tension forces occur at any gas-liquid interface (or even interfaces between two immiscible liquids) and are generated by the cohesive forces between the molecules of the liquid. These cohesive forces balance each other within the liquid phase but are unopposed at the surface of the liquid. Surface tension is what causes water to bead and form droplets. It causes a liquid to shrink to form the smallest possible surface area. The unit of measurement of surface tension is dynes per centimeter (dyn/cm).

The role of the surface tension forces in the elastic recoil of the lung can be demonstrated in an experiment such as that shown in Figure 2–8.

In this experiment, a pressure-volume curve for an excised lung was generated as was done in Figure 2–6. Because the lung was inflated with air, an air-liquid interface was present in the lung, and surface tension forces contributed to alveolar elastic recoil. Then, all the gas was removed from the lung, and it was inflated again,

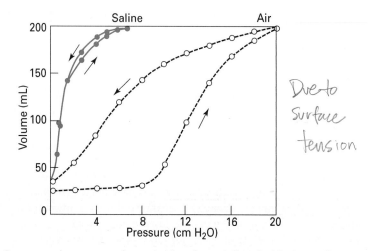

Figure 2–8. Pressure-volume curves for excised cat lungs inflated with air or saline. (Reproduced with permission form Clements, 1965.)

this time with saline instead of with air. In this situation, surface tension forces are absent because there is no air-liquid interface. The elastic recoil is due only to the elastic recoil of the lung tissue itself. Note that there is no hysteresis with saline inflation. Whatever causes the hysteresis appears to be related to surface tension in the lung. To recapitulate, the curve at left (saline inflation) represents the elastic recoil due to only the lung tissue itself. The curve at right demonstrates the recoil due to both the lung tissue and the surface tension forces. The difference between the two curves is the recoil due to surface tension forces.

The demonstration of the large role of surface tension forces in the recoil pressure of the lung led to consideration of how surface tension affects the alveoli. One traditional way of thinking about this has been to consider the alveolus to be a sphere

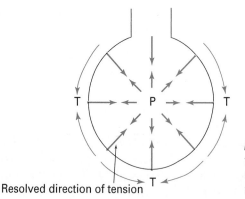

$T \propto Pr$

Resolved direction of tension

Figure 2–9. Relationship between the pressure inside a distensible sphere, such as an alveolus, and its wall tension.

hanging from the airway, as in Figure 2–9. The relationship between the pressure inside the alveolus and the wall tension of the alveolus would then be given by Laplace's law (units in parentheses).

$$\text{Pressure (dyn/cm}^2) = \frac{2 \times \text{tension (dyn/cm)}}{\text{radius (cm)}}$$

This can be rearranged as

$$T = \frac{P \times r}{2}$$

The surface tension of most liquids (such as water) is constant and not dependent on the area of the air-liquid interface. Consider what this would mean in the lung, where alveoli of different sizes are connected to each other by common airways and collateral ventilation pathways (described in Chapter 1). If two alveoli of different sizes are connected by a common airway (Figure 2–10) and the surface tension of the two alveoli is equal, then according to Laplace's law, the pressure in the small alveolus must be greater than that in the larger alveolus and the smaller alveolus will empty into the larger alveolus. If surface tension is independent of surface area, the smaller the alveolus on the right becomes, the higher the pressure in it.

Thus, if the lung were composed of interconnected alveoli of different sizes (which it is) with a *constant surface tension* at the air-liquid interface, it would be expected to be inherently unstable, with a tendency for smaller alveoli to collapse into larger ones. Normally, this is not the case, which is fortunate because collapsed alveoli require very great distending pressures to reopen, partly because of the cohesive forces at the liquid-liquid interface of collapsed alveoli. At least two factors

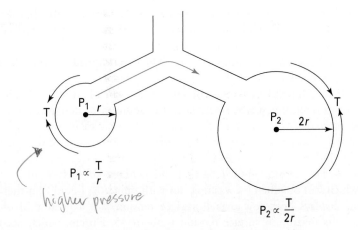

higher pressure

Figure 2–10. Schematic representation of two alveoli of different sizes connected to a common airway. If the surface tension is the same in both alveoli, then the smaller alveolus will have a higher pressure and will empty into the larger alveolus.

↳ As w/ H₂O

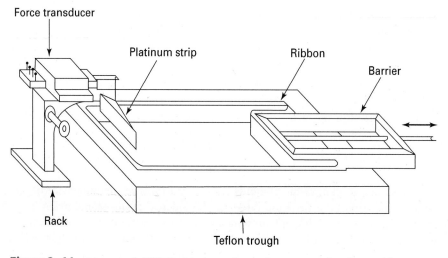

Figure 2–11. A Langmuir-Wilhelmy balance for measurement of surface tension. (Reproduced with permission from Clements, 1965.)

cause the alveoli to be more stable than this prediction based on constant surface tension. The first factor is a substance called *pulmonary surfactant,* which is produced by specialized alveolar cells, and the second is the structural interdependence of the alveoli.

Pulmonary Surfactant

The surface tension of a liquid can be measured with an apparatus like that shown in Figure 2–11.

The liquid to be inspected is placed in the trough. The movable barrier (denoted by the arrow at right) allows a determination of the role of the surface area of the air-liquid interface on surface tension. The surface tension is measured by the downward force on the platinum strip, which is suspended from the force transducer.

The results of a series of such experiments are shown in Figure 2–12. The surface tension properties of water, water after the addition of detergent, and lung extract are plotted with respect to the relative surface area of the trough seen in Figure 2–11. Water has a relatively high surface tension (about 72 dyn/cm) that is completely independent of surface area. Addition of detergent to the water decreases the surface tension, but it is still independent of surface area. "Lung extract," which was obtained by washing out with saline the liquid film that lines the alveoli, displays both low overall surface tension and a great deal of area dependence. Its maximum surface tension is about 45 dyn/cm, which occurs at high relative areas. At low relative areas, the surface tension falls to nearly 0 dyn/cm. Furthermore, the lung extract also displays a great deal of hysteresis, similar to that seen in Figures 2–6 and 2–8.

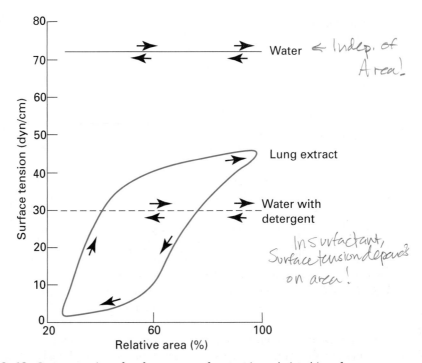

Figure 2–12. Representation of surface area–surface tension relationships of water, water with detergent, and lung extract. (Reproduced with permission after Clements, 1965.)

From these data, it can be concluded that the alveolar surface contains a component fluid that lowers the elastic recoil due to surface tension, even at high lung volumes. This increases the compliance of the lungs above that predicted by an air-water interface and thus decreases the inspiratory work of breathing.

Because the surface tension decreased dramatically at low relative areas, it is reasonable to assume that the surface tension of different-sized alveoli is *not constant* and that smaller alveoli have lower surface tensions. This helps equalize alveolar pressures throughout the lung (so the end-expiratory pressure of all the alveoli is 0 cm H_2O) and to stabilize alveoli. Finally, the hysteresis seen in lung pressure-volume curves like those in Figure 2–6 appears to be a property of the fluid lining the alveoli, although the precise physicochemical reason for this is not yet fully understood.

The surface-active component of the lung extract is called _pulmonary surfactant_. It is a complex consisting of about 85% to 90% lipids and 10% to 15% proteins. The lipid portion is about 85% phospholipid, approximately 75% of which is dipalmitoyl phosphatidylcholine. There are four specific surfactant proteins: SP-A, SP-B, SP-C, and SP-D. This complex is manufactured by specialized alveolar cells known as type II alveolar epithelial cells (see Chapters 1 and 10). Pulmonary surfactant appears to be continuously produced in the lung, but it is also continuously used up in or cleared from the lung. Some pulmonary surfactant is taken back into the type II cells (reuptake), where it is recycled and secreted again, or it is degraded and used to synthesize other phospholipids. Other surfactant is cleared from the alveoli by alveolar macrophages, absorption into the lymphatics, or migration up to the small airways and the mucociliary escalator (see Chapter 10). Although the alveolar surface is usually considered to be completely lined with liquid, some studies have shown that the surface consists of both dry areas and wet areas. Type II alveolar epithelial cells may also help remove liquid from the alveolar surface by actively pumping sodium and water from the alveolar surface into the interstitium.

The clinical consequences of a lack of functional pulmonary surfactant can be seen in several conditions. Surfactant is not produced by the fetal lung until about the fourth month of gestation, and it may not be fully functional until the seventh month or later. Prematurely born infants who do not have functional pulmonary surfactant experience great difficulty in inflating their lungs, especially on their first breaths. Even if their alveoli are inflated for them, the tendency toward spontaneous collapse is great because their alveoli are much less stable without pulmonary surfactant. Therefore, the lack of functional pulmonary surfactant in a prematurely born neonate may be a major factor in the *infant respiratory distress syndrome.* Pulmonary surfactant may also be important in maintaining the stability of small airways.

Hypoxia or hypoxemia (low oxygen in the arterial blood), or both, may lead to a decrease in surfactant production or an increase in surfactant destruction. This condition may be a contributing factor in the *acute respiratory distress syndrome* (also known as adult respiratory distress syndrome or "shock-lung syndrome") seen in patients after trauma or surgery. One thing that can be done to help maintain patients with acute or infant respiratory distress syndrome is to ventilate their lungs with positive-pressure ventilators and to keep their alveolar pressure above atmospheric pressure during expiration (this is known as positive end-expiratory pressure [PEEP]). This process opposes the increased elastic recoil of the alveoli and the tendency for spontaneous atelectasis to occur because of a lack of pulmonary surfactant. Exogenous pulmonary surfactant is now administered directly into the airway of neonates with infant respiratory distress syndrome.

In summary, pulmonary surfactant helps decrease the work of inspiration by lowering the surface tension of the alveoli, thus reducing the elastic recoil of the lung and making the lung more compliant. Surfactant also helps stabilize the alveoli by lowering even further the surface tension of smaller alveoli, equalizing the pressure inside alveoli of different sizes.

Alveolar Interdependence

A second factor tending to stabilize the alveoli is their mechanical interdependence, which was discussed at the beginning of this chapter. Alveoli do not hang from the airways like a "bunch of grapes" (the translation of the Latin word "acinus"), and they are not spheres. They are mechanically interdependent polygons with flat walls shared by adjacent alveoli. Alveoli are not normally held open by positive airway pressure, as shown in Figures 2–9 and 2–10; they are held open by the chest wall pulling on the outer surface of the lung, as shown in Figure 2–2. If an alveolus, such as the one in the middle of Figure 2–13, were to begin to collapse, it would

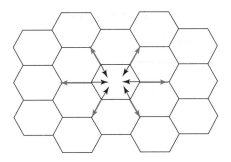

Figure 2–13. Representation of alveolar interdependence helping to prevent an alveolus from collapsing spontaneously.

increase the stresses on the walls of the adjacent alveoli, which would tend to hold it open. This process would oppose a tendency for isolated alveoli suffering from a relative lack of pulmonary surfactant to collapse spontaneously. Conversely, if a whole subdivision of the lung (such as a lobule) has collapsed, as soon as the first alveolus is reinflated, it helps to pull other alveoli open by its mechanical interdependence with them. Thus both pulmonary surfactant and the mechanical interdependence of the alveoli help stabilize the alveoli and oppose alveolar collapse (atelectasis).

INTERACTION OF LUNG & CHEST WALL: THE STATIC PRESSURE-VOLUME CURVE

The interaction between the lung and the chest wall was discussed earlier in this chapter. The inward elastic recoil of the lung normally opposes the outward elastic recoil of the chest wall, and vice versa. If the integrity of the lung–chest wall system is disturbed by breaking the seal of the chest wall (for example, by a penetrating knife wound), the inward elastic recoil of the lung can no longer be opposed by the outward recoil of the chest wall, and their interdependence ceases. Lung volume decreases, and alveoli have a much greater tendency to collapse, especially if air moves in through the wound until intrapleural pressure equalizes with atmospheric pressure and abolishes the transpulmonary pressure gradient. At this point nothing is tending to hold the alveoli open and their elastic recoil is causing them to collapse. Similarly, the chest wall tends to expand because its outward recoil is no longer opposed by the inward recoil of the lung.

When the lung–chest wall system is intact and the respiratory muscles are relaxed, the volume of gas left in the lungs is determined by the balance of these two forces. The volume of gas in the lungs at the end of a normal tidal expiration, when no respiratory muscles are actively contracting, is known as the *functional residual capacity* (FRC). For any given situation, the FRC will be that lung volume at which the outward recoil of the chest wall is equal to the inward recoil of the lungs. The relationship between lung elastic recoil and chest wall elastic recoil is illustrated in static (or "relaxation") pressure-volume curves (Figure 2–14).

In the studies from which these data were taken, participants breathed air from a spirometer so that lung volumes could be measured. Intrapleural pressure was measured with an esophageal balloon, and pressure was also measured at the person's nose or mouth. The subjects were instructed to breathe air into or from the spirometer to

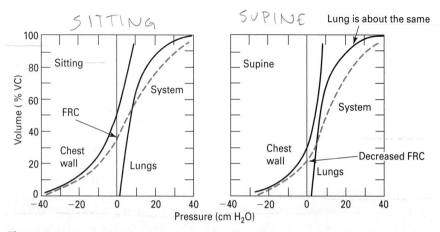

Figure 2–14. Static pressure-volume curves of the lung, chest wall, and total system in the sitting and supine positions. VC = vital capacity; FRC = functional residual capacity. (Reproduced with permission from Agostoni, 1972.)

attain different lung volumes. A stopcock in the spirometer tubing near the subject's mouth was then closed, and the subject was instructed to suddenly relax his or her respiratory muscles. The pressure then measured at the nose or mouth (which is equal to alveolar pressure at this point when no airflow is occurring) is the sum of the recoil pressure of both lungs and the chest wall. It is represented by the dotted line labeled "system" (respiratory system) in Figure 2–14. The individual recoil pressures of the lung and the chest wall can be calculated because the intrapleural pressure is known. Lung recoil pressure is labeled "lungs" on the graphs; chest wall recoil pressure is labeled "chest wall" on the graphs. The graph on the left was drawn from data obtained when participants were sitting up; the graph on the right was drawn from data obtained when participants were lying on their backs.

The left graph in Figure 2–14 shows that the pressure measured at the mouth (system) is equal to 0 cm H_2O at the point where lung recoil pressure is equal and opposite to chest wall recoil pressure. Therefore, alveolar pressure is also 0 cm H_2O. The lung volume at this point is the person's FRC.

As the person increases his or her lung volume, the total system recoil pressure becomes positive because of two factors: the increased inward elastic recoil of the lung and the decreased outward elastic recoil of the chest wall. In fact, at high lung volumes the recoil pressure of the chest wall is also positive (note the point where the chest wall line crosses the 0 pressure line). This is because at high lung volumes, above about 70% of the total lung capacity (TLC), when a person is in an upright posture, the chest wall also has inward elastic recoil. Seventy percent of the TLC is approximately equal to 60% of the vital capacity (VC—defined later in this chapter) seen in the left panel of Figure 2–14. In other words, if one could imagine a relaxed intact chest wall with no lungs in it, the resting volume of the thorax would be about 70% of the volume of the thorax when the lungs are maximally (voluntarily) expanded. At thoracic volumes below about 70% of the TLC, the chest wall elastic recoil is outward; at thoracic volumes above 70% of the TLC, the recoil is inward. Therefore, at high lung volumes the mouth pressure is highly positive because both lung and chest wall elastic recoil are inward.

At lung volumes below the FRC, the relaxation pressure measured at the mouth is negative because the outward recoil of the chest wall is greater than the reduced inward recoil of the lungs.

The point of this discussion can be seen in the right-hand graph of Figure 2–14, in which the data collected were from supine subjects. Although the elastic recoil curve for the lung is relatively unchanged, the recoil curves for the chest wall and the respiratory system are shifted to the right. The reason for this shift is the effect of gravity on the mechanics of the chest wall, especially the diaphragm. When a person is standing up or sitting, the contents of the abdomen are being pulled away from the diaphragm by gravity. When the same person lies down, the abdominal contents are pushing inward against the relaxed diaphragm. This occurrence decreases the overall outward recoil of the chest wall and displaces the chest wall elastic recoil curve to the right. Because the respiratory system curve is the sum of the lung and chest wall curves, it is also shifted to the right.

The lung volume at which the outward recoil of the chest wall is equal to the inward recoil of the lung is much lower in the supine subject, as can be seen

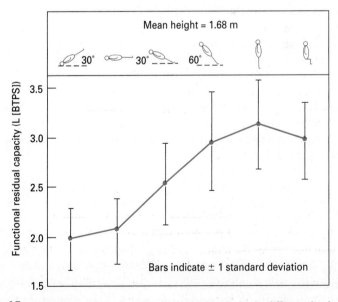

Figure 2–15. Alterations of the functional residual capacity in different body positions. (From Nunn's *Applied Respiratory Physiology*, 4th edition by J.F. Nunn. Reprinted by permission of Elsevier Science Limited.)

at the point where the system line crosses the 0 recoil pressure line. In other words, the FRC decreased appreciably just because the person changed from the sitting to the supine position. Figure 2–15 shows the effect of body position on the FRC.

AIRWAYS RESISTANCE

Several factors besides the elastic recoil of the lungs and the chest wall must be overcome to move air into or out of the lungs. These factors include the inertia of the respiratory system, the frictional resistance of the lung and chest wall tissue, and the frictional resistance of the airways to the flow of air. The inertia of the system is negligible. Pulmonary tissue resistance is caused by the friction encountered as the lung tissues move against each other as the lung expands. The airways resistance plus the pulmonary tissue resistance is often referred to as the *pulmonary resistance*. Pulmonary tissue resistance normally contributes about 20% of the pulmonary resistance, with airways resistance responsible for the other 80%. Pulmonary tissue resistance can be increased in such conditions as pulmonary sarcoidosis and fibrosis. Because *airways resistance* is the major component of the total resistance and because it can increase tremendously both in healthy people and in those suffering from various diseases, the remainder of this chapter will concentrate on airways resistance.

Laminar, Turbulent, & Transitional Flow

Generally, the relationship among pressure, flow, and resistance is stated as

$$\text{Pressure difference} = \text{flow} \times \text{resistance}$$

Therefore,

$$\text{Resistance} = \frac{\text{pressure difference (cm } H_2O)}{\text{flow (liters/s)}}$$

This means that resistance is a meaningful term only during flow. When airflow is considered, the units of resistance are usually cm H_2O/L/s.

The resistance to airflow is analogous to electrical resistance in that resistances in *series* are added directly:

$$R_{tot} = R_1 + R_2 + \cdots$$

Resistances in *parallel* are added as reciprocals:

$$\frac{1}{R_{tot}} = \frac{1}{R_1} + \frac{1}{R_2} + \cdots$$

Understanding and quantifying the resistance to airflow in the conducting system of the lungs is difficult because of the nature of the airways themselves. It is relatively easy to inspect the resistance to airflow in a single, unbranched, indistensible tube; however, the ever-branching, narrowing, distensible, and compressible system of airways makes analysis of the factors contributing to airways

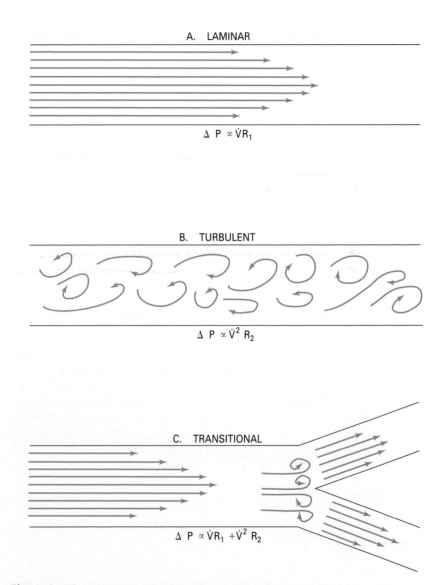

A. LAMINAR

$$\Delta P \propto \dot{V} R_1$$

B. TURBULENT

$$\Delta P \propto \dot{V}^2 R_2$$

C. TRANSITIONAL

$$\Delta P \propto \dot{V} R_1 + \dot{V}^2 R_2$$

Figure 2–16. Illustration of laminar, turbulent, and transitional airflow.

resistance especially complicated. Therefore, equations can only approximate what is really happening clinically.

Airflow, like that of other fluids, can occur as either laminar or turbulent flow.

As seen in Figure 2–16, *laminar flow* (or streamline flow) consists of a number of concentrically arranged cylinders of air flowing at different rates. This telescopelike arrangement is such that the cylinder closest to the wall of the vessel has the slowest velocity because of frictional forces with the wall; the pathway in the center of the vessel has the highest velocity.

When a fluid such as air flows through rigid, smooth-bore tubes, its behavior is governed by Poiseuille's law. The pressure difference is directly proportional to the flow times the resistance:

$$\Delta P \propto \dot{V} R_1$$

where ΔP = pressure difference
$\dot{V}$ = airflow
R_1 = resistance

According to Poiseuille's law, the resistance is directly proportional to the viscosity of the fluid and the length of the tube and is inversely proportional to the *fourth power* of the radius of the tube:

$$R = \frac{8\eta l}{\pi r^4} \quad \leftarrow \text{FOURTH POWER!}$$

where η = viscosity of fluid
l = length of tube
r = radius of tube

Note that if the radius is cut in half, the resistance is multiplied by 16 because the resistance is inversely proportional to the radius to the fourth power.

Flow changes from *laminar* to *turbulent* when Reynolds' number exceeds 2000. Reynolds' number is a dimensionless number equal to the density of the fluid times the velocity of the fluid times the diameter of the tube divided by the viscosity of the fluid:

$$\text{Reynolds' number} = \frac{\rho \times Ve \times D}{\eta}$$

Reynolds > 2000 ⟹ TURBULENT

where ρ = density of fluid
Ve = linear velocity of fluid
D = diameter of tube
η = viscosity of fluid

During turbulent flow, the relationship among the pressure difference, flow, and resistance changes. Because the pressure difference is proportional to the flow squared, much greater pressure differences are required to generate the same airflow. The resistance term is influenced more by the density than it is by the viscosity during turbulent flow:

$$\Delta P \propto \dot{V}^2 R_2$$

Transitional flow is a mixture of laminar and turbulent flow. This type of flow often occurs at branch points or points distal to partial obstructions.

Turbulent flow tends to occur if airflow is high, gas density is high, the tube radius is large, or all three conditions exist. True laminar flow probably occurs only in the smallest airways, where the linear velocity of airflow is extremely low. Linear velocity (cm/s) is equal to the flow (cm^3/s) divided by the cross-sectional area. The total cross-sectional area of the smallest airways is very large (see Chapter 1), and so the linear velocity of airflow is very low. The airflow in the trachea and larger airways is usually either turbulent or transitional.

Distribution of Airways Resistance

About 25–40% of the total resistance to airflow is located in the upper airways: the nose, nasal turbinates, oropharynx, nasopharynx, and larynx. Resistance is higher when one breathes through the nose than when one breathes through the mouth.

The vocal cords open slightly during normal inspirations and close slightly during expirations. During deep inspirations, they open widely. The muscles of the oropharynx also contract during normal inspirations, which dilates and stabilizes the upper airway. During deep forced inspirations, the development of negative pressure could cause the upper airway to be pulled inward and partly or completely obstruct airflow. Reflex contraction of these *pharyngeal dilator muscles* normally keeps the airway open (see Figure 2–25).

As for the tracheobronchial tree, the component with the highest individual resistance is obviously the smallest airway, which has the smallest radius. Nevertheless, because the smallest airways are arranged in parallel, their resistances add as reciprocals, so that the total resistance to airflow offered by the numerous small airways is extremely low during normal, quiet breathing. Therefore, under normal circumstances the greatest resistance to airflow resides in the medium-sized bronchi.

Control of Bronchial Smooth Muscle

The smooth muscle of the airways from the trachea down to the alveolar ducts is under the control of efferent fibers of the autonomic nervous system. Stimulation of the cholinergic *parasympathetic* postganglionic fibers causes *constriction* of bronchial smooth muscle as well as increased glandular mucus secretion. The preganglionic fibers travel in the vagus. Stimulation of the adrenergic *sympathetic* fibers causes dilation of bronchial and bronchiolar smooth muscle as well as inhibition of glandular secretion. This dilation of the airways smooth muscle is mediated by beta$_2$ (β_2) receptors, which predominate in the airways. Selective stimulation of the alpha (α) receptors with pharmacologic agents causes bronchoconstriction. Adrenergic transmitters carried in the blood may be as important as those released from the sympathetic nerves in causing bronchodilation. The bronchial smooth muscle is normally under greater parasympathetic than sympathetic tone.

Inhalation of chemical irritants, smoke, or dust; stimulation of the arterial chemoreceptors; and substances such as histamine cause *reflex constriction* of the airways. Decreased CO_2 in the branches of the conducting system causes a *local* constriction of the smooth muscle of the nearby airways; increased CO_2 or decreased O_2 causes a local dilation. This may help balance ventilation and perfusion (see Chapter 5). Many other substances can have direct or indirect effects on airway smooth muscle (Table 2–2). Leukotrienes usually cause bronchoconstriction, as do some prostaglandins.

Table 2–2. Active Control of the Airways.

Constrict
Parasympathetic stimulation
Acetylcholine
Histamine
Leukotrienes
Thromboxane A_2
Serotonin
α-Adrenergic agonists
Decreased P_{CO_2} in small airways

Dilate
Sympathetic stimulation (β_2 receptors)
Circulating β_2 agonists
Nitric oxide
Increased P_{CO_2} in small airways
Decreased P_{O_2} in small airways

Lung Volume & Airways Resistance

Airways resistance *decreases* with increasing lung volume, as shown in Figure 2–17 (normal curve). This relationship is still present in an emphysematous lung, although in emphysema the resistance is higher than that in a healthy lung, especially at low lung volumes.

There are two reasons for this relationship; both mainly involve the small airways which, as described in Chapter 1, have little or no cartilaginous support. The

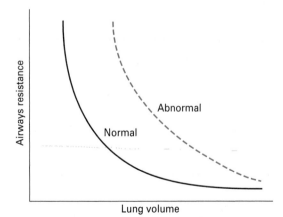

Figure 2–17. Relationship between lung volume and airways resistance. Total lung capacity is at right; residual volume is at left. Solid line = normal lung; dashed line = abnormal (emphysematous) lung. (Reproduced with permission from Murray, 1972.)

small airways are therefore rather distensible and also *compressible.* Thus the transmural pressure gradient across the wall of the small airways is an important determinant of the radius of the airways: Since resistance is inversely proportional to the radius to the *fourth power,* changes in the radii of small airways can cause dramatic changes in airways resistance, even with so many parallel pathways. To increase lung volume, a person breathing normally takes a "deep breath," that is, makes a strong inspiratory effort. This effort causes intrapleural pressure to become much more negative than the -7 or -10 cm H_2O seen in a normal, quiet breath. The transmural pressure gradient across the wall becomes much more positive, and small airways are distended.

A second reason for the decreased airways resistance seen at higher lung volumes is that the so-called traction on the small airways increases. As shown in the schematic drawing in Figure 2–18 (see also the alveolar duct in Figure 1–2), the small airways traveling through the lung form attachments to the walls of alveoli. As the alveoli expand during the course of a deep inspiration, the elastic recoil in their walls increases; this elastic recoil is transmitted to the attachments at the airway, pulling it open.

Dynamic Compression of Airways

Airways resistance is extremely high at low lung volumes, as can be seen in Figure 2–17. To achieve low lung volumes, a person must make a forced expiratory effort by contracting the muscles of expiration, mainly the abdominal and internal intercostal muscles. This effort generates *positive* intrapleural pressure, which can be as high as 120 cm H_2O during a maximal forced expiratory effort. (Maximal inspiratory intrapleural pressures can be as low as -80 cm H_2O.)

The effect of this high positive intrapleural pressure on the transmural pressure gradient during a forced expiration can be seen at right in Figure 2–19, a schematic drawing of a single alveolus and airway.

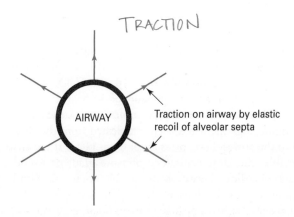

Figure 2–18. Representation of "traction" of the alveolar septa on a small distensible airway. Compare this figure with the picture of the alveolar duct in Figure 1–2.

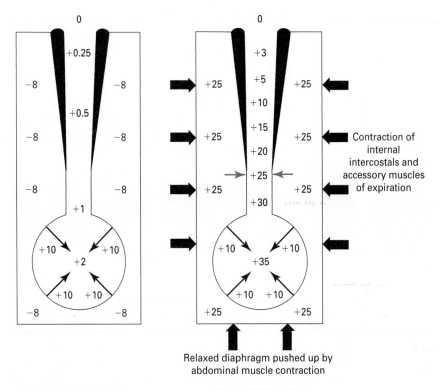

Figure 2–19. Schematic diagram illustrating dynamic compression of airways and the equal pressure point hypothesis during a forced expiration. *Left:* Passive (eupneic) expiration. Intrapleural pressure is −8 cm H_2O, alveolar elastic recoil pressure is +10 cm H_2O, and alveolar pressure is +2 cm H_2O. *Right:* Forced expiration *at the same lung volume.* Intrapleural pressure is +25 cm H_2O, alveolar elastic recoil pressure is +10 cm H_2O, and alveolar pressure is +35 cm H_2O.

The muscles of expiration are generating a positive intrapleural pressure of +25 cm H_2O. Pressure in the alveolus is higher than intrapleural pressure because of the alveolar elastic recoil pressure of +10 cm H_2O, which together with intrapleural pressure, gives an alveolar pressure of +35 cm H_2O. The alveolar elastic recoil pressure decreases at lower lung volumes because the alveolus is not as distended. In the figure, a gradient has been established from the alveolar pressure of +35 cm H_2O to the atmospheric pressure of 0 cm H_2O. If the airways were rigid and incompressible, the large expiratory pressure gradient would generate very high rates of airflow. However, the airways are not uniformly rigid and the smallest airways, which have no cartilaginous support and rely on the traction of alveolar septa to help keep them open, may be compressed or may even collapse. Whether or not they actually collapse depends on the transmural pressure gradient across the walls of the smallest airways.

The situation during a normal *passive* expiration at the same lung volume (note the same alveolar elastic recoil pressure) is shown in the left part of Figure 2–19. The transmural pressure gradient across the smallest airways is

$$+1 \text{ cm } H_2O - (-8)\text{cm } H_2O = +9 \text{ cm } H_2O$$

tending to hold the airway open. During the forced expiration at right, the transmural pressure gradient is 30 cm H_2O − 25 cm H_2O, or only 5 cm H_2O holding the airway open. The airway may then be slightly compressed, and its resistance to airflow will be even greater than during the passive expiration. This increased resistance during a forced expiration is called *dynamic compression* of airways.

Consider what must occur during a maximal forced expiration. As the expiratory effort is increased to attain a lower and lower lung volume, intrapleural pressure is getting more and more positive, and more and more dynamic compression will occur. Furthermore, as lung volume decreases, there will be less alveolar elastic recoil pressure and the difference between alveolar pressure and intrapleural pressure will decrease.

One way of looking at this process is the *equal pressure point hypothesis.* (Another explanation of flow limitation during forced expiration, *the wave speed flow-limiting mechanism,* is too complex to discuss here.) At any instant during a forced expiration, there is a point along the airways where the pressure inside the airway is just equal to the pressure outside the airway. At that point the transmural pressure gradient is 0 (note the arrows in Figure 2–19). Above that point, the transmural pressure gradient is *negative:* The pressure outside the airway is greater than the pressure inside it, and the airway will collapse if cartilaginous support or alveolar septal traction is insufficient to keep it open.

As the forced expiratory effort continues, the equal pressure point is likely to *move down the airway* from larger to smaller airways. This movement happens because, as the muscular effort increases, intrapleural pressure increases and because, as lung volume decreases, alveolar elastic recoil pressure decreases. As the equal pressure point moves down the airway, dynamic compression increases and the airways ultimately begin to collapse. This airways closure can be demonstrated only at especially low lung volumes in healthy subjects, but the *closing volume* may occur at higher lung volumes in patients with emphysema, which will be discussed at the end of this chapter. The closing volume test itself will be discussed in Chapter 3.

It is important to consider the pressure gradient for airflow when thinking about a forced expiration. During a passive expiration the pressure gradient for airflow (the ΔP in $\Delta P = \dot{V}R$) is simply alveolar pressure minus atmospheric pressure. But if dynamic compression occurs, the effective pressure gradient is *alveolar pressure minus intrapleural pressure* (which equals the alveolar elastic recoil pressure) because intrapleural pressure is higher than atmospheric pressure and because intrapleural pressure can exert its effects on the compressible portion of the airways.

Thus, during a forced expiration, when intrapleural pressure becomes positive and dynamic compression occurs, the effective driving pressure for airflow from the lung is the alveolar elastic recoil pressure. Alveolar elastic recoil is also important in *opposing* dynamic compression of the airways because of its role in the traction of the alveolar septa on small airways, as shown in Figure 2–18. The effects of alveolar elastic recoil on airflow during a forced expiration are illustrated in Figure 2–20.

Assessment of Airways Resistance

The resistance to airflow cannot be measured directly but must be calculated from the pressure gradient and airflow during a breath:

$$R = \frac{\Delta P}{\dot{V}}$$

This formula is an approximation because it presumes that all airflow is laminar, which is not true. But there is a second problem: How can the pressure gradient be determined? To know the pressure gradient, the alveolar pressure—which also cannot be measured directly—must be known. Alveolar pressure can be calculated using a body plethysmograph, an expensive piece of equipment described in detail in the next chapter, but this procedure is not often done. Instead, airways resistance is usually assessed indirectly. The assessment of airways resistance during expiration will be emphasized because that factor is of interest in patients with emphysema, chronic bronchitis, and asthma.

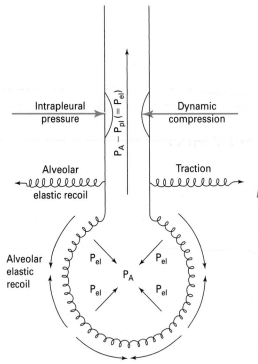

Figure 2–20. Representation of the effects of alveolar elastic recoil on airflow during a forced expiration. When dynamic compression occurs, alveolar elastic recoil helps to oppose it by traction on the small airways. The alveolar elastic recoil pressure becomes the effective driving pressure for airflow from the lung. P_A = alveolar pressure; P_{pl} = intrapleural pressure; P_{el} = alveolar elastic recoil pressure.

Forced Vital Capacity

One way of assessing expiratory airways resistance is to look at the results of a forced expiration into a spirometer, as shown in Figure 2–21. This measurement is called a *forced vital capacity* (FVC). The *vital capacity* (VC) is the volume of air a subject is able to expire after a maximal inspiration to the total lung capacity (TLC). A FVC means that a maximal expiratory effort was made during this maneuver.

In a FVC test, a person makes a maximal inspiration to the TLC. After a moment, he or she makes a maximal forced expiratory effort, blowing as much air as possible out of the lungs. At this point, only a *residual volume* (RV) of air is left in the lungs. (The lung volumes will be described in detail in the next chapter.) This procedure takes only a few seconds, as can be seen on the time scale.

The part of the curve most sensitive to changes in expiratory airways resistance is the first second of expiration. The volume of air expired in the first second of expiration (the FEV_1, or forced expiratory volume in 1 second), especially when expressed as a ratio with the total amount of air expired during the FVC, is a good index of expiratory airways resistance. In normal subjects, the FEV_1/FVC is greater than 0.80; that is, at least 80% of the FVC is expired in the first second. A patient with airway obstruction caused by an episode of asthma, for example, would be expected to have an FEV_1/FVC far below 0.80, as shown in the middle and bottom panels in Figure 2–21.

The bottom panel of Figure 2–21 shows similar FVC curves that would be obtained from a commonly used rolling seal spirometer. The curves are reversed right to left and upside down if they are compared with those in the top and middle panels. The TLC is at the bottom left, and the RVs are at the top right. The time scale is left to right. Note the calculations of the FEV_1 to FVC ratios.

Another way of expressing the same information is the $FEF_{25-75\%}$, or forced (mid) expiratory flow rate (formerly called the MMFR, or maximal midexpiratory flow rate). This variable is simply the slope of a line drawn between the points on the expiratory curve at 25% and 75% of the FVC. In cases of airway obstruction, this line is not nearly as steep as it is on a curve obtained from someone with normal airways resistance. Thus, *elevated airways resistance takes time to overcome.*

Isovolumetric Pressure-Flow Curve

This technique is not often used clinically because the data obtained are tedious to plot. Analysis of the results obtained from this test, however, demonstrates several points we have already discussed. Isovolumetric pressure-flow curves are obtained by having a subject make repeated expiratory maneuvers with different degrees of effort. Intrapleural pressures are determined with an esophageal balloon, lung volumes are determined with a spirometer, and airflow rates are determined by using a pneumotachograph. The pressure-flow relationship for each of the expiratory maneuvers of various efforts is plotted on a curve for a particular lung volume. For example, the middle curve of Figure 2–22 was constructed by determining the intrapleural pressure and airflow for each expiratory maneuver as the subject's lung volume passed through 50% of the VC. Therefore, none of the three curves in

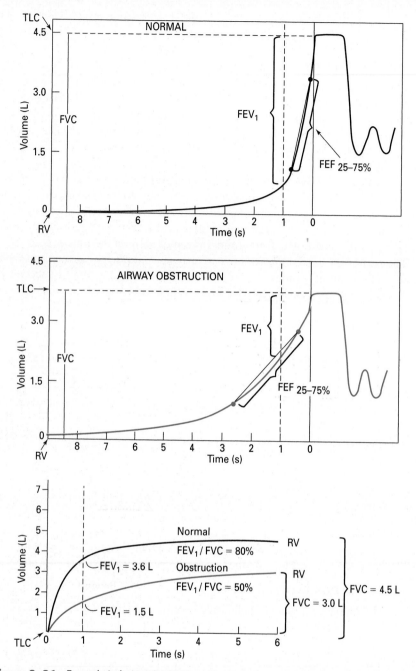

Figure 2–21. Forced vital capacity (FVC maneuver using a spirometer). (See Figure 3–4 for a diagram of a spirometer.) *Upper trace:* FVC from a normal subject. *Lower trace:* FVC from a patient with obstructive disease. FEV_1 = forced expiratory volume in the first second; $FEF_{25-75\%}$ = forced expiratory flow between 25% and 75% of the forced vital capacity. *Bottom traces:* Similar curves obtained from a more commonly used rolling seal spirometer. Note that the total lung capacity (TLC) is at the bottom of the curves and the residual volumes (RVs) are at the top; volume therefore refers to the volume exhaled into the spirometer in the bottom trace. The time scale is from left to right.

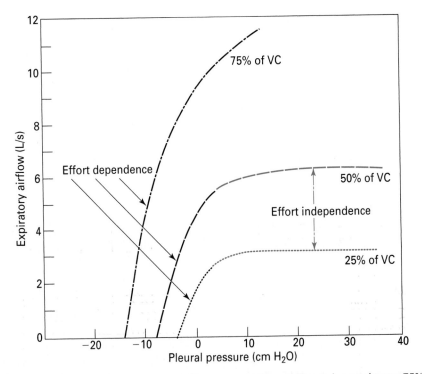

Figure 2–22. Isovolumetric pressure-flow curves at three different lung volumes: 75%, 50%, and 25% of the vital capacity (VC). (Reproduced with permission from Hyatt, 1965.)

Figure 2–22 is really a continuous line; each curve is constructed from individual data points.

The middle curve in Figure 2–22 demonstrates dynamic compression and supports the equal pressure point hypothesis. At this lung volume, at which elastic recoil of the alveoli should be the same no matter what the expiratory effort, with increasing expiratory effort airflow increases *up to a point.* Beyond that point, generating more positive intrapleural pressure does not increase airflow: It is *effort-independent.* Airways resistance must be increasing with increasing expiratory effort. Airflow has become independent of effort because of greater dynamic compression with more positive intrapleural pressures. The equal pressure point has moved to compressible small airways and is fixed there. Note that at even lower lung volumes (25% of the VC), at which there is less alveolar elastic recoil, this occurs with lower maximal airflow rates. In other words, because alveolar pressure equals the sum of the intrapleural pressure and the alveolar elastic recoil pressure during a forced expiration at a given lung volume, the driving pressure for airflow becomes independent of expiratory muscle effort because increasing the intrapleural pressure increases the alveolar pressure by the same amount. Only the alveolar elastic recoil, which is constant at a given lung volume, drives air out of the lung.

At high lung volumes (75% of VC), airflow increases steadily with increasing effort. It is entirely *effort-dependent* because alveolar elastic recoil pressure is high (which increases both the alveolar septal traction on small airways and the pressure gradient for airflow) and because highly positive intrapleural pressures cannot be attained at such high lung volumes with the airway wide open.

FLOW-VOLUME CURVES

These same principles are demonstrated in the expiratory portion of flow-volume curves (Figure 2–23).

A family of flow-volume curves such as those depicted in Figure 2–23 is obtained in the same way as were the data in Figure 2–22, only in this case flow rates are plotted against lung volume for expiratory efforts of different intensities. Intrapleural pressures are not necessary. Because such curves can be plotted instantaneously if one has an X–Y plotter, this test is often used clinically. There are two interesting points about this family of curves, which corresponds to the three curves in Figure 2–22. At high lung volumes, the airflow rate is effort-dependent, which can be seen in the left-hand portion of the curves. At low lung volumes, however, the expiratory efforts of different initial intensities all merge into the same effort-independent curve, as seen in the right-hand portion of the curve. Again, this difference is because intrapleural pressures high enough to cause dynamic compression are necessary to attain very low lung volumes, no matter what the initial expiratory effort. Also, at low lung volumes there is less alveolar elastic recoil pressure, and so there is less traction on the same airways and a smaller pressure gradient for airflow.

The maximal flow-volume curve is often used as a diagnostic tool, as shown in Figure 2–24, because it helps distinguish between two major classes of pulmonary diseases—airway *obstructive* diseases and *restrictive* diseases, such as fibrosis. Obstructive diseases are those diseases that interfere with airflow; restrictive diseases are those diseases that restrict the expansion of the lung (see the pulmonary function test decision tree in the Appendix).

Figure 2–24 shows that both obstruction and restriction can cause a decrease in the maximal flow rate that the patient can attain, the *peak expiratory flow* (PEF; shown in Figure 2–23), but that this decrease occurs for different reasons. Restrictive diseases, which usually entail elevated alveolar elastic recoil, may have decreased PEF because the TLC (and thus the VC) is decreased. The effort-independent part of the curve is similar to that obtained from a person with normal lungs. In fact, the FEV_1/FVC is usually normal or even above normal since *both* the FEV_1 and FVC are decreased because the lung has a low volume and because alveolar elastic recoil pressure may be increased. On the other hand, in patients with obstructive diseases, the PEF and FEV_1/FVC are both low.

Obstructive diseases—such as asthma, bronchitis, and emphysema—are often associated with high lung volumes, which is helpful because the high volumes increase the alveolar elastic recoil pressure. The RV may be greatly increased if airway closure occurs at relatively high lung volumes. A second important feature of the flow-volume curve of a patient with obstructive disease is the

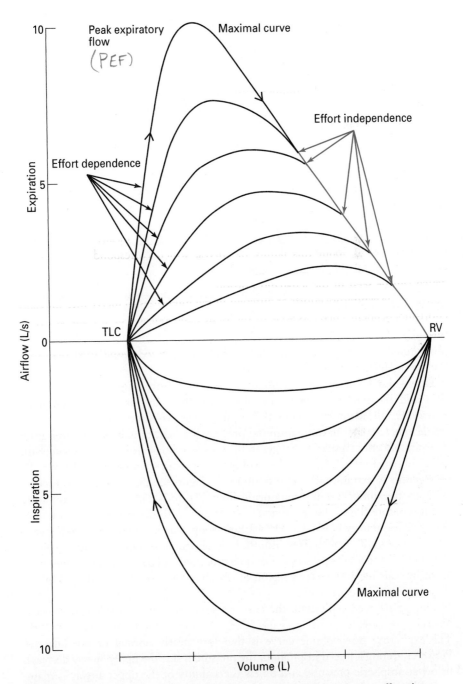

Figure 2–23. Flow-volume curves of varying intensities, demonstrating effort dependence at high lung volumes and effort independence at low lung volumes. Note that there is no effort independence in inspiration. The peak expiratory flow (PEF) is labeled for the maximal expiratory curve. TLC = total lung capacity; RV = residual volume.

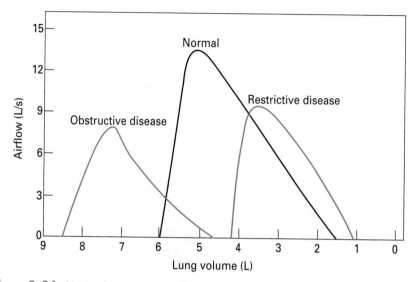

Figure 2–24. Maximal expiratory flow-volume curves representative of obstructive and restrictive diseases.

effort-independent portion of the curve, which is depressed inward: Flow rates are *low* for any relative volume.

Flow-volume curves are very useful in assessing obstructions of the upper airways and the trachea. Flow-volume loops can help distinguish between *fixed obstructions* (those not affected by the inspiratory or expiratory effort) and *variable obstructions* (changes in the transmural pressure gradient caused by the inspiratory or expiratory effort result in changes in the cross-sectional area of the obstruction). If the obstruction is variable, flow-volume loops can demonstrate whether the obstruction is extrathoracic or intrathoracic (Figure 2–25). A fixed obstruction affects both expiratory and inspiratory airflow (Figure 2–25A). Both the expiratory and inspiratory flow-volume curves are truncated, with decreased peak expiratory and peak inspiratory flows. The flow-volume loop is unable to distinguish between a fixed extrathoracic and a fixed intrathoracic obstruction, which would usually be determined with a bronchoscope. Fixed obstructions can be caused by foreign bodies or by scarring that makes a region of the airway too stiff to be affected by the transmural pressure gradient.

During a forced expiration, the cross-sectional area of a variable extrathoracic obstruction increases as the pressure inside the airway increases (Figure 2–25B). The expiratory flow-volume curve is therefore nearly normal or not affected. However, during a forced inspiration, the pressure inside the upper airway decreases below atmospheric pressure, and unless the stability of the upper airway is maintained by reflex contraction of the pharyngeal muscles or by other structures, the cross-sectional area of the upper airway will decrease. Therefore, the inspiratory flow-volume curve is truncated in patients with variable extrathoracic obstructions.

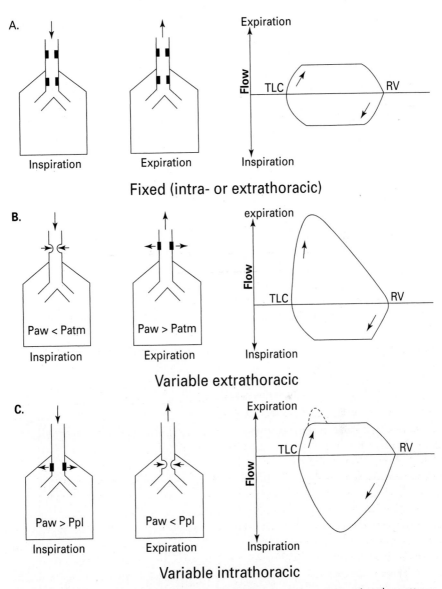

A.

Inspiration Expiration

Fixed (intra- or extrathoracic)

B.

Paw < Patm Paw > Patm

Inspiration Expiration

Variable extrathoracic

C.

Paw > Ppl Paw < Ppl

Inspiration Expiration

Variable intrathoracic

Figure 2–25. Inspiratory and expiratory flow-volume curves representing the patterns in: **A:** Fixed intra- or extrathoracic obstruction. **B:** Variable extrathoracic obstruction. **C:** Variable intrathoracic obstruction. TLC = total lung capacity; RV = residual volume; Paw = airway pressure; Patm = atmospheric pressure; Ppl = intrapleural pressure. (Reproduced with permission from Burrows B, Knudson RJ, Quan SF, Kettel LJ: *Respiratory Disorders: A Pathophysiologic Approach,* 2nd ed. Copyright © 1983 by Year Book Medical Publishers, Chicago.)

Variable extrathoracic obstructions can be caused by tumors, fat deposits, weakened or flabby pharyngeal muscles (as in obstructive sleep apnea), paralyzed vocal cords, enlarged lymph nodes, or inflammation.

During a forced expiration, positive intrapleural pressure decreases the transmural pressure gradient across a variable intrathoracic tracheal obstruction, decreasing its cross-sectional area and decreasing the peak expiratory flow (PEF) (Figure 2–25C). During a forced inspiration, as large negative intrapleural pressures are generated, the transmural pressure gradient across the variable intrathoracic obstruction increases and its cross-sectional area increases. Thus, the inspiratory flow-volume curve is nearly normal or not affected. Variable intrathoracic obstructions of the trachea are most commonly caused by tumors.

Dynamic Compliance

At this point, the *dynamic compliance* of the lungs, which is the change in the volume of the lungs divided by the change in the alveolar-distending pressure *during the course of a breath*, can be considered. At low breathing frequencies, around 15 breaths per minute and lower, dynamic compliance is about equal to static compliance, and the ratio of dynamic compliance to static compliance is 1 (Figure 2–26).

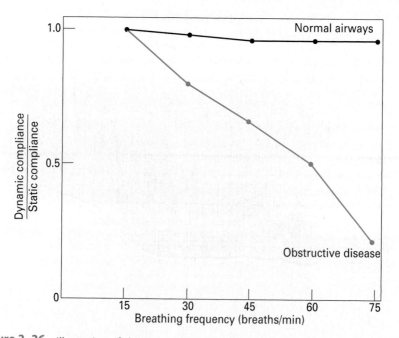

Figure 2–26. Illustration of changes in the ratio of dynamic compliance to static compliance with increasing breathing frequencies. The ratio changes little in normal subjects but decreases dramatically in patients with obstructive diseases of the small airways.

In normal persons, this ratio stays near 1 even at much higher breathing frequencies. However, in patients with elevated resistance to airflow in some of their small airways, the ratio of dynamic compliance to static compliance falls dramatically as breathing frequency is increased. This indicates that changes in dynamic compliance reflect changes in airways resistance as well as changes in the compliance of alveoli.

The effects of increased breathing frequency on dynamic compliance can be explained by thinking of a pair of hypothetical alveoli supplied by the same airway. Consider the time courses of their changes in volume in response to an abrupt increase in airway pressure (a "step" increase) in a situation in which the compliance of each alveolus or the resistance in the branch of the airway supplying it can be arbitrarily altered.

If the resistances and compliances of the two units were equal, the two alveoli would fill with identical time courses. If the resistances were equal, but the compliance of one were half that of the other, then it would be expected that the alveoli would fill with nearly identical time courses but that the less compliant one would receive only half the volume received by the other. If the compliances of the two units were equal but one was supplied by an airway with twice the resistance to airflow of the one supplying the other, then it would be expected that the two units would ultimately fill to the same volume. However, the one supplied by the airway with elevated resistance fills more slowly than the other because of its elevated resistance. This difference means that at high breathing frequencies the one that fills more quickly than the other will accommodate a larger volume of air per breath.

This situation may also lead to a redistribution of alveolar air after the inflating pressure has ceased because one alveolus has more air in it than the other. But both have equal compliance characteristics. The more distended one therefore has a higher elastic recoil pressure, and because they are joined by a common airway, some air is likely to follow the pressure gradient and move to the other.

Now let's extrapolate this two-unit situation to a lung with millions of airways supplying millions of alveoli. In a patient with small-airways disease, many alveoli may be supplied by airways with higher resistance to airflow than normal. These alveoli are sometimes referred to as "slow alveoli" or alveoli with long "time constants." As the patient increases the breathing frequency, the slowest alveoli will not have enough time to fill and will contribute nothing to the dynamic compliance. As the frequency increases, more and more slow alveoli will drop out and dynamic compliance will continue to fall.

THE WORK OF BREATHING

The major points discussed in this chapter can be summarized by considering the work of breathing. The work done in breathing is proportional to the pressure change times the volume change. The volume change is the volume of air moved into and out of the lung—the *tidal volume*. The pressure change is the change in transpulmonary pressure necessary to overcome the *elastic* work of breathing and the *resistive* work of breathing.

Elastic Work

The elastic work of breathing is the work done to overcome the elastic recoil of the chest wall and the pulmonary parenchyma and the work done to overcome the surface tension of the alveoli. Restrictive diseases are those diseases in which the elastic work of breathing is increased. For example, the work of breathing is elevated in obese patients (who have increased inward chest wall elastic recoil) and in patients with pulmonary fibrosis or a relative lack of pulmonary surfactant (who have increased elastic recoil of the alveoli).

Resistive Work

The resistive work of breathing is the work done to overcome the tissue resistance and the airways resistance. The tissue resistance may be elevated in conditions such as sarcoidosis. Elevated airways resistance is much more common and is seen in obstructive diseases such as asthma, bronchitis, and emphysema; upper airway obstruction; and accidental aspirations of foreign objects. Normally, most of the resistive work is that done to overcome airways resistance.

The resistive work of breathing can be extremely great during a *forced expiration,* when dynamic compression occurs. This is especially true in patients who already have elevated airways resistance during normal, quiet breathing. For example, in patients with emphysema, a disease that attacks and obliterates alveolar walls, the work of breathing can be tremendous because of the destruction of the elastic tissue support of their small airways, which allows dynamic compression to occur unopposed. Also, the decreased elastic recoil of alveoli leads to a decreased pressure gradient for expiration.

The oxygen cost of normal, quiet (eupneic) breathing is normally less than 5% of the total body oxygen uptake. This percentage can increase to as much as 30% in normal persons during maximal exercise. In patients with obstructive lung disease, however, the work of breathing can be the factor that limits exercise.

KEY CONCEPTS

A pressure gradient between the atmosphere and the alveoli must be established to move air into or out of the alveoli.

*During inspiration, alveoli expand passively in response to an increased **transmural pressure gradient;** during normal quiet expiration, the elastic recoil of the alveoli returns them to their original volume.*

*The volume of gas in the lungs at the end of a normal tidal expiration (the **FRC**), when no respiratory muscles are actively contracting, is determined by the balance point of the inward recoil of the lungs and the outward recoil of the chest wall.*

At the FRC, intrapleural pressure is **negative** because the pleural liquid is between the opposing forces of the inward recoil of the lungs and the outward recoil of the chest wall.

Alveoli are more compliant (and have less elastic recoil) at low volumes; alveoli are less compliant (and have more elastic recoil) at high volumes.

Pulmonary surfactant increases alveolar compliance and helps prevent atelectasis by reducing surface tension in the alveoli.

During forced expiration, when intrapleural pressure becomes positive, small airways are compressed (**dynamic compression**) and may even collapse.

The two main components of the **work of breathing** are the elastic recoil of the lungs and chest wall and the resistance to air flow.

CLINICAL PROBLEMS

2–1. A woman inspires 500 mL from a spirometer. The intrapleural pressure, determined using an esophageal balloon, was -5 cm H_2O before the inspiratory effort and -10 cm H_2O at the end of the inspiration. What is the pulmonary compliance?

2–2. A postoperative patient whose respiratory muscles have been paralyzed with pancuronium bromide, a curare-like drug, is maintained by a positive-pressure respirator. At end expiration (when alveolar pressure equals 0), intrapleural pressure, as measured by an esophageal balloon, is equal to -3 cm H_2O. At the peak of inspiration, alveolar pressure is $+20$ cm H_2O and intrapleural pressure is $+10$ cm H_2O. Tidal volume is 500 mL.

  a. What is the patient's pulmonary compliance?

  b. What is the patient's total compliance?

  c. What is the patient's chest wall compliance?

2–3. Which of the following conditions are reasonable explanations for a patient's decreased static pulmonary compliance (the pressure-volume curve for the lungs shifted to the right)?

  a. Decreased functional pulmonary surfactant

  b. Fibrosis of the lungs

  c. Surgical removal of one lobe

  d. Pulmonary vascular congestion

  e. All of the above

2–4. Which of the following tend to increase airways resistance?

  a. Stimulation of the parasympathetic postganglionic fibers innervating the bronchial and bronchiolar smooth muscle

  b. Low lung volumes

  c. Forced expirations

  d. Breathing through the nose instead of the mouth

  e. All of the above

2–5. Which of the following statements concerning alveolar pressure is/are correct?

    a. Alveolar pressure is lower than atmospheric pressure during a normal negative-pressure inspiration.

    b. Alveolar pressure is greater than atmospheric pressure during a forced expiration.

    c. Alveolar pressure equals the sum of the intrapleural pressure plus the alveolar elastic recoil pressure.

    d. Alveolar pressure equals atmospheric pressure at the end of a normal tidal expiration.

    e. All of the above.

2–6. Which of the following statements concerning small airways is/are true?

    a. The total resistance to airflow decreases with successive generations of airways because there are increasing numbers of units arranged in parallel.

    b. The linear velocity of airflow decreases as the airways decrease in size because their total cross-sectional area increases.

    c. Alveolar elastic recoil plays an important role in determining the resistance to airflow in small airways because alveolar septal traction helps to oppose dynamic compression.

    d. Airflow in small airways is usually laminar.

    e. All of the above.

2–7. Which of the following statements concerning pulmonary mechanics during the early portion of a forced expiration, when lung volume is still high, is/are correct?

    a. There is less alveolar elastic recoil at high lung volumes than there is at low lung volumes.

    b. Airways resistance is greater at high lung volumes than it is at low lung volumes.

    c. There is more dynamic compression of airways at high lung volumes than there is at low lung volumes.

    d. The effective pressure gradient for airflow is greater at high lung volumes than it is at low lung volumes.

SUGGESTED READINGS

Agostoni E. Mechanics of the pleural space. *Physiol Rev.* 1972;52:57–128.

Agostoni E, Hyatt RE. Static behavior of the respiratory system. In: Macklem PT, Mead J, eds. *Mechanics of Breathing, part 1, Handbook of Physiology, sec 3: The Respiratory System.* Bethesda, Md: American Physiological Society; 1986;3:113–130.

Boggs DS, Kinasewitz GT. Review: pathophysiology of the pleural space. *Am J Med Sci.* 1995;309:53–59.

Burrows B, Knudson RJ, Quan SF, Kettel LJ. *Respiratory Disorders: A Pathophysiologic Approach.* 2nd ed. Chicago, Ill: Year Book; 1983:78–93.

Carney D, DiRocco J, Nieman G. Dynamic alveolar mechanics and ventilator-induced lung injury. *Crit Care Med.* 2005;33[Suppl]:S122–S128.

Clements JA, Tierney DF. Alveolar instability associated with altered surface tension. In: Fenn WO, Rahn H, eds. *Handbook of Physiology, sec 3: Respiration.* Washington, DC: American Physiological Society; 1965;2:1567–1568.

Comroe JH. *Physiology of Respiration.* 2nd ed. Chicago: Year Book; 1974:94–141.

Decramer M. The respiratory muscles. In: Fishman AP et al, eds. *Pulmonary Diseases and Disorders,* 3rd ed. New York: McGraw-Hill; 1998:63–71.

De Troyer A, Kirkwood PA, Wilson TA. Respiratory action of the intercostal muscles. *Physiol Rev.* 2005;85:717–756.

Dorrington KL, Young JD. Development of a concept of a liquid pulmonary alveolar lining layer (editorial). *Brit J Anaesth.* 2001;86:614–617.

Griese M. Pulmonary surfactant in health and human lung diseases: state of the art. *Eur Respir J.* 1999;13:1455–1476.

Hyatt RE. Dynamic lung volumes. In: Fenn WO, Rahn H, eds. *Handbook of Physiology, sec 3: Respiration.* Washington, DC: American Physiological Society; 1965;2:1381–1398.

Hyatt RE. Forced expiration. In: Macklem PT, Mead J, eds. *Mechanics of Breathing, part 1, Handbook of Physiology, sec 3: The Respiratory System.* Bethesda, Md: American Physiological Society; 1986;3:295–314.

Ingram RH Jr, Pedley TJ. Pressure-flow relationships in the lungs. In: Macklem PT, Mead J, eds. *Mechanics of Breathing, part 1, Handbook of Physiology, sec 3: The Respiratory System.* Bethesda, Md: American Physiological Society; 1986;3:277–293.

Lai-Fook SJ. Pleural mechanics and fluid exchange. *Physiol Rev.* 2004;84:385–410.

Levitzky MG, Cairo JM, Hall SM. *Introduction to Respiratory Care.* Philadelphia, PA: WB Saunders and Company; 1990.

Mead J, Takashima T, Leith D. Stress distribution in lungs: A model of pulmonary elasticity. *J Appl Physiol.* 1970;28:596–608.

Mead J, Turner JM, Macklem PT, Little JB. Significance of the relationship between lung recoil and maximum expiratory flow. *J Appl Physiol.* 1967;22:95–108.

Murray JF. *The Normal Lung.* 2nd ed. Philadelphia, PA: WB Saunders and Company; 1986:83–138.

Murray JF, Greenspan RH, Gold WM, Cohen AB. Early diagnosis of chronic obstructive lung disease. *Calif Med.* 1972;116:37–55.

Nunn JF. *Nunn's Applied Respiratory Physiology.* 4th ed. Oxford: Butterworth-Heinemann; 1993:36–90, 117–134.

Osmond DG. Functional anatomy of the chest wall. In: Roussos C, Macklem PT, eds. *The Thorax, part A.* New York: Marcel Dekker; 1985:199–233.

Poole DC, Sexton WL, Farkas GA, Powers SK, Reid MB. Diaphragm structure and function in health and disease. *Med Sci Sports Exerc.* 1997;29:738–754.

Prange HD. Laplace's law and the alveolus: A misconception of anatomy and a misapplication of physics. *Adv Physiol Educ.* 2003;27:34–40.

Weibel ER. *The Pathway for Oxygen: Structure and Function in the Mammalian Respiratory System.* Cambridge, Mass: Harvard University Press; 1984.

Wetzel RC, Herold CJ, Zerhouni EA, Robotham JL. Hypoxic bronchodilation. *J Appl Physiol.* 1992;73:1202–1206.

Alveolar Ventilation

3

OBJECTIVES

The reader understands the ventilation of the alveoli.
- *Defines alveolar ventilation.*
- *Defines the standard lung volumes and understands their measurement.*
- *Predicts the effects of alterations in lung and chest wall mechanics, due to normal or pathologic processes, on the lung volumes.*
- *Defines anatomic dead space and relates the anatomic dead space and the tidal volume to alveolar ventilation.*
- *Understands the measurement of the anatomic dead space and the determination of alveolar ventilation.*
- *Defines physiologic and alveolar dead space and understands their determination.*
- *Predicts the effects of alterations of alveolar ventilation on alveolar carbon dioxide and oxygen levels.*
- *Describes the regional differences in alveolar ventilation found in the normal lung and explains these differences.*
- *Predicts the effects of changes in lung volume, aging, and disease processes on the regional distribution of alveolar ventilation.*
- *Defines the closing volume and explains how it can be demonstrated.*
- *Predicts the effects of changes in pulmonary mechanics on the closing volume.*

Alveolar ventilation is the exchange of gas between the alveoli and the external environment. It is the process by which oxygen is brought into the lungs from the atmosphere and by which the carbon dioxide carried into the lungs in the mixed venous blood is expelled from the body. Although alveolar ventilation is usually defined as the volume of fresh air *entering* the alveoli per minute, a similar volume of alveolar air *leaving* the body per minute is implicit in this definition.

THE LUNG VOLUMES

The volume of gas in the lungs at any instant depends on the mechanics of the lungs and chest wall and the activity of the muscles of inspiration and expiration. The lung volume under any specified set of conditions can be altered by pathologic and normal physiologic processes. Standardization of the conditions under which lung volumes are measured allows comparisons to be made among subjects or patients. The size of a person's lungs depends on his or her height and weight or body surface area, as well as on his or her age and sex. Therefore, the lung volumes for a patient are usually compared with data in a table of "predicted" lung volumes matched to age, sex, and body size. The lung volumes are normally expressed at the body temperature and ambient pressure and saturated with water vapor (BTPS).

The Standard Lung Volumes & Capacities

There are four standard lung *volumes* (which are not subdivided) and four standard lung capacities, which consist of two or more standard lung volumes in combination (Figure 3–1).

THE TIDAL VOLUME

The tidal volume (VT) is the volume of air entering or leaving the nose or mouth per breath. It is determined by the activity of the respiratory control centers in the brain as they affect the respiratory muscles and by the mechanics of the lung and the chest wall. During normal, quiet breathing (eupnea) the VT of a 70-kg adult is about 500 mL per breath, but this volume can increase dramatically, for example, during exercise.

THE RESIDUAL VOLUME

The residual volume (RV) is the volume of gas left in the lungs after a maximal forced expiration. It is determined by the force generated by the muscles of expiration and the inward elastic recoil of the lungs as they oppose the outward elastic recoil of the chest wall. Dynamic compression of the airways during the forced expiratory effort may also be an important determinant of the RV as airway collapse occurs, thus trapping gas in the alveoli. The RV of a healthy 70-kg adult is about 1.5 L, but it can be much greater in a disease state such as emphysema, in which inward alveolar elastic recoil is diminished and much airway collapse and gas trapping occur. The RV is important to a healthy person because it prevents the lungs from collapsing at very low lung volumes. Such collapsed alveoli would require extremely great inspiratory efforts to reinflate.

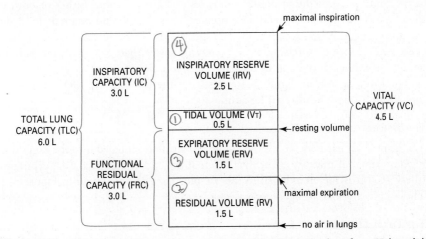

Figure 3–1. The standard lung volumes and capacities. Typical values for a 70-kg adult are shown.

3) ### THE EXPIRATORY RESERVE VOLUME

The expiratory reserve volume (ERV) is the volume of gas that is expelled from the lungs during a maximal forced expiration that *starts* at the end of a normal tidal expiration. It is therefore determined by the difference between the functional residual capacity (FRC) and the RV. The ERV is about 1.5 L in a healthy 70-kg adult.

4) ### THE INSPIRATORY RESERVE VOLUME

The inspiratory reserve volume (IRV) is the volume of gas that is inhaled into the lungs during a maximal forced inspiration *starting* at the end of a normal tidal inspiration. It is determined by the strength of contraction of the inspiratory muscles, the inward elastic recoil of the lung and the chest wall, and the starting point, which is the FRC plus the VT. The IRV of a normal 70-kg adult is about 2.5 L.

THE FUNCTIONAL RESIDUAL CAPACITY

The functional residual capacity (FRC) is the volume of gas remaining in the lungs at the end of a normal tidal expiration. Because it was traditionally assumed that no muscles of respiration are contracting at the end of a normal tidal expiration, the FRC is usually considered to represent the balance point between the inward elastic recoil of the lungs and the outward elastic recoil of the chest wall, as discussed in Chapter 2.

However, the respiratory muscles may have significant tone at the FRC, and in certain circumstances the FRC may be greater than or even less than the lung volume of the totally relaxed respiratory system. Thus, the lung volume at which the inward elastic recoil of the lungs is equal and opposite to the outward elastic recoil of the chest wall is sometimes referred to as the *relaxation volume* of the respiratory system. The FRC may be greater than the relaxation volume if the next inspiration occurs before the relaxation volume is reached, either because of high breathing rates or high resistance to expiratory airflow in the larynx or peripheral airways; or active contraction of the inspiratory muscles at end expiration. Either or both of these may occur in babies, who have higher FRCs than would be predicted from the great inward elastic recoil of their lungs and the small outward recoil of their chest walls. During exercise, the FRC may be lower than the relaxation volume because of active contraction of the expiratory muscles.

The FRC, as seen in Figure 3–1, consists of the RV plus the ERV. It is therefore about 3 L in a healthy 70-kg adult.

THE INSPIRATORY CAPACITY

The inspiratory capacity (IC) is the volume of air that is inhaled into the lungs during a maximal inspiratory effort that *begins* at the end of a normal tidal expiration (the FRC). It is therefore equal to the VT plus the IRV, as shown in Figure 3–1. The IC of a normal 70-kg adult is about 3 L.

THE TOTAL LUNG CAPACITY

The total lung capacity (TLC) is the volume of air in the lungs after a maximal inspiratory effort. It is determined by the strength of contraction of the inspiratory muscles and the inward elastic recoil of the lungs and the chest wall. The TLC consists of all four lung volumes: the RV, the VT, the IRV, and the ERV. The TLC is about 6 L in a healthy 70-kg adult.

THE VITAL CAPACITY

The vital capacity (VC), discussed in Chapter 2, is the volume of air expelled from the lungs during a maximal forced expiration starting after a maximal forced inspiration. The VC is therefore equal to the TLC minus the RV, or about 4.5 L in a healthy 70-kg adult. The VC is also equal to the sum of the VT and the IRV and ERV. It is determined by the factors that determine the TLC and RV.

MEASUREMENT OF THE LUNG VOLUMES

Measurement of the lung volumes is important clinically because many pathologic states can alter specific lung volumes or their relationships to one another. The lung volumes, however, can also change for normal physiologic reasons. Changing from a standing to a supine posture decreases the FRC because gravity is no longer pulling the abdominal contents away from the diaphragm. This decreases the outward elastic recoil of the chest wall, as noted in Chapter 2, Figure 2–14. The RV and TLC do not change significantly when a person changes from standing to the supine position. If the FRC is decreased, then the ERV will also decrease (Figure 3–2), and the IRV will increase. The VC, RV, and TLC may decrease slightly because some of the venous blood that collects in the lower extremities and

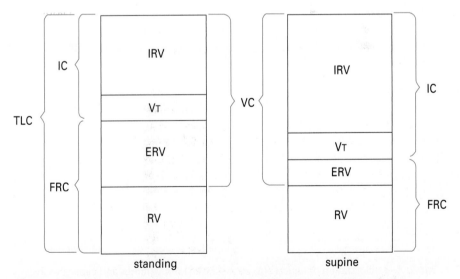

Figure 3–2. Illustration of alterations in the lung volumes and capacities that occur when a subject changes from the standing to the supine position. IC = inspiratory capacity; TLC = total lung capacity; FRC = functional residual capacity; IRV = inspiratory reserve volume; VT = tidal volume; ERV = expiratory reserve volume; RV = residual volume; VC = vital capacity.

the abdomen when a person is standing returns to the thoracic cavity when that person lies down.

Determination of the lung volumes can be useful diagnostically in differentiating between two major types of pulmonary disorders—the restrictive diseases and the obstructive diseases. Restrictive diseases like alveolar fibrosis, which reduce the compliance of the lungs, lead to compressed lung volumes (Figure 3–3). The increased elastic recoil of the lungs leads to a lower FRC, a lower TLC, a lower VC, and lower IRV and ERV, and it may even decrease the RV. The V_T may also be decreased, with a corresponding increase in breathing frequency, to minimize the work of breathing.

Obstructive diseases such as emphysema and chronic bronchitis cause increased resistance to airflow. Airways may become completely obstructed because of mucous plugs as well as because of the high intrapleural pressures generated to overcome the elevated airways resistance during a forced expiration. This is especially a problem in emphysema, in which destruction of alveolar septa leads to decreased elastic recoil of the alveoli and less radial traction, which normally help hold small airways open. For these reasons, the RV, the FRC, and the TLC may

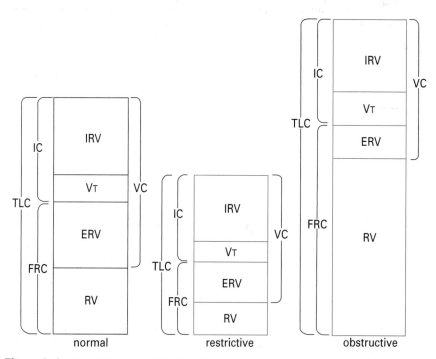

Figure 3–3. Illustration of typical alterations in the lung volumes and capacities in restrictive and obstructive diseases. The pattern shown for obstructive diseases is more characteristic for emphysema and asthma than for chronic bronchitis. IC = inspiratory capacity; TLC = total lung capacity; FRC = functional residual capacity; IRV = inspiratory reserve volume; V_T = tidal volume; ERV = expiratory reserve volume; RV = residual volume; VC = vital capacity.

be greatly increased in obstructive diseases, as seen in Figure 3–3. The VC and ERV are usually decreased. The breathing frequency may be decreased to reduce the work expended overcoming the airways resistance, with a corresponding increase in the V_T.

Spirometry

The spirometer is a simple device for measuring gas volumes. The frequently used water spirometer, shown in Figure 3–4, consists of an inverted canister, or "bell," floating in a water-filled space between two concentrically arranged cylinders. The space inside the inner drum, which is closed off from the atmosphere by the bell, is connected to tubing that extends to a mouthpiece into which the person breathes. As the person breathes in and out, gas enters and leaves the spirometer, and the bell then floats higher (during expiration) and lower (during inspiration). The top of the bell is connected by a pulley to a pen that writes on a rotating drum, thus tracing the person's breathing pattern.

As is evident from Figure 3–4, the spirometer can measure only the lung volumes that the subject can exchange with it. As is the case with many pulmonary function tests, the subject must be conscious and cooperative and understand the instructions for performing the test. The V_T, IRV, ERV, IC, and VC can all be measured with a spirometer (as can the forced expiratory volume in 1 second [FEV_1], forced vital capacity [FVC], and forced expiratory flow [$FEF_{25-75\%}$], as discussed in Chapter 2). The RV, the FRC, and the TLC, however, cannot be determined with a spirometer because the subject cannot exhale all the gas in the lungs. The gas in a spirometer is at ambient temperature, pressure, and water vapor saturation, and the volumes of gas collected in a spirometer must be converted to equivalent volumes in the body. Other kinds of spirometers include rolling seal and bellows spirometers. These spirometers are not water-filled and are more portable.

Measurement of Lung Volumes Not Measurable with Spirometry

The lung volumes not measurable with spirometry can be determined by the nitrogen-washout technique, by the helium-dilution technique, and by body plethysmography. The FRC is usually determined, and RV (which is equal to FRC minus ERV) and the TLC (which is equal to VC plus RV) are then calculated from volumes obtained by spirometry.

NITROGEN-WASHOUT TECHNIQUE

In the nitrogen-washout technique, the person breathes 100% oxygen through a one-way valve so that all the *expired* gas is collected. The concentration of nitrogen in the expired air is monitored with a nitrogen analyzer until it reaches zero. At this point all the nitrogen is washed out of the person's lungs. The total volume of *all* the gas the person expired is determined, and this amount is multiplied by the percentage of nitrogen in the mixed expired air, which can be determined with the nitrogen analyzer. The total volume of nitrogen in the person's lungs *at the beginning of the test* can thus be determined. Nitrogen constitutes about 80% of the

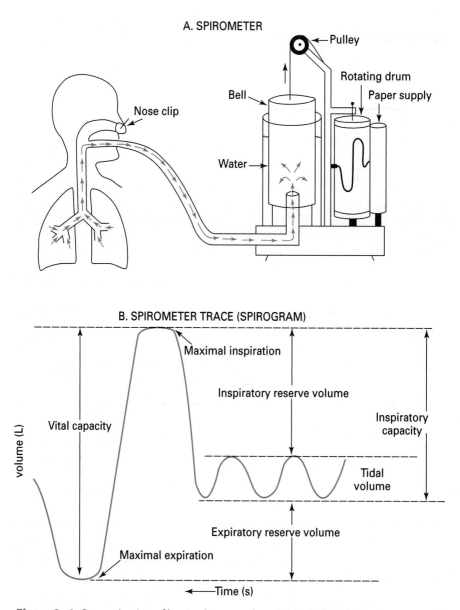

Figure 3–4. Determination of lung volumes and capacities with a spirometer.
A: Schematic representation of a water-filled spirometer. **B:** Determination of the tidal volume, vital capacity, inspiratory capacity, inspiratory reserve volume, and expiratory reserve volume from a spirometer trace.

person's initial lung volume, and so multiplying the initial nitrogen volume by 1.25 gives the person's initial lung volume. If the test is *begun* at the end of a normal tidal expiration, the volume determined is the FRC:

$$\text{Total volume expired} \times \% N_2 = \text{original volume of } N_2 \text{ in lungs}$$
$$\text{Original volume of } N_2 \text{ in lungs} \times 1.25 = \text{original lung volume}$$

HELIUM-DILUTION TECHNIQUE

The helium-dilution technique makes use of the following relationship: If the total *amount* of a substance dissolved in a volume is known and its *concentration* can be measured, the *volume* in which it is dissolved can be determined. For example, if a known amount of a solute is dissolved in an unknown volume of solvent, and the concentration of the solute can be determined, then the volume of solvent can be calculated:

$$Q = CV$$

$$\text{Amount of solute (mg)} = \text{concentration of solute (mg/mL)}$$
$$\times \text{volume of solvent (mL)}$$

In the helium-dilution technique, helium is dissolved in the gas in the lungs and its concentration is determined with a helium meter, allowing calculation of the lung volume. Helium is used for this test because it is not taken up by the pulmonary capillary blood and because it does not diffuse out of the blood, and so the total *amount* of helium does not change during the test. The person breathes in and out of a spirometer filled with a mixture of helium and oxygen, as shown in Figure 3–5. The helium concentration is monitored continuously with a helium meter until its concentration in the inspired air equals its concentration in the person's expired air. At this point, the concentration of helium is the same in the person's lungs as it is in the spirometer, and the test is *stopped* at the end of a normal tidal expiration, in other words, at the FRC.

The FRC can then be determined by the following formula (total amount of He before test = total amount of He at end of test):

$$F_{HE_i} \, Vsp_i = F_{HE_f} (Vsp_f + V_{L_f})$$

That is, the *total* amount of helium in the system initially is equal to its initial fractional concentration (F_{HE_i}) times the initial volume of the spirometer (Vsp_i). This must be equal to the *total* amount of helium in the lungs and the spirometer at the end of the test, which is equal to the final (lower) fractional concentration of helium (F_{HE_f}) times the final volume of the spirometer (Vsp_f) *and* the volume of the lungs at the end of the test (V_{L_f}). Since it may take several minutes for the helium concentration to equilibrate between the lungs and the spirometer, in practice, CO_2 is absorbed from the system and oxygen is added to the spirometer at the rate at which it is used by the person. Both the nitrogen-washout and helium-dilution methods can be used on unconscious patients.

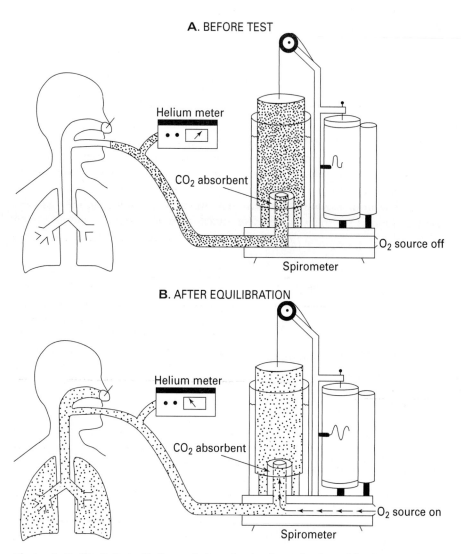

A. BEFORE TEST

Helium meter

CO_2 absorbent

O_2 source off

Spirometer

B. AFTER EQUILIBRATION

Helium meter

CO_2 absorbent

O_2 source on

Spirometer

Figure 3–5. The helium-dilution technique for the determination of the functional residual capacity. **A:** Before the test, the spirometer is filled with a mixture of helium (denoted by the dots) and oxygen. The concentration of helium is determined by the helium meter. **B:** The subject breathes from the spirometer until the helium concentration in the lungs equilibrates with that in the spirometer. During the equilibration period, the subject's expired carbon dioxide is absorbed and oxygen is added to the spirometer at the subject's oxygen consumption rate. The helium concentration and spirometer volume are determined after equilibration, when the subject is at functional residual capacity.

Body Plethysmography

A problem common to both the nitrogen-washout technique and the helium-dilution technique is that neither can measure trapped gas because nitrogen trapped in alveoli supplied by closed airways cannot be washed out and because the helium cannot enter alveoli supplied by closed airways. Furthermore, if the patient's lungs have many alveoli served by airways with high resistance to airflow (the "slow alveoli" discussed at the end of Chapter 2), it may take a very long time for all the nitrogen to wash out of the patient's lungs or for the inspired and expired helium concentrations to equilibrate. In such patients, measurements of the lung volumes with a body plethysmograph are much more accurate because they do include trapped gas.

The body plethysmograph makes use of Boyle's law, which states that for a closed container at a constant temperature, the pressure times the volume is constant. The body plethysmograph, an expensive piece of equipment, is shown schematically in Figure 3–6.

As can be seen from the figure, the body plethysmograph is an airtight chamber large enough so that the patient can sit inside it. The patient sits in the closed plethysmograph, or "box," and breathes through a mouthpiece and tubing. The tubing contains a sidearm connected to a pressure transducer ("mouth pressure"), an electrically controlled shutter that can occlude the airway when activated by the person conducting the test, and a pneumotachograph to measure airflow, allowing the operator to follow the subject's breathing pattern. A second pressure transducer, which must be very sensitive, monitors the pressure in the plethysmograph ("box pressure").

After the subject breathes through the open tube for a while to establish a normal breathing pattern, the operator closes the shutter in the airway at the end of a normal tidal expiration. At this point the subject *breathes in* for an instant against a closed airway. As the subject breathes in against the closed airway, the chest continues to expand and the pressure measured by the transducer in the plethysmograph (P_{box}) *increases* because the volume of air in the plethysmograph (V_{box}) decreases by the amount the patient's chest volume increased (ΔV):

$$P_{boxi} \times V_{boxi} = P_{boxf} \times (V_{boxi} - \Delta V) \qquad (1)$$

where $(V_{boxi} - \Delta V) = V_{boxf}$

That is, the product of the initial box pressure times the initial box volume must equal the final box pressure times the final box volume (the initial box volume minus a change in volume), according to Boyle's law. Of course, direct measurement of box volume, which is really equal to the volume of the plethysmograph *minus the volume occupied by the patient,* is impossible, and so the plethysmograph is calibrated with the patient in it by injecting known volumes of air into the plethysmograph and determining the increase in pressure. After such a graph of pressure changes with known changes in volume has been constructed, the ΔV in Equation (1) can be determined.

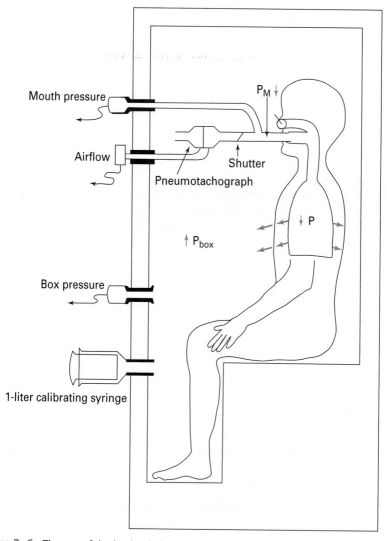

Figure 3–6. The use of the body plethysmograph for the determination of the functional residual capacity. The subject is seated in the small airtight chamber and breathes through the apparatus shown. By monitoring the subject's airflow with a pneumotachograph, the operator can briefly occlude the subject's airway at end expiration. As the subject makes an inspiratory effort against the closed airway, the pressure in the chamber (P_{box}) increases and the pressure at the subject's mouth (P_M) decreases. The subject's functional residual capacity can then be calculated.

The product of the pressure measured at the mouth (P_M) times the volume of the patient's lungs (V_L) must also be constant during the inspiration against a closed airway. As the patient breathes in, the volume of the lungs increases by the same amount as the decrease in the volume of the box determined in Equation (1) above (ΔV). As the lung volume increases, the pressure measured at the mouth decreases, as predicted by Boyle's law:

$$P_{M_i} \times V_{L_i} = P_{M_f} \times (V_{L_i} + \Delta V) \tag{2}$$

where $(V_{L_i} + \Delta V) = V_{L_f}$

The ΔV in Equation (2) is equal to that solved for in Equation (1) and V_{L_i} is now solved for. It is the FRC, since the airway was occluded at the end of a normal tidal expiration. In current practice the patient makes several panting inspiratory efforts against the closed airway, and all the calculations described above are made automatically by a computer receiving inputs from the pressure transducers.

ANATOMIC DEAD SPACE & ALVEOLAR VENTILATION

The volume of air entering and leaving the nose or mouth per minute, the *minute volume,* is not equal to the volume of air entering and leaving the alveoli per minute. *Alveolar ventilation* is *less* than the minute volume because the last part of each inspiration remains in the conducting airways and does not reach the alveoli. Similarly, the last part of each expiration remains in the conducting airways and is not expelled from the body. No gas exchange occurs in the conducting airways for anatomic reasons: The walls of the conducting airways are too thick for much diffusion to take place; mixed venous blood does not come into contact with the air. The conducting airways are therefore referred to as the *anatomic dead space.*

The anatomic dead space is illustrated in Figure 3–7. A subject breathes in from a balloon filled with 500 mL of a test gas such as helium that is not taken up by or liberated from the pulmonary capillary blood. Initially (Figure 3–7A), there is no test gas in the subject's airways or lungs. The subject then (Figure 3–7B) breathes in all 500 mL of the gas. However, not all the gas reaches the alveoli. The final portion of the inspired gas remains in the conducting airways, completely filling them. The volume of the test gas reaching the alveoli is equal to the volume breathed in from the balloon minus the volume of the anatomic dead space, in this case 500 mL − 150 mL, or 350 mL. The 350 mL of test gas mixes with the air already in the alveoli and is diluted. During expiration (Figure 3–7C) the first gas breathed back into the balloon is the undiluted test gas that remained in the anatomic dead space. Following the undiluted test gas is part of the gas that reached the alveoli and was diluted by the alveolar air. The last 150 mL of alveolar gas breathed out remains in the anatomic dead space. The concentration of test gas collected in the balloon after expiration is lower than it was before the breath but higher than the concentration left in the alveoli and conducting airways because it is composed of pure test gas from the anatomic dead space and diluted test gas from the alveoli.

Therefore, for any respiratory cycle, not all the tidal volume reaches the alveoli because the last part of each inspiration and each expiration remains in the dead space. The relationship among the V_T breathed in and out through the nose or

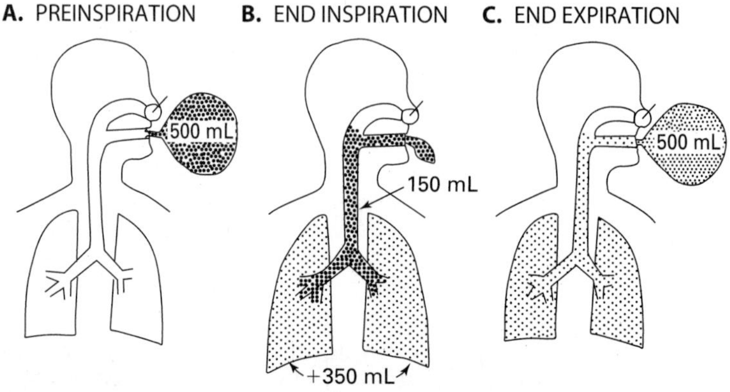

A. PREINSPIRATION   **B.** END INSPIRATION   **C.** END EXPIRATION

Figure 3–7. Illustration of the anatomic dead space. **A:** The subject inspires 500 mL from a balloon filled with a high concentration of a test gas (denoted by the dots). **B:** At the end of the inspiration, only 350 mL of the test gas has reached the alveoli. This 350 mL is added to the 2 to 3 L of alveolar gas already in the lungs at the functional residual capacity, and so its concentration is diluted. The other 150 mL of test gas remains virtually unchanged in the subject's anatomic dead space. **C:** At end expiration, diluted test gas remains virtually unchanged in the subject's anatomic dead space, and it remains equally concentrated in alveolar air and in the anatomic dead space. The test gas in the balloon is a mixture of undiluted gas from the dead space and diluted alveolar gas.

mouth, the dead space volume (V_D), and the volume of gas entering and leaving the alveoli per breath (V_A) is:

$$V_T = V_D + V_A$$
$$\text{or} \quad V_A = V_T - V_D$$

Thus, if a person with an anatomic dead space of 150 mL has a V_T of 500 mL per breath, then only 350 mL of gas enters and leaves the alveoli per breath.

The alveolar ventilation (per minute) can be determined by multiplying both sides of the above equation by the breathing frequency (n) in breaths per minute:

$$n(V_A) = n(V_T) - n(V_D)$$

Thus, if $n = 12$ breaths per minute in the example above:

$$4200 \frac{mL}{min} = 6000 \frac{mL}{min} - 1800 \frac{mL}{min}$$

The alveolar ventilation ($\dot{V}_A$) in liters per minute is equal to the minute volume ($\dot{V}_E$) minus the volume wasted ventilating the dead space per minute ($\dot{V}_D$):

$$\dot{V}_A = \dot{V}_E - \dot{V}_D$$

The dot over the letter V indicates *per minute*. The symbol $\dot{V}_E$ is used because expired gas is usually collected. There is a difference between the volume of gas inspired and the volume of gas expired because as air is inspired, it is heated to body temperature and humidified and also because normally less carbon dioxide is produced than oxygen is consumed.

MEASUREMENT OF ALVEOLAR VENTILATION

Alveolar ventilation cannot be measured directly but must be determined from the V_T, the breathing frequency, and the dead space ventilation, as noted in the previous section.

Measurement of Anatomic Dead Space

For a normal, healthy subject, the anatomic dead space can be estimated by referring to a table of standard values matched to sex, age, height, and weight or body surface area. A reasonable estimate of anatomic dead space is 1 mL of dead space per pound of ideal body weight. Nevertheless, it may be important to determine the anatomic dead space in a particular patient. This can be done by using Fowler's method. This method uses a nitrogen meter to analyze the expired nitrogen concentration after a single inspiration of 100% oxygen. The expired gas volume is measured simultaneously. Fowler's method is summarized in Figure 3–8.

The subject breathes in a single breath of 100% oxygen through a one-way valve, holds it in for a second, and then exhales through the one-way valve. *Nitrogen concentration* at the mouth and the *volume expired* are monitored simultaneously. Initially, the nitrogen concentration at the mouth is 80%, the same as that of the ambient atmosphere. As the stopcock is turned and the subject begins to inspire 100% oxygen, the nitrogen concentration at the mouth falls to zero. The subject holds his or her breath for a second or so and then exhales through the valve into a spirometer or pneumotachograph. The first part of the expired gas registers 0% nitrogen because it is undiluted 100% oxygen from the anatomic dead space. In the transitional period that follows, the expired gas registers a slowly rising nitrogen concentration. During this time, the expired gas is a mixture of dead space gas and alveolar gas because of a gradual transition between the conducting pathways and the respiratory bronchioles, as was seen in Figure 1–5. The final portion of expired gas comes solely from the alveoli and is called the *alveolar plateau*. Its nitrogen concentration is less than 80% because some of the breath of 100% oxygen reached the alveoli and diluted the alveolar nitrogen concentration, as shown in Figure 3–7. The volume of the anatomic dead space is the volume expired between the beginning of the expiration and the midpoint of the transitional phase, as shown in Figure 3–8.

Physiologic Dead Space: The Bohr Equation

Fowler's method is especially useful for the determination of the *anatomic* dead space. It does not, however, permit the calculation of another form of wasted ventilation in the lung—the *alveolar dead space.* The alveolar dead space is the volume of gas that enters *unperfused* alveoli per breath. Alveolar dead space is therefore ventilated but not perfused. No gas exchange occurs in these

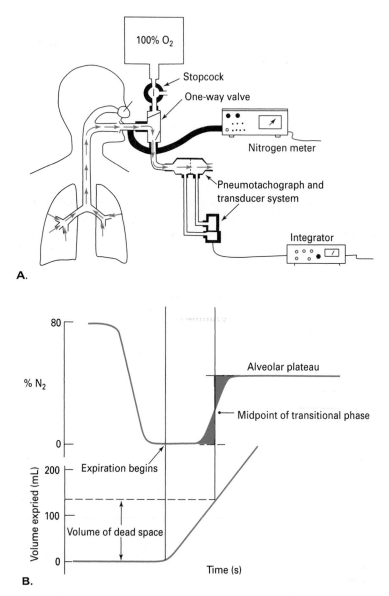

Figure 3–8. Fowler's method for the determination of anatomic dead space. **A:** The subject takes a single breath of 100% oxygen, holds his or her breath for a second, and then exhales. Nitrogen concentration is monitored along with the volume of gas expired, in this case by integrating with time the airflow (L/s) determined by a pneumo-tachograph-differential air pressure transducer system. **B:** The volume of gas expired between the beginning of the exhalation and the midpoint of the rising phase of the expired nitrogen concentration trace is the anatomic dead space. (The midpoint is determined such that the two shaded areas are equal.)

alveoli for physiologic, rather than anatomic, reasons. A healthy person has little or no alveolar dead space, but a person with a low cardiac output might have a great deal of alveolar dead space, for reasons explained in the next chapter.

The Bohr equation permits the determination of the sum of the anatomic and the alveolar dead space. The anatomic dead space *plus* the alveolar dead space is known as the *physiologic dead space:*

Physiologic dead space = anatomic dead space + alveolar dead space

The Bohr equation makes use of a simple concept: Any measurable volume of carbon dioxide found in the mixed *expired* gas must come from alveoli that are *both ventilated and perfused* because there are negligible amounts of carbon dioxide in inspired air. Inspired air remaining in the anatomic dead space or entering unperfused alveoli will leave the body as it entered (except for having been heated to body temperature and humidified), contributing little or no carbon dioxide to the mixed expired air:

$$\underset{\substack{\text{Volume of } CO_2 \\ \text{in mixed expired air}}}{F_{\bar{E}_{CO_2}} \times V_T} \quad = \quad \underset{\substack{\text{Volume of } CO_2 \\ \text{coming from dead space}}}{F_{I_{CO_2}} \times V_{D_{CO_2}}} \quad + \quad \underset{\substack{\text{Volume of } CO_2 \\ \text{coming from alveoli}}}{F_{A_{CO_2}} \times V_A}$$

where F = fractional concentration
$\bar{E}$ = mixed expired
I = inspired
A = alveolar
$V_{D_{CO_2}}$ = dead space for CO_2 (physiologic dead space)
$F_{A_{CO_2}}$ = fractional concentration of CO_2 in alveoli that are both ventilated and perfused

Since $F_{I_{CO_2}}$ is approximately equal to zero, the $F_{I_{CO_2}} \times V_{D_{CO_2}}$ term drops out. Substituting $(V_T - V_{D_{CO_2}})$ for V_A:

$$F_{\bar{E}_{CO_2}} \times V_T = F_{A_{CO_2}}(V_T - V_{D_{CO_2}})$$
$$F_{\bar{E}_{CO_2}} \times V_T = F_{A_{CO_2}} \times V_T - F_{A_{CO_2}} \times V_{D_{CO_2}}$$
$$V_{D_{CO_2}} \times F_{A_{CO_2}} = V_T(F_{A_{CO_2}} - F_{\bar{E}_{CO_2}})$$
$$\frac{V_{D_{CO_2}}}{V_T} = \frac{F_{A_{CO_2}} - F_{\bar{E}_{CO_2}}}{F_{A_{CO_2}}}$$
$$\text{Since } F_{CO_2} = \frac{P_{CO_2}}{P_{tot}}$$
$$\text{then } \frac{V_{D_{CO_2}}}{V_T} = \frac{P_{A_{CO_2}} - P_{\bar{E}_{CO_2}}}{P_{A_{CO_2}}}$$

The P_{CO_2} of the collected mixed expired gas can be determined with a CO_2 meter. The CO_2 meter is often also used to estimate the alveolar P_{CO_2} by analyzing the gas expelled at the end of a normal tidal expiration, the "end-tidal CO_2" (Figure 3–9). But in a person with significant alveolar dead space, the estimated alveolar P_{CO_2} obtained in this fashion may not reflect the P_{CO_2} of alveoli that are ventilated and perfused because some of this mixed end-tidal gas comes from unperfused alveoli. This gas dilutes the CO_2 coming from alveoli that are both ventilated and perfused. There is, however, an equilibrium between the P_{CO_2} of *perfused* alveoli and their end-capillary P_{CO_2} (see Chapter 6 for detailed discussion), so that in patients without significant venous-to-arterial shunts, the *arterial* P_{CO_2} represents the mean P_{CO_2} of the *perfused* alveoli. Therefore, the Bohr equation should be rewritten as:

$$\frac{V_{D_{CO_2}}}{V_T} = \frac{Pa_{CO_2} - P\bar{E}_{CO_2}}{Pa_{CO_2}}$$

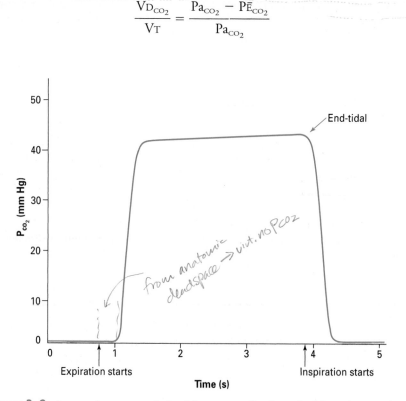

Figure 3–9. A normal capnograph: Partial pressure of carbon dioxide at the mouth as determined by an infrared carbon dioxide meter or mass spectrometer. During *inspiration* the P_{CO_2} rapidly decreases to near zero (0.3 mm Hg). The first expired gas comes from the anatomic dead space and therefore also has a P_{CO_2} near zero. After exhalation of a mixture of gas from alveoli and anatomic dead space, the gas expired is a mixture from all ventilated alveoli. The slope of the alveolar plateau normally rises slightly because the alveolar P_{CO_2} increases a few mm Hg between inspirations. The last alveolar gas expired before inspiration is called *end-tidal*.

The V_T is determined with a spirometer, and the physiologic dead space is then calculated. If the arterial P_{CO_2} is greater than the mixed alveolar P_{CO_2} determined by sampling the end-tidal CO_2, then the physiologic dead space is probably greater than the anatomic dead space; that is, a significant *arterial-alveolar CO_2 difference* means that there is significant alveolar dead space. As already noted, this difference is determined from the P_{CO_2} from an arterial blood gas sample and from the end-tidal P_{CO_2}. Situations in which alveoli are ventilated but not perfused include those in which portions of the pulmonary vasculature have been occluded by blood clots in the venous blood (pulmonary emboli), situations in which there is low venous return leading to low right ventricular output (hemorrhage), and situations in which alveolar pressure is high (positive-pressure ventilation with positive end-expiratory pressure).

The anatomic dead space can be altered by bronchoconstriction, which decreases V_D; bronchodilation, which increases V_D; or traction or compression of the airways, which increases and decreases V_D, respectively.

ALVEOLAR VENTILATION & ALVEOLAR OXYGEN & CARBON DIOXIDE LEVELS

The levels of oxygen and carbon dioxide in alveolar gas are determined by the alveolar ventilation, the oxygen consumption ($\dot{V}O_2$) of the body, and the carbon dioxide production of the body ($\dot{V}CO_2$). Each inspiration brings into the 3 L of gas already in the lungs approximately 350 mL of fresh air containing about 21% oxygen, and each expiration removes about 350 mL of air containing about 5 to 6% carbon dioxide. Meanwhile, about 250 mL of carbon dioxide per minute diffuses from the pulmonary capillary blood into the alveoli, and about 300 mL of oxygen per minute diffuses from the alveolar air into the pulmonary capillary blood.

Partial Pressures of Respiratory Gases

According to Dalton's law, in a gas mixture, the pressure exerted by each individual gas is independent of the pressures of other gases in the mixture. The partial pressure of a particular gas is equal to its fractional concentration times the total pressure of all the gases in the mixture. Thus for any gas in a mixture (gas$_1$) its partial pressure is

$$P_{gas_1} = \% \text{ total gas} \times P_{tot}$$

Oxygen constitutes 20.93% of dry atmospheric air. At a standard barometric pressure of 760 mm Hg,

$$P_{O_2} = 0.2093 \times 760 \text{ mm Hg} = 159 \text{ mm Hg}$$

(The units mm Hg are also expressed as torr, in honor of Evangelista Torricelli, the inventor of the barometer.) Carbon dioxide constitutes only about 0.04% of dry atmospheric air, and so,

$$P_{CO_2} = 0.0004 \times 760 \text{ mm Hg} = 0.3 \text{ mm Hg}$$

Dry Atmospheric Gas at Standard Barometric Pressure	
P_{O_2}	159.0 mm Hg
P_{CO_2}	0.3 mm Hg
P_{N_2}	600.6 mm Hg

As air is inspired through the upper airways, it is heated and humidified, as will be discussed in Chapter 10. The partial pressure of water vapor is a relatively constant 47 mm Hg at body temperature, and so the humidification of 1 L of dry gas *in a closed container* at 760 mm Hg would increase its total pressure to 760 mm Hg + 47 mm Hg = 807 mm Hg. In the body, the gas will simply expand, according to Boyle's law, so that 1 L of gas at 760 mm Hg is *diluted* by the added water vapor. The P_{O_2} of inspired air, or PI_{O_2} (saturated with water vapor at a standard barometric pressure), then is equal to the fractional concentration of inspired oxygen (the FI_{O_2}) times the barometric pressure minus the water vapor pressure:

$$PI_{O_2} = FI_{O_2} (P_B - P_{H_2O})$$

where P_B = barometric pressure and P_{H_2O} = the water vapor pressure

$$0.2093 (760 - 47) \text{ mm Hg} = 149 \text{ mm Hg}$$

The P_{CO_2} of inspired air (the PI_{CO_2}) is equal to the $FI_{CO_2} (P_B - P_{H_2O})$ or 0.0004 (760 − 47) mm Hg = 0.29 mm Hg. This rounds back up to 0.3 mm Hg.

Inspired Gas at Standard Barometric Pressure	
PI_{O_2}	149.0 mm Hg
PI_{CO_2}	0.3 mm Hg
PI_{N_2}	564.0 mm Hg
PI_{H_2O}	47.0 mm Hg

Alveolar gas is composed of the 2.5 to 3 L of gas already in the lungs at the FRC and the approximately 350 mL per breath entering and leaving the alveoli. About 300 mL of oxygen is continuously diffusing from the alveoli into the pulmonary capillary blood per minute at rest and is being replaced by alveolar ventilation.

Similarly, about 250 mL of carbon dioxide is diffusing from the mixed venous blood in the pulmonary capillaries into the alveoli per minute and is then removed by alveolar ventilation. (The P_{O_2} and P_{CO_2} of mixed venous blood are about 40 mm Hg and 45 to 46 mm Hg, respectively.) Because of these processes, the partial pressures of oxygen and carbon dioxide in the alveolar air are determined by the alveolar ventilation, the pulmonary capillary perfusion, the oxygen consumption, and the carbon dioxide production. Alveolar ventilation is normally adjusted by the respiratory control center in the brain to keep mean arterial and alveolar P_{CO_2} at about 40 mm Hg (see Chapter 9). Mean alveolar P_{O_2} is about 104 mm Hg.

Alveolar Gas at Standard Barometric Pressure	
PA_{O_2}	104 mm Hg
PA_{CO_2}	40 mm Hg
PA_{N_2}	569 mm Hg
PA_{H_2O}	47 mm Hg

The alveolar P_{O_2} increases by 2 to 4 mm Hg with each normal tidal inspiration and falls slowly until the next inspiration. Similarly, the alveolar P_{CO_2} falls 2 to 4 mm Hg with each inspiration and increases slowly until the next inspiration. Expired air is a mixture of about 350 mL of alveolar air and 150 mL of air from the dead space. Therefore, the P_{O_2} of mixed expired air is higher than alveolar P_{O_2} and lower than the inspired P_{O_2}, or approximately 120 mm Hg. Similarly, the P_{CO_2} of mixed expired air is much higher than the inspired P_{CO_2} but lower than the alveolar P_{CO_2}, or about 27 mm Hg.

Mixed Expired Air at Standard Barometric Pressure	
PE_{O_2}	120 mm Hg
PE_{CO_2}	27 mm Hg
PE_{N_2}	566 mm Hg
PE_{H_2O}	47 mm Hg

Alveolar Ventilation & Carbon Dioxide

The concentration of carbon dioxide in the alveolar gas is, as already discussed, dependent on the alveolar ventilation and on the rate of carbon dioxide production by the body (and its delivery to the lung in the mixed venous blood). The volume of carbon dioxide expired per unit of time ($\dot{V}E_{CO_2}$) is equal to the alveolar ventilation ($\dot{V}A$) times the alveolar fractional concentration of CO_2 (FA_{CO_2}). No carbon dioxide comes from the dead space:

$$\dot{V}E_{CO_2} = \dot{V}A \times FA_{CO_2}$$

Similarly, the fractional concentration of carbon dioxide in the alveoli is directly proportional to the carbon dioxide production by the body ($\dot{V}_{CO_2}$) and inversely proportional to the alveolar ventilation:

$$F_{A_{CO_2}} \propto \frac{\dot{V}_{CO_2}}{\dot{V}_A}$$

Since $F_{A_{CO_2}} \times (P_B - P_{H_2O}) = P_{A_{CO_2}}$

then $P_{A_{CO_2}} \propto \dfrac{\dot{V}_{CO_2}}{\dot{V}_A}$

 In healthy people, alveolar P_{CO_2} is in equilibrium with arterial P_{CO_2} (Pa_{CO_2}). Thus, if alveolar ventilation is doubled (and carbon dioxide production is unchanged), then the alveolar and arterial P_{CO_2} are reduced by one-half. If alveolar ventilation is cut in half, near 40 mm Hg, then alveolar and arterial P_{CO_2} will double. This can be seen in the upper part of Figure 3–10.

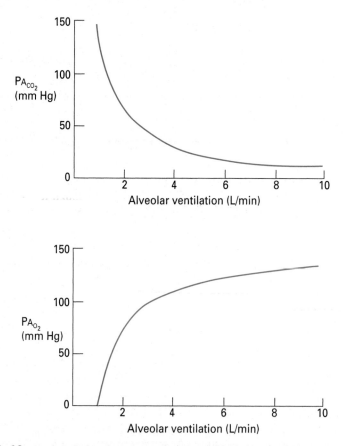

Figure 3–10. Predicted alveolar gas tensions for different levels of alveolar ventilation. (From Nunn's *Applied Respiratory Physiology, 4th edition* by J.F. Nunn, 1993. Reprinted by permission of Elsevier Science Limited.)

Alveolar Ventilation & Oxygen

It is evident that as alveolar ventilation increases, the alveolar P_{O_2} will also increase. Doubling alveolar ventilation, however, cannot double PA_{O_2} in a person whose alveolar P_{O_2} is already 104 mm Hg because the highest PA_{O_2} one could possibly achieve (breathing air at sea level) is the inspired P_{O_2} of about 149 mm Hg. The alveolar P_{O_2} can be calculated by using the *alveolar air equation.* (The derivation of this formula is outside the scope of this book.)

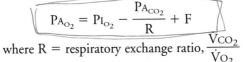

$$PA_{O_2} = PI_{O_2} - \frac{PA_{CO_2}}{R} + F$$

where R = respiratory exchange ratio, $\dfrac{\dot{V}_{CO_2}}{\dot{V}_{O_2}}$

F = a small correction factor

As already noted, $PI_{O_2} = FI_{O_2} (P_B - P_{H_2O})$. The F is usually ignored. Therefore:

$$PA_{O_2} = FI_{O_2} (P_B - P_{H_2O}) - \frac{PA_{CO_2}}{R}$$

As alveolar ventilation increases, the alveolar P_{CO_2} decreases, bringing the alveolar P_{O_2} closer to the inspired P_{O_2}, as can be seen in the lower part of Figure 3–10. Note that the alveolar P_{O_2} obtained using the alveolar air equation is a calculated idealized average alveolar P_{O_2}. It represents what alveolar P_{O_2} *should be,* not necessarily what it is.

REGIONAL DISTRIBUTION OF ALVEOLAR VENTILATION

As previously discussed, a 70-kg person has about 2.5 to 3 L of gas in the lungs at the FRC. Each breath brings about 350 mL of fresh gas into the alveoli and removes about 350 mL of alveolar air from the lung. Although it is reasonable to assume that the alveolar ventilation is distributed fairly evenly to alveoli throughout the lungs, this is not the case. Studies performed on normal subjects seated upright have shown that alveoli in the lower regions of the lungs receive more ventilation per unit volume than do those in the upper regions of the lung.

Demonstration of Differences between Dependent & Nondependent Regions

If a normal subject, seated in the upright posture and breathing normally (inspiring from the FRC), takes a single breath of a mixture of oxygen and radioactive ^{133}Xe, the relative ventilation of various regions of the lung can be determined by placing scintillation counters over appropriate areas of the thorax, as shown in Figure 3–11.

It is assumed that if the oxygen and ^{133}Xe are well mixed, then the amount of radioactivity measured by the scintillation counters in each region will be directly proportional to the relative ventilation (the ventilation per unit volume) in each region.

The results of a series of such experiments are shown on the graph on the right side of Figure 3–11. In a subject seated in the upright posture and breathing normally

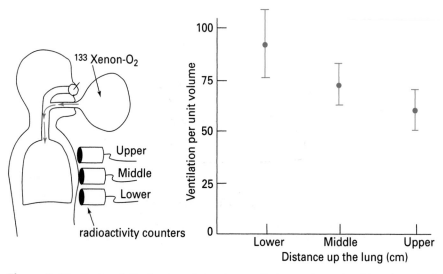

Figure 3–11. Regional distribution of alveolar ventilation as determined by a breath of a mixture of ^{133}Xe and O_2. (Data of Bryan, 1964. Reproduced with permission.)

from the FRC, the lower regions of the lung are relatively better ventilated than the upper regions of the lung.

If a similar study is done on a subject lying on his or her left side, the regional differences in ventilation between the *anatomic* upper, middle, and lower regions of the lung disappear, although there is better relative ventilation of the left lung than of the right lung. The regional differences in ventilation thus appear to be influenced by gravity, with regions of the lung lower with respect to gravity (the *"dependent"* regions) relatively better ventilated than those regions above them (the *"nondependent"* regions).

Explanation for Differences in Regional Alveolar Ventilation

In Chapter 2, the intrapleural surface pressure was discussed as if it were uniform throughout the thorax. Precise measurements made of the intrapleural surface pressures of intact chests in the upright position have shown that this is not the case: The intrapleural surface pressure is *less negative* in the lower, gravity-dependent regions of the thorax than it is in the upper, nondependent regions. There is a gradient of the intrapleural surface pressure such that for every centimeter of vertical displacement down the lung (from nondependent to dependent regions) the intrapleural surface pressure increases by about +0.2 to +0.5 cm H_2O. This gradient is apparently caused by gravity and by mechanical interactions between the lung and the chest wall.

The influence of this gradient of intrapleural surface pressure on regional alveolar ventilation can be explained by predicting its effect on the transpulmonary pressure gradients in upper and lower regions of the lung. The left side of Figure 3–12 shows that *alveolar* pressure is zero in both regions of the lung at

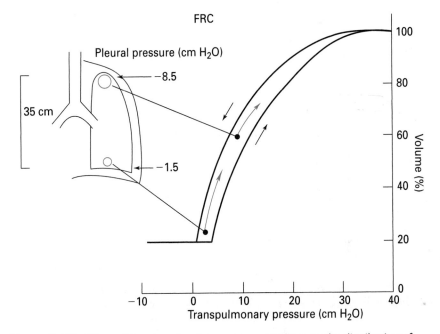

Figure 3–12. Effect of the pleural surface pressure gradient on the distribution of inspired gas at the *functional residual capacity (FRC)*. (After Milic-Emili, 1977.)

the FRC. Since the intrapleural pressure is *more negative in upper regions* of the lung than it is in lower regions of the lung, the *transpulmonary pressure* (alveolar minus intrapleural) is greater in upper regions of the lung than it is in lower regions of the lung. Because the alveoli in upper regions of the lung are subjected to greater distending pressures than those in more dependent regions of the lung, they have greater *volumes* than the alveoli in more dependent regions.

It is this difference in *volume* that leads to the difference in *ventilation* between alveoli located in dependent and nondependent regions of the lung. This can be seen on the hypothetical pressure-volume curve shown on the right side of Figure 3–12. This curve is similar to the pressure-volume curve for a whole lung shown in Figure 2–6, except that this curve is drawn with the pressure-volume characteristics of single alveoli in mind. The abscissa is the transpulmonary pressure (alveolar pressure minus intrapleural pressure). The ordinate is the volume of the alveolus expressed as a percent of its maximum.

The alveolus in the upper, nondependent region of the lung has a larger transpulmonary pressure than does the alveolus in a more dependent region because the intrapleural pressure in the upper, nondependent regions of the lung is more negative than it is in more dependent regions. Because of this greater transpulmonary pressure, the alveolus in the upper region of the lung has a greater volume than the alveolus in a more gravity-dependent region of the lung. At the FRC, the alveolus in the upper part of the lung is on a *less steep portion* of the alveolar

UPPER LUNG = ↑ Volume (due to ↑ transpulm P)
↓ compliance

pressure-volume curve (i.e., it is *less compliant*) in Figure 3–12 than is the more compliant alveolus in the lower region of the lung. Therefore, any change in the transpulmonary pressure during a normal respiratory cycle will cause a greater *change in volume* in the alveolus in the lower, gravity-dependent region of the lung than it will in the alveolus in the nondependent region of the lung, as shown by the arrows in the figure. Because the alveoli in the lower parts of the lung have a greater change in volume per inspiration and per expiration, they are better *ventilated* than those alveoli in nondependent regions (during eupneic breathing from the FRC).

A second effect of the intrapleural pressure gradient in a person seated upright is on regional static lung volume, as is evident from the above discussion. At the FRC, most of the alveolar air is in upper regions of the lung because those alveoli have larger volumes. Most of the ERV is also in upper portions of the lung. On the other hand, most of the IRV and IC are in lower regions of the lung.

Alterations of Distribution at Different Lung Volumes

As discussed in the previous section, most of the air inspired during a tidal breath begun at the FRC enters the dependent alveoli. If a slow inspiration is begun at the RV, however, the initial part of the breath (inspiratory volume less than the ERV) enters the nondependent upper alveoli, and dependent alveoli begin to fill later in the breath. The intrapleural pressure gradient from the upper parts of the lung to the lower parts of the lung is also the cause of this preferential ventilation of non-dependent alveoli at low lung volumes.

Positive intrapleural pressures are generated by the expiratory muscles during a forced expiration to the RV. This results in dynamic compression of small airways, as described in Chapter 2. At the highest intrapleural pressures these airways close, and gas is trapped in their alveoli. Because of the gradient of intrapleural pressure found in the upright lung, at low lung volumes the pleural surface pressure is more positive in lower regions of the lung than it is in upper regions. Also, alveoli in lower lung regions have less alveolar elastic recoil to help hold small airways open because they have smaller volumes than do the alveoli in upper regions. This means that airway closure will occur *first* in airways in lower regions of the lung, as can be seen in the hypothetical alveolar pressure-volume curve at the RV shown in Figure 3–13. The expiratory effort has ended and the inspiratory effort has just begun. Airways in the lowest regions of the lung are still closed, and the local pleural surface pressure is still slightly positive. No air enters these alveoli during the first part of the inspiratory effort (as indicated by the horizontal arrow) until sufficient negative pressure is generated to open these closed airways.

In contrast to the situation at the FRC, at the RV the alveoli in the upper regions of the lungs are now on a much steeper portion of the pressure-volume curve. They now have a much greater change in volume per change in transpulmonary pressure—they are more compliant at this lower lung volume. Therefore, they receive more of the air initially inspired from the RV.

It has already been noted that even at low lung volumes the upper alveoli are larger in volume than are the lower gravity-dependent alveoli. They therefore constitute most of the RV.

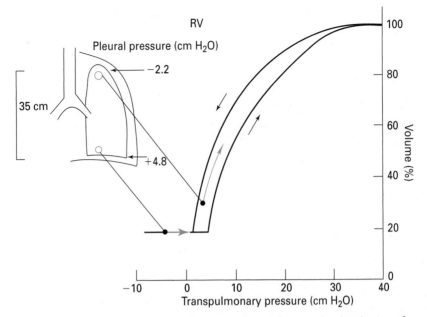

Figure 3–13. Effect of the pleural surface pressure gradient on the distribution of inspired gas at the *residual volume (RV)*. (After Milic-Emili, 1977.)

Patients with emphysema have greatly decreased alveolar elastic recoil, leading to high FRCs, extremely high RVs, and airway closure in dependent parts of the lung even at high lung volumes. They therefore have relatively more ventilation of nondependent alveoli.

THE CLOSING VOLUME

The lung volume at which airway closure *begins* to occur is known as the *closing volume*. It can be demonstrated by utilizing the same equipment used in Fowler's method for the quantification of the anatomic dead space seen in Figure 3–8. This method can also demonstrate certain maldistributions of alveolar ventilation.

The subject, seated upright, *starts from the RV* and inspires a single breath of 100% oxygen all the way up to the TLC. The person then exhales all the way back down to the RV. Nitrogen concentration at the mouth and the volume of gas expired are monitored simultaneously throughout the second expiration.

Consider what occurs during the *first* expiration to the RV. Because of the gradient of intrapleural pressure from the top of the lung to the bottom of the lung, the alveoli in upper parts of the lung are larger than those in lower regions of the lung. Any gas left in the lungs at the end of this initial forced expiration to the RV is about 80% nitrogen, and so most of the nitrogen (and most of the RV) are in upper parts of the lung. Alveoli in lower portions of the lung have smaller volumes and thus contain less nitrogen. At the bottom part of the lung, airways are closed, trapping whatever small volume of gas remains in these alveoli.

The subject then inspires 100% oxygen to the TLC. Although the initial part of this breath will probably enter the upper alveoli, as described previously, most of the 100% oxygen will enter the more dependent alveoli. (The *very* first part, which does enter the upper alveoli, is dead-space gas, which is 80% nitrogen anyway.) If the nitrogen concentration of alveoli in different parts of the lung could be measured at this point, the nitrogen concentration would be highest in the upper regions of the lung and the lowest in the lower regions of the lung.

The subject then exhales to the RV as the expired nitrogen concentration and gas volume are monitored. The expired nitrogen concentration trace is shown in Figure 3–14.

The first gas the subject exhales (phase I) is pure gas from the anatomic dead space. It is still virtually 100% oxygen or 0% nitrogen. The second portion of gas exhaled by the subject (phase II) is a mixture of dead-space gas and alveolar gas. The third portion of gas expired by the subject is mixed alveolar gas from the upper and lower regions (phase III, or the "alveolar plateau").

Note that in a healthy person the slope of phase III is nearly horizontal. In patients with certain types of airways-resistance maldistribution, the phase III slope rises rapidly. This is because those alveoli that are supplied by high-resistance airways fill more slowly than those supplied by the normal airways during the 100%

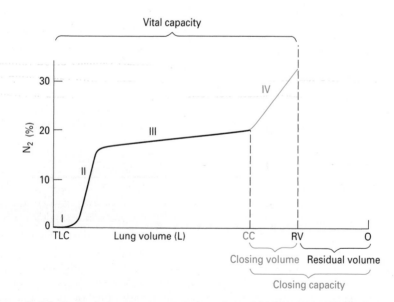

Figure 3–14. Expired nitrogen concentration after inhalation of a single breath of 100% oxygen from the residual volume to the total lung capacity. Subject exhales to the residual volume. *Phase I:* 0% nitrogen from anatomic dead space. *Phase II:* mixture of gas from anatomic dead space and alveoli. *Phase III:* "alveolar plateau" gas from alveoli. A steep slope of phase III indicates nonuniform distribution of alveolar gas. *Phase IV:* closing volume. Takeoff point (closing capacity) of phase IV denotes beginning of airway closure in dependent portions of the lung.

oxygen inspiration. Thus, they have a relatively higher nitrogen concentration. During expiration they empty more slowly, and when they do, the expired nitrogen concentration rises.

As the expiration to the RV continues, the positive pleural surface pressure causes dynamic compression and ultimately airway closure. Because of the intrapleural pressure gradient from the upper parts of the lung to the lower parts of the lung and because the smaller alveoli in lower parts of the lung have less elastic recoil, the airway closure first occurs in lower regions of the lung where the nitrogen concentration is the lowest. Thus, as airway closure begins, the expired nitrogen concentration rises abruptly because more and more of the expired gas is coming from alveoli in upper regions of the lung. These alveoli have the highest nitrogen concentration. The point at which the expired nitrogen concentration trace rises abruptly is the volume at which airway closure in dependent parts of the lung begins. At this point, the subject is at his or her *closing capacity,* which is equal to the RV plus the volume expired between the beginning of airway closure and the RV. This volume is called the *closing volume.* (Unfortunately, many people, the author included, commonly use the terms closing volume and closing capacity interchangeably.)

THE EFFECTS OF AGING

Aging causes important changes in the structure and function of the respiratory system. These include a loss of alveolar elastic recoil, alterations in chest wall structure causing it to have increased outward elastic recoil, decreased respiratory muscle strength, and a loss of alveolar surface area and pulmonary capillary blood volume.

The progressive loss of alveolar elastic recoil, combined with calcification of costal cartilages, decreased spaces between the spinal vertebrae, and a greater degree of spinal curvature, leads to increased static lung compliance and decreased chest wall compliance. This usually leads to an increase in the FRC with aging, as shown in Figure 3–15. The TLC, if adjusted for the decrease in height seen in older people, stays fairly constant with age.

Loss of alveolar elastic recoil results in decreased traction on small airways to oppose dynamic compression during forced expirations, as well as decreased driving pressures for airflow. This leads to airway closure at higher lung volumes, as shown by the rising closing capacity illustrated in Figure 3–15, and, combined with a decrease in the strength of the expiratory muscles, leads to an increase in the RV and decreased maximal expiratory airflow rates such as the $FEF_{25-75\%}$ and FEV_1. As shown in Figure 3–15, airway closure may occur in dependent airways of the elderly even at lung volumes above the FRC. Such older persons may therefore have relatively more ventilation of upper airways than do younger individuals. If blood flow to these poorly ventilated dependent regions is not reduced, this will lead to decreased arterial oxygen tension, which will be discussed in Chapter 5. The loss of alveolar surface area and decreased pulmonary capillary blood volume result in a decreased pulmonary diffusing capacity, which will be discussed in Chapter 6. This can also contribute to a progressive decrease in arterial oxygen tension with aging.

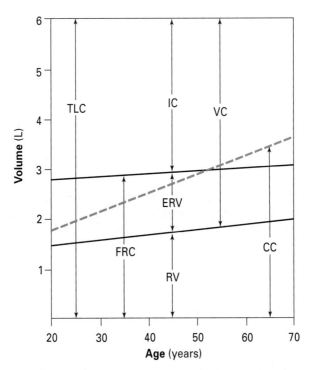

Figure 3–15. Illustration of the alterations in the standard lung volumes and capacities occurring with age. TLC = total lung capacity; FRC = functional residual capacity; ERV = expiratory reserve volume; RV = residual volume; IC = inspiratory capacity; VC = vital capacity; CC = closing capacity. (Reproduced with permission from Levitzky, 1984.)

KEY CONCEPTS

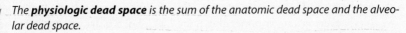

① *Alveolar ventilation is less than the volume of air entering or leaving the nose or mouth per minute (the minute volume) because the last part of each inspiration remains in the conducting airways (the **anatomic dead space**).*

② *Alveoli that are ventilated but not perfused constitute **alveolar dead space**.*

③ *The **physiologic dead space** is the sum of the anatomic dead space and the alveolar dead space.*

④ *At constant carbon dioxide production, alveolar P_{CO_2} is approximately inversely proportional to alveolar ventilation; alveolar P_{O_2} must be calculated with the **alveolar air equation**.*

⑤ *At or near the functional residual capacity, alveoli in lower regions of the upright lung are relatively better ventilated than those in upper regions of the lung.*

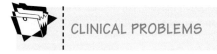

CLINICAL PROBLEMS

3–1. Which of the following conditions are reasonable explanations for a patient's functional residual capacity that is significantly less than predicted?

    a. Third trimester of pregnancy

    b. Pulmonary fibrosis

    c. Obesity

    d. Emphysema

    e. All of the above

    f. a, b, and c

3–2. What is the effect on each of the following standard lung volumes and capacities of changing from a supine to an upright position?

Functional residual capacity (FRC)

Residual volume (RV)

Expiratory reserve volume (ERV)

Total lung capacity (TLC)

Tidal volume V_T

Inspiratory reserve volume (IRV)

Inspiratory capacity (IC)

Vital capacity (VC)

3–3. How would the predicted values for the standard lung volumes and capacities and the closing capacity of a healthy elderly person differ from those of a young healthy person?

3–4. A volume of 1 L of gas is measured in a spirometer at 23°C (296 K; P_{H_2O} is 21 mm Hg), and barometric pressure is 770 mm Hg.

    a. What would the volume be under STPD conditions?

    b. What would the volume be under BTPS conditions?

3–5. A subject starts at her FRC and breathes 100% O_2 through a one-way valve. The expired air is collected in a very large spirometer (called a Tissot spirometer). The test is continued until the expired N_2 concentration, as measured by a nitrogen analyzer, is virtually zero. At this time there are 36 L of gas in the spirometer, of which 5.6% is N_2. What is the subject's FRC?

3–6. A 63-year-old-woman who is 5 ft 5 in tall and weighs 100 lb complains of dyspnea. During the determination of her lung volumes, she rebreathes the gas in a 20-L-capacity spirometer that originally contained 10 L of 15% helium. After a number of breaths, the concentration of helium in her lungs is equal to that now in the spirometer, which is 11% helium. (During the equilibration period, the expired CO_2 was absorbed by an absorbent chemical in the spirometer and O_2 was added to the spirometer at the subject's $\dot{V}_{O_2}$.) At the end of a normal expiration, the spirometer contains 10.64 L when corrected to BTPS. What is her FRC?

3–7. The same patient discussed in the previous problem, now in a body plethysmograph, breathes normally through a mouthpiece. At the end of a normal expiration, a valve in the mouthpiece is closed. The next inspiratory effort is made against the closed valve. Additional air cannot enter the lungs; instead, the inspiratory effort lowers the pressure at the mouth by 10 mm Hg and expands the gas in the lungs by 50 mL, as determined by the increase in the plethysmograph pressure and its calibration curve with the subject in the box. What is the patient's FRC measured with this technique?

3-8. How do you explain the difference between the two FRCs obtained for this patient?

3-9. A patient on a ventilator has a rate of 10 breaths per minute and a tidal volume (V_T) of 500 mL.

   a. What is the patient's $\dot{V}_E$?

   b. If the patient's anatomic dead space is estimated to be 150 mL, what is his $\dot{V}_A$?

   c. If his rate is increased to 15 breaths per minute with V_T remaining at 500 mL, what will his new $\dot{V}_E$ and $\dot{V}_A$ be?

   d. If his V_T is increased to 750 mL, with his rate remaining at 10 breaths per minute, what will his new $\dot{V}_E$ and $\dot{V}_A$ be?

3-10. The following measurements were made on a patient when the barometric pressure was 747 mm Hg:

$$P_{A_{CO_2}} = 40 \text{ mm Hg}$$
$$F\bar{E}_{CO_2} = 0.04$$
$$\dot{V}_E = \frac{6 \text{ L}}{\text{min}}$$
$$\text{breathing frequency} = \frac{12 \text{ breaths}}{\text{min}}$$

where $F\bar{E}_{CO_2}$ = fractional concentration of CO_2 in the subject's mixed expired air.
   What is the patient's V_D/V_T? What is the patient's physiologic dead space? Assuming the patient's anatomic dead space is 100 mL, what is her alveolar dead space? Is this patient's arterial P_{CO_2} likely to be lower than, greater than, or equal to her end-tidal P_{CO_2}?

3-11. A person with a $P_{A_{CO_2}}$ of 40 mm Hg, a $P_{A_{O_2}}$ of 104 mm Hg, and a respiratory exchange ratio of 0.8 breathing room air at a barometric pressure of 760 mm Hg doubles alveolar ventilation. What will this person's new steady-state $P_{A_{CO_2}}$ and $P_{A_{O_2}}$ be (assuming no change in oxygen consumption and carbon dioxide production and assuming that the correction factor [F] = 0)?

3-12. A normal person, seated upright, begins to inspire from the residual volume. The first 100 mL of inspired gas is labeled with xenon 133. Most of this radioactive gas (i.e., the first 100 mL of gas inspired after the dead space) will probably be found:

   a. in alveoli in lower portions of the lung.

   b. in alveoli in upper portions of the lung.

   c. uniformly distributed to all alveoli.

SUGGESTED READINGS

Bryan AC, Bentivoglio LG, Beerel F, MacLeish H, Zidulka A, Bates DV. Factors affecting regional distribution of ventilation and perfusion in the lung. *J Appl Physiol.* 1964;19:395–402.

Cotes JE. *Lung Function: Assessment and Application in Medicine.* 4th ed. Oxford: Blackwell; 1979.

Forster RE II, Dubois AB, Briscoe WA, Fisher AB. *The Lung: Physiologic Basis of Pulmonary Function Tests.* 3rd ed. Chicago, Ill: Year Book; 1986.

Levitzky MG. The effect of aging on the respiratory system. *Physiologist.* 1984;27:102–107.

Macklem PT, Murphy BR. The forces applied to the lung in health and disease. *Am J Med.* 1974;57:371–377.

Milic-Emili J. Ventilation. In: West JB, ed. *Regional Differences in the Lung.* New York, NY: Academic Press; 1977:167–199.

Milic-Emili J. Pulmonary statics. In: Widdicombe JG, ed. *MTP International Review of Sciences: Respiratory Physiology.* London, England: Butterworth; 1974:105–137.

Milic-Emili J. Static distribution of lung volumes. In: Macklem PT, Mead J, eds. *Mechanics of Breathing, part 2, Handbook of Physiology, sec 3: The Respiratory System.* Bethesda, Md: American Physiological Society; 1986;3:561–574.

Murray JF. *The Normal Lung.* 2nd ed. Philadelphia, Pa: WB Saunders and Company; 1986:108–117, 339–358.

Palecek F. Hyperinflation: Control of Functional Residual Capacity. *Physiol Res.* 2001;50:221–230.

Nunn JF. *Nunn's Applied Respiratory Physiology.* 4th ed. Oxford: Butterworth-Heinemann; 1993:117–134, 156–163.

Watson RA, Pride NB. Postural changes in lung volumes and respiratory resistance in subjects with obesity. *J Appl Physiol.* 2005;98:512–517.

West JB. *Ventilation/Blood Flow and Gas Exchange.* 5th ed. Oxford: Blackwell; 1990:25–29.

Blood Flow to the Lung

4

OBJECTIVES

The reader knows the structure, function, distribution, and control of the blood supply of the lung.

▶ *Compares and contrasts the bronchial circulation and the pulmonary circulation.*

▶ *Describes the anatomy of the pulmonary circulation, and explains its physiologic consequences.*

▶ *Compares and contrasts the pulmonary circulation and the systemic circulation.*

▶ *Describes and explains the effects of lung volume on pulmonary vascular resistance.*

▶ *Describes and explains the effects of elevated intravascular pressures on pulmonary vascular resistance.*

▶ *Lists the neural and humoral factors that influence pulmonary vascular resistance.*

▶ *Describes the effect of gravity on pulmonary blood flow.*

▶ *Describes the interrelationships of alveolar pressure, pulmonary arterial pressure, and pulmonary venous pressure, as well as their effects on the regional distribution of pulmonary blood flow.*

▶ *Predicts the effects of alterations in alveolar pressure, pulmonary arterial and venous pressure, and body position on the regional distribution of pulmonary blood flow.*

▶ *Describes hypoxic pulmonary vasoconstriction and discusses its role in localized and widespread alveolar hypoxia.*

▶ *Describes the causes and consequences of pulmonary edema.*

The lung receives blood flow via both the bronchial circulation and the pulmonary circulation. *Bronchial blood flow* constitutes a very small portion of the output of the left ventricle and supplies part of the tracheobronchial tree with systemic arterial blood. *Pulmonary blood flow* constitutes the entire output of the right ventricle and supplies the lung with the mixed venous blood draining all the tissues of the body. It is this blood that undergoes gas exchange with the alveolar air in the pulmonary capillaries. Because the right and left ventricles are arranged in series in normal adults, pulmonary blood flow is approximately equal to 100% of the output of the left ventricle. That is, pulmonary blood flow is equal to the cardiac output—normally about 3.5 L/min/m^2 of body surface area at rest.

There is about 250 to 300 mL of blood per square meter of body surface area in the pulmonary circulation. About 60 to 70 mL/m^2 of this blood is located in the pulmonary capillaries. It takes a red blood cell about 4 to 5 seconds to travel through the pulmonary circulation at resting cardiac outputs; about 0.75 of a second of this time is spent in pulmonary capillaries. Pulmonary capillaries have average diameters of around 6 μm; that is, they are slightly smaller than the average erythrocyte, which has a diameter of about 8 μm. Erythrocytes must therefore change their shape slightly as they pass through the pulmonary capillaries. An erythrocyte passes through a number of pulmonary capillaries as it travels through the lung. Gas exchange starts to take place in smaller pulmonary arterial vessels, which are not truly capillaries by histologic standards. These arterial segments and successive capillaries may be thought of as *functional pulmonary capillaries.* In most cases in this book, *pulmonary capillaries* refer to functional pulmonary capillaries rather than to anatomic capillaries.

About 280 billion pulmonary capillaries supply the approximately 300 million alveoli, resulting in a potential surface area for gas exchange estimated to be 50 to 100 m^2. As was shown in Figure 1–3, the alveoli are completely enveloped in pulmonary capillaries. The capillaries are so close to one another that some researchers have described pulmonary capillary blood flow as resembling blood flowing through two parallel sheets of endothelium held together by occasional connective tissue supports.

THE BRONCHIAL CIRCULATION

The bronchial arteries arise variably, either directly from the aorta or from the intercostal arteries. They supply arterial blood to the tracheobronchial tree and to other structures of the lung down to the level of the terminal bronchioles. They also provide blood flow to the hilar lymph nodes, visceral pleura, pulmonary arteries and veins, vagus, and esophagus. Lung structures distal to the terminal bronchioles, including the respiratory bronchioles, alveolar ducts, alveolar sacs, and alveoli, receive oxygen directly by diffusion from the alveolar air and nutrients from the mixed venous blood in the pulmonary circulation. The bronchial circulation may be important in the "air-conditioning" of inspired air, which is discussed in Chapter 10.

The blood flow in the bronchial circulation constitutes about 2% of the output of the left ventricle. Blood pressure in the bronchial arteries is the same as that in the other systemic arteries (disregarding differences due to hydrostatic effects, which will be discussed later in this chapter). This is much higher than the blood pressure in the pulmonary arteries (Figure 4–1). The reasons for this difference will be discussed in the next section.

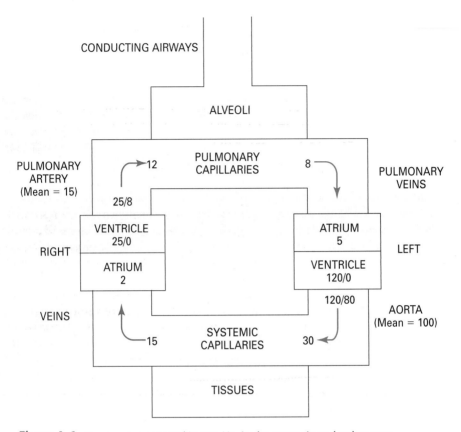

Figure 4–1. Pressures, expressed in mm Hg, in the systemic and pulmonary circulations.

The venous drainage of the bronchial circulation is unusual. Although some of the bronchial venous blood enters the azygos and hemiazygos veins, a substantial portion of bronchial venous blood enters the *pulmonary* veins. The blood in the pulmonary veins has undergone gas exchange with the alveolar air—that is, the pulmonary veins contain "arterial" blood. Therefore, the bronchial venous blood entering the pulmonary venous blood is part of the normal anatomic right-to-left shunt, which will be discussed in Chapter 5. Histologists have also identified *anastomoses,* or connections, between some bronchial capillaries and pulmonary capillaries and between bronchial arteries and branches of the pulmonary artery. These connections probably play little role in a healthy person but may open in pathologic states, such as when either bronchial or pulmonary blood flow to a portion of lung is occluded. For example, if pulmonary blood flow to an area of the lung is blocked by a pulmonary embolus, bronchial blood flow to that area increases. The main anatomic features of the bronchial circulation are illustrated in Figure 4–2.

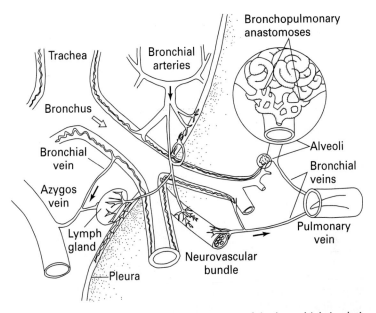

Figure 4–2. Illustration of the main anatomic features of the bronchial circulation. Note that the bronchial circulation supplies blood flow to the tracheobronchial tree down to the level of the terminal bronchioles as well as to the pulmonary blood vessels, the visceral pleura, the hilar lymph nodes, and branches of nerves, including the vagus. A bronchopulmonary anastomosis is shown at right and is enlarged in the inset. Venous drainage is to both the right side of the circulation via the azygos (and hemiazygos) vein and the left side of the circulation via the pulmonary veins. (Reproduced with permission from Deffebach, Charan, Lakshminarayan, and Butler, 1987.)

THE FUNCTIONAL ANATOMY OF THE PULMONARY CIRCULATION

The pulmonary circulation, from beginning to end, is much thinner-walled than corresponding parts of the systemic circulation. This is particularly true of the main pulmonary artery and its branches. The pulmonary artery rapidly subdivides into terminal branches that have thinner walls and greater internal diameters than do corresponding branches of the systemic arterial tree. There is much less vascular smooth muscle in the walls of the vessels of the pulmonary arterial tree, and there are no highly muscular vessels that correspond to the systemic arterioles. The pulmonary arterial tree rapidly subdivides over a short distance, ultimately branching into the approximately 280 billion pulmonary capillaries, where gas exchange occurs.

 The thin walls and small amount of smooth muscle found in the pulmonary arteries have important physiologic consequences. The pulmonary vessels offer much less resistance to blood flow than do the systemic arterial vessels. They are also much more *distensible* and *compressible* than systemic arterial vessels. These factors lead to much lower intravascular pressures than those found in the systemic arteries. The pulmonary vessels are located in the thorax and are subject to alveolar and intrapleural pressures that can change greatly. Therefore, factors other than the tone of the pulmonary vascular smooth muscle may have profound effects on pulmonary vascular resistance (PVR).

Determination of Pulmonary Vascular Resistance

PVR cannot be measured directly but must be calculated. Poiseuille's law, which states that for a Newtonian fluid flowing steadily through a nondistensible tube, $P_1 - P_2 = \dot{Q} \times R$, is usually used to estimate PVR. This can be rearranged to:

$$R = \frac{P_1 - P_2}{\dot{Q}}$$

where P_1 = pressure at the beginning of the tube (in millimeters of mercury)
$\quad P_2$ = pressure at the end of the tube
$\quad \dot{Q}$ = flow (in milliliters per minute)
$\quad R$ = resistance (in millimeters of mercury per milliliter per minute)

For the pulmonary circulation, then,

$$PVR = \frac{MPAP - MLAP}{PBF}$$

That is, the PVR is equal to the mean pulmonary artery pressure (MPAP) minus the mean left atrial pressure (MLAP), with the result divided by pulmonary blood flow (PBF), which is equal to the cardiac output.

This formula, however, is only an *approximation* because blood is not a Newtonian fluid, because pulmonary blood flow is *pulsatile* (and may also be turbulent), because the pulmonary circulation is *distensible* (and *compressible*), and because the pulmonary circulation is a very complex branching structure. (Remember that resistances in series add directly; resistances in parallel add as reciprocals.) Furthermore, the mean left atrial pressure may not be the effective downstream pressure for the calculation of PVR under all lung conditions (see the section on zones of the lung later in this chapter).

The intravascular pressures in the pulmonary circulation are lower than those in the systemic circulation (Figure 4–1). This is particularly striking with respect to the arterial pressures of the two circuits.

Because the right and left circulations are in series, the outputs of the right and left ventricles must be approximately equal to each other over the long run. (If they are not, blood and fluid will build up in the lungs or periphery.) If the two outputs are the same and the measured pressure drops across the systemic circulation and the pulmonary circulation are about 98 and 10 mm Hg, respectively, then the PVR must be about one tenth that of the systemic vascular resistance (SVR) (see Figure 4–1). (SVR is sometimes called TPR for *total peripheral resistance.*) This low resistance to blood flow offered by the pulmonary circulation is due to the *structural* aspects of the pulmonary circulation already discussed. The pulmonary vasculature is thinner walled, has much less vascular smooth muscle, and is generally more distensible than the systemic circulation.

Distribution of Pulmonary Vascular Resistance

The distribution of pulmonary vascular resistance (PVR) can be seen by looking at the pressure drop across each of the three major components of the pulmonary vasculature: the pulmonary arteries, the pulmonary capillaries, and the pulmonary veins. In Figure 4–1, the resistance is fairly evenly distributed among the three components. At rest, about one third of the resistance to blood flow is located in the pulmonary arteries, about one third is located in the pulmonary capillaries, and about one third is located in the pulmonary veins. This is in contrast to the systemic circulation, in which about 70% of the resistance to blood flow is located in the systemic arteries, mostly in the highly muscular systemic arterioles.

Consequences of Differences in Pressure between the Systemic & Pulmonary Circulations

The pressure at the bottom of a column of a liquid is proportional to the height of the column times the density of the liquid times gravity. Thus, when the normal mean systemic arterial blood pressure is stated to be about 100 mm Hg, the pressure developed in the aorta is equivalent to the pressure at the bottom of a column of mercury that is 100 mm high (it will push a column of mercury up 100 mm). Mercury is chosen for pressure measurement when high pressures are expected because it is a very dense liquid. Water is used when lower pressures are to be measured because mercury is 13.6 times as dense as water. Therefore, lower pressures, such as alveolar and pleural pressures, are expressed in centimeters of water.

Nevertheless, when mean arterial blood pressure is stated to be 100 mm Hg, this is specifically with reference to the level of the left atrium. Blood pressure in the feet of a person who is standing is much higher than 100 mm Hg because of the additional pressure exerted by the "column" of blood from the heart to the feet. In fact, blood pressure in the feet of a standing person of average height with a mean arterial blood pressure of 100 mm Hg is likely to be about 180 mm Hg. Because venous pressure is similarly increased in the feet (about 80 mm Hg), the pressure *difference* between arteries and veins is unaffected. Conversely, pressure decreases with distance above the heart ("above" with respect to gravity), so that blood pressure at the top of the head may only be 40 to 50 mm Hg.

The left ventricle, then, must maintain a relatively high mean arterial pressure because such high pressures are necessary to overcome hydrostatic forces and pump blood "uphill" to the brain. The apices of the lungs are a much shorter distance above the right ventricle, and so such high pressures are unnecessary.

A second consequence of the high arterial pressure in the systemic circulation is that it allows the redistribution of left ventricular output and the control of blood flow to different tissues. Because the left ventricle is supplying all the tissues of the body with blood, it must be able to meet varying demands for blood flow in different tissues under various circumstances. For example, during exercise the blood vessels supplying the exercising muscle dilate in response to the increased local metabolic demand (and blood flow to the skin also increases to aid in thermoregulation). Blood pressure is partly maintained by increasing the resistance to blood flow in other vascular beds. A high pressure head is thus necessary to allow such redistributions by altering the vascular resistance to blood flow in different organs; also, these redistributions help maintain the pressure head. In the pulmonary circulation, redistributions of right ventricular output are usually unnecessary because all alveolar-capillary units that are participating in gas exchange are performing the same function. The pressure head is low and the small amount of smooth muscle in the pulmonary vessels (which is in large part *responsible* for the low pressure head) makes such local redistributions unlikely. An exception to this will be seen in the section on hypoxic pulmonary vasoconstriction.

A final consequence of the pressure difference between the systemic and pulmonary circulations is that the workload of the left ventricle (stroke work equals stroke volume times arterial pressure) is much greater than that of the right ventricle. The metabolic demand of the left ventricle is also much greater than that of the right ventricle. The difference in wall thickness of the left and right ventricles of the adult is a reminder of the much greater workload of the left ventricle.

PULMONARY VASCULAR RESISTANCE

The relatively small amounts of vascular smooth muscle, low intravascular pressures, and high distensibility of the pulmonary circulation lead to a much greater importance of extravascular effects ("passive factors") on PVR. Gravity, body position, lung volume, alveolar and intrapleural pressures, intravascular pressures, and right ventricular output all can have profound effects on PVR without any alteration in the tone of the pulmonary vascular smooth muscle.

The Concept of a Transmural Pressure Gradient

For distensible-compressible vessels, the *transmural pressure gradient* is an important determinant of the vessel diameter (see discussion of airways resistance in Chapter 2). As the transmural pressure gradient (which is equal to pressure inside minus pressure outside) increases, the vessel diameter increases and resistance falls; as the transmural pressure decreases, the vessel diameter decreases and the resistance increases. *Negative* transmural pressure gradients lead to compression or even collapse of the vessel.

Lung Volume & Pulmonary Vascular Resistance

Two different groups of pulmonary vessels must be considered when the effects of lung volume changes on PVR are analyzed—namely, the alveolar and extraalveolar vessels (Figure 4–3).

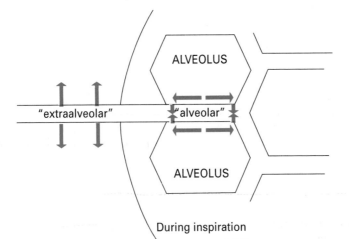

Figure 4–3. Illustration of alveolar and extraalveolar pulmonary vessels during an inspiration. The alveolar vessels (pulmonary capillaries) are exposed to the expanding alveoli and elongated. The extraalveolar vessels, here shown exposed to the intrapleural pressure, expand as the intrapleural pressure becomes more negative and as radial traction increases during the inspiration.

As lung volume increases during a normal negative-pressure inspiration, the alveoli increase in volume. While the alveoli expand, the vessels found between them, mainly pulmonary capillaries, are elongated. As these vessels are stretched, their diameters decrease, just as stretching a rubber tube causes its diameter to narrow. Resistance to blood flow through the alveolar vessels increases as the alveoli expand because the alveolar vessels are longer (resistance is directly proportional to length) and because their radii are smaller (resistance is inversely proportional to radius to the *fourth* power). At high lung volumes, then, the resistance to blood flow offered by the alveolar vessels increases greatly; at low lung volumes, the resistance to blood flow offered by the alveolar vessels decreases. This can be seen in the "alveolar" curve in Figure 4–4.

One group of the *extraalveolar* vessels, the larger arteries and veins, is exposed to the intrapleural pressure. As lung volume is increased by making the intrapleural pressure more negative, the transmural pressure gradient of the larger arteries and veins increases and they distend. Another factor tending to decrease the resistance to blood flow offered by the extraalveolar vessels at higher lung volumes is *radial traction* by the connective tissue and alveolar septa holding the larger vessels in place in the lung. (Look at the small branch of the pulmonary artery at the bottom of Figure 1–2.) Thus, at high lung volumes (attained by normal negative-pressure breathing), the resistance to blood flow offered by the extraalveolar vessels decreases (Figure 4–4). During a forced expiration to low lung volumes, however, intrapleural pressure becomes very positive. Extraalveolar vessels are compressed, and as the alveoli decrease in size, they exert less radial traction on the extraalveolar

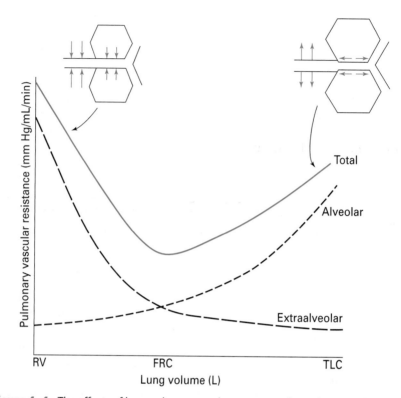

Figure 4–4. The effects of lung volume on pulmonary vascular resistance (PVR). PVR is lowest near the functional residual capacity (FRC) and increases at both high and low lung volumes because of the combined effects on the alveolar and extraalveolar vessels. To achieve low lung volumes, one must generate positive intrapleural pressures so that the extraalveolar vessels are compressed, as seen at left in the figure. RV = residual volume; TLC = total lung capacity. (Graph after Murray, 1976, 1986. Reproduced with permission.)

vessels. The resistance to blood flow offered by the extraalveolar vessels increases greatly (see left side of Figure 4–4).

Because the alveolar and extraalveolar vessels may be thought of as two groups of resistances in series with each other, the resistances of the alveolar and extraalveolar vessels are additive at any lung volume. Thus, the effect of changes in lung volume on the *total* PVR gives the U-shaped curve seen in Figure 4–4. PVR is lowest near the functional residual capacity and increases at both high and low lung volumes.

A second type of extraalveolar vessel is the so-called corner vessel, or extraalveolar capillary (see the circled asterisk in Figure 1–3). Although these vessels are found between alveoli, their locations at junctions of alveolar septa give them different mechanical properties. Expansion of the alveoli during inspiration increases the wall tension of the alveolar septa, and the corner vessels are distended by increased radial traction, whereas the alveolar capillaries are compressed.

TEST Q!
→

Also note that during *mechanical* positive-pressure ventilation, alveolar pressure (P_A) and intrapleural pressure are *positive* during inspiration. In this case, both the alveolar and extraalveolar vessels are compressed as lung volume increases, and the resistance to blood flow offered by both alveolar and extraalveolar vessels increases during lung inflation. This is especially a problem during mechanical positive-pressure ventilation with positive end-expiratory pressure (PEEP). During PEEP, airway pressure (and thus alveolar pressure) is kept positive at end expiration to help prevent atelectasis. In this situation, alveolar pressure and intrapleural pressure are positive during both inspiration and expiration. PVR is elevated in both alveolar and extraalveolar vessels throughout the respiratory cycle. In addition, because intrapleural pressure is always positive, the other intrathoracic blood vessels are subjected to decreased transmural pressure gradients; the venae cavae, which have low intravascular pressure, are also compressed. If cardiovascular reflexes are unable to adjust to this situation, cardiac output may fall precipitously because of decreased venous return and high PVR.

Recruitment & Distention

During exercise, cardiac output can increase several-fold without a correspondingly great increase in mean pulmonary artery pressure. Although the mean pulmonary artery pressure does increase, the increase is only a few millimeters of mercury, even if cardiac output has doubled or tripled. Since the pressure drop across the pulmonary circulation is proportional to the cardiac output times the PVR (i.e., $\Delta P = \dot{Q} \times R$), this must indicate a decrease in PVR.

Like the effects of lung volume on PVR, this decrease appears to be *passive*—that is, it is not a result of changes in the tone of pulmonary vascular smooth muscle caused by neural mechanisms or humoral agents. In fact, a fall in PVR in response to increased blood flow or even an increase in perfusion pressure can be demonstrated in a vascularly isolated perfused lung, as was used to obtain the data summarized in Figure 4–5.

In this experiment, the blood vessels of the left lung of a dog were isolated, cannulated, and perfused with a pump. The lung was ventilated with a mechanical respirator. Blood flow to the lung and mean pulmonary artery pressure were elevated by increasing the pump output. As can be seen from the graph, increasing the blood flow to the lung caused a decrease in the calculated PVR. Increasing the left atrial pressure also decreased PVR in these studies.

 There are two different mechanisms that can explain this decrease in PVR in response to elevated blood flow and perfusion pressure: recruitment and distention (Figure 4–6).

RECRUITMENT

As indicated in the diagram, at resting cardiac outputs, not all the pulmonary capillaries are perfused. A substantial number of capillaries are probably unperfused because of hydrostatic effects that will be discussed later in this chapter. Others may be unperfused because they have a relatively high *critical opening pressure*.

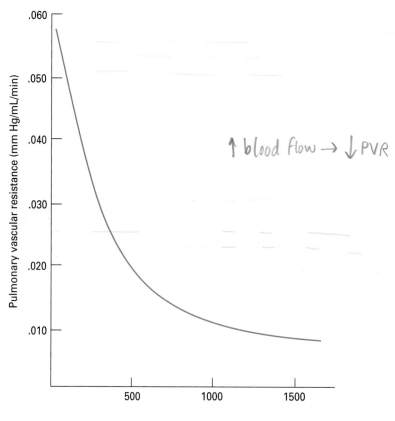

Figure 4–5. The effect of blood flow on pulmonary vascular resistance. Increased blood flow decreases pulmonary vascular resistance. (After Borst, 1956. Reproduced by permission of the American Heart Association, Inc.)

That is, these vessels, because of their high vascular smooth muscle tone or other factors such as positive alveolar pressure, require a higher perfusion pressure than that solely necessary to overcome hydrostatic forces. Under normal circumstances, it is not likely that the critical opening pressures for pulmonary blood vessels are very great because they have so little smooth muscle.

Increasing blood flow increases the mean pulmonary artery pressure, which opposes hydrostatic forces and exceeds the critical opening pressure in previously unopened vessels. This series of events opens new parallel pathways for blood flow, which lowers the PVR. This opening of new pathways is called *recruitment*. Note that *decreasing* the cardiac output or pulmonary artery pressure can result in a *derecruitment* of pulmonary capillaries.

DISTENTION

The distensibility of the pulmonary vasculature has already been discussed in this chapter. As perfusion pressure increases, the transmural pressure gradient of the

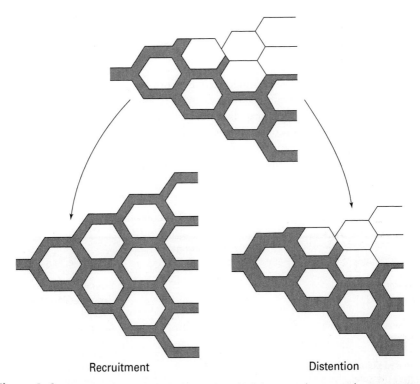

Recruitment   Distention

Figure 4–6. Illustration of the mechanisms by which increased mean pulmonary artery pressure may decrease pulmonary vascular resistance. The upper figure shows a group of pulmonary capillaries, some of which are perfused. At left, the previously unperfused capillaries are recruited (opened) by the increased perfusion pressure. At right, the increased perfusion pressure has distended those vessels already open.

pulmonary blood vessels increases, causing distention of the vessels. This increases their radii and decreases their resistance to blood flow.

RECRUITMENT OR DISTENTION?

The answer to the question of whether it is recruitment or distention that causes the decreased PVR seen with elevated perfusion pressure is probably *both*. Perhaps *recruitment* of pulmonary capillaries occurs with small increases in pulmonary vascular pressures and *distention* at higher pressures. Note that recruitment increases the surface area for gas exchange and may decrease alveolar dead space. Derecruitment caused by low right ventricular output or high alveolar pressures decreases the surface area for gas exchange and may increase alveolar dead space.

Control of Pulmonary Vascular Smooth Muscle

Pulmonary vascular smooth muscle is responsive to both *neural* and *humoral* influences. These produce "active" alterations in PVR, as opposed to those "passive" factors discussed in the previous section. A final passive factor, *gravity*, will be discussed later in this chapter. The main "passive" and "active" factors that influence PVR are summarized in Tables 4–1 and 4–2.

NEURAL EFFECTS

The pulmonary vasculature is innervated by both sympathetic and parasympathetic fibers of the autonomic nervous system. The innervation of pulmonary vessels is relatively sparse in comparison with that of systemic vessels. There is relatively more innervation of the larger vessels and less of the smaller, more muscular vessels. There appears to be no innervation of vessels smaller than 30 μm in diameter. There does not appear to be much innervation of intrapulmonary veins and venules.

Table 4–1. Passive Influences on Pulmonary Vascular Resistance

Cause	Effect on Pulmonary Vascular Resistance	Mechanism
Increased lung volume (above FRC)	Increases	Lengthening and compression of alveolar vessels
Decreased lung volume (below FRC)	Increases	Compression of and less traction on extraalveolar vessels
Increased pulmonary artery pressure; increased left atrial pressure; increased pulmonary blood volume; increased cardiac output	Decreases	Recruitment and distention
Gravity; body position	Decreases in gravity-dependent regions of the lungs	Hydrostatic effects lead to recruitment and distention
Increased (more positive) interstitial pressure	Increases	Compression of vessels
Increased blood viscosity	Increases	Viscosity directly increases resistance
Positive-pressure ventilation: Increased alveolar pressure	Increases	Compression and derecruitment of alveolar vessels
Positive intrapleural pressure	Increases	Compression of extraalveolar vessels; compression of vena cava decreases pulmonary blood flow and leads to derecruitment

FRC = functional residual capacity.

Table 4–2. Active Influences on Pulmonary Vascular Resistance

Increase	Decrease
Stimulation of sympathetic innervation (may have greater effect by decreasing large vessel distensibility)	Stimulation of parasympathetic innervation (if vascular tone is already elevated)
Norepinephrine, epinephrine	Acetylcholine
α-Adrenergic agonists	β-Adrenergic agonists
$PGF_{2\alpha}$, PGE_2	PGE_1
Thromboxane	Prostacyclin (PGI_2)
Endothelin	Nitric oxide
Angiotensin	Bradykinin
Histamine (primary a pulmonary venoconstrictor)	
Alveolar hypoxia	
Alveolar hypercapnia	
Low pH of mixed venous blood	

PG = prostaglandin.

The effects of stimulation of the sympathetic innervation of the pulmonary vasculature are somewhat controversial. Some investigators have demonstrated an increase in PVR with sympathetic stimulation of the innervation of the pulmonary vasculature, whereas others have shown only a decreased *distensibility* with no change in calculated PVR. Stimulation of the parasympathetic innervation of the pulmonary vessels generally causes vasodilation, although its physiologic function is not known.

HUMORAL EFFECTS

The catecholamines epinephrine and norepinephrine both increase PVR when injected into the pulmonary circulation. Histamine, found in the lung in mast cells, is a pulmonary vasoconstrictor. Certain prostaglandins and related substances, such as $PGF_{2\alpha}$, PGE_2, and thromboxane, are also pulmonary vasoconstrictors, as is endothelin, a 21 amino acid peptide synthesized by the vascular endothelium. Alveolar hypoxia and hypercapnia also cause pulmonary vasoconstriction, as will be discussed later in this chapter. Acetylcholine, the β-adrenergic agonist isoproterenol, nitric oxide (NO), and certain prostaglandins, such as PGE_1 and PGI_2 (prostacyclin), are pulmonary vasodilators.

THE REGIONAL DISTRIBUTION OF PULMONARY BLOOD FLOW: THE ZONES OF THE LUNG

Determinations of the regional distribution of pulmonary blood flow have shown that *gravity* is another important "passive" factor affecting local PVR and the relative perfusion of different regions of the lung. The interaction of the effects of gravity and extravascular pressures may have a profound influence on the relative perfusion of different areas of the lung.

Measurement of Total Pulmonary Blood Flow

The total pulmonary blood flow (which is the cardiac output) can currently be determined clinically in several ways, each of which has the disadvantage of being *invasive* to the patient (i.e., requiring minor surgery).

THE FICK PRINCIPLE

In 1870, Adolf Fick pointed out the following relationship, now known as the Fick principle: The total amount of oxygen absorbed by the body per minute ($\dot{V}_{O_2}$) must be equal to the cardiac output in milliliters per minute ($\dot{Q}t$) times the difference in oxygen *content,* in milliliters of oxygen per 100 mL of blood, between the arterial and mixed venous blood ($Ca_{O_2} - C\bar{v}_{O_2}$):

$$\dot{V}_{O_2} = \dot{Q}t \times (Ca_{O_2} - C\bar{v}_{O_2})$$
$$\dot{Q}t = \frac{\dot{V}_{O_2}}{Ca_{O_2} - C\bar{v}_{O_2}}$$

Both arterial and mixed venous (which is equal to pulmonary artery) blood must be sampled in this method.

THE INDICATOR DILUTION TECHNIQUE

In this method, a known amount of an indicator dye that stays in the blood vessels, such as indocyanine green, is injected intravenously as a bolus. The systemic arterial dye concentration is monitored continuously with a densitometer as the dye passes through the aorta. Correction must be made for recirculating dye because the concentration change of interest is that which occurs in a single pass through the pulmonary circulation. A curve of the dye concentration as it changes with time is constructed, and then the area under the curve is determined by integration. Dividing this amount by the time of passage of the dye gives the average concentration of dye through the passage. If the cardiac output is high, the dye concentration falls rapidly, and so the area under the curve is small and the average dye concentration is low. If the cardiac output is low, the area under the curve is large and the average dye concentration is high. The cardiac output ($\dot{Q}t$) is equal to the amount of dye injected in milligrams (I) divided by the mean dye concentration in milligrams per milliliter (c) times the time of passage (t) in seconds:

$$\dot{Q}t = \frac{I}{ct}$$

The calculations are usually done automatically in newer densitometers. Both arterial and venous catheters are necessary for this technique.

THE THERMAL DILUTION TECHNIQUE

This method is similar in principle to the indicator dilution technique. Cold fluid, for example, saline, is injected into a central vein, and the change in temperature of the blood downstream is monitored continuously with a thermistor. With high cardiac outputs, the temperature returns to normal rapidly; with low cardiac outputs, the temperature rises slowly. The advantage of this method is that the insertion of a single intravenous catheter is the only necessary surgical procedure. A type of catheter known as a quadruple-lumen Swan-Ganz catheter is used. One lumen is connected to a tiny inflatable balloon at the end of the catheter. During the insertion of the catheter, the balloon is inflated so that the tip of the catheter "floats" in the direction of blood flow: through the right atrium and ventricle and into the pulmonary artery. The balloon is then deflated. A second lumen carries the thermistor wire to the end of the catheter. A third lumen travels only part of the way down the catheter so that it opens into a central vein. This lumen is used for the injection of the cold solution. The final lumen, at the end of the catheter, is open to the pulmonary artery, and it allows pulmonary artery pressure to be monitored. (It can also be used to sample mixed venous blood.) This monitoring is necessary because the only way the physician knows that the catheter is placed properly is by recognizing the characteristic pulmonary artery pressure trace (unless a fluoroscope is used).

The temperature change after the injection is monitored by a cardiac output "computer" that automatically calculates the cardiac output from the volume and temperature of the injected substance, the original blood temperature, and the temperature change of the blood with time.

If the Swan-Ganz catheter is advanced, with the balloon inflated, until it completely occludes a branch of the pulmonary artery, it is said to be "wedged." The pressure measured at the tip of the catheter with the balloon still inflated is approximately equal to the pressure in the vascular segment immediately distal to it, the pulmonary capillary pressure. Because there are no valves between the pulmonary capillaries and the lumen of the left atrium, this *"pulmonary capillary wedge pressure"* is similar to left atrial pressure. When the balloon is deflated, the pressure measured at the tip of the catheter is pulmonary artery pressure. Figure 4–7 shows a pressure

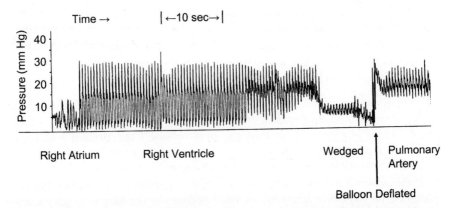

Figure 4–7. Pressure trace obtained from an anesthetized dog as a Swan-Ganz catheter is advanced through the right atrium, the right ventricle, through the main pulmonary artery, and into a branch of the pulmonary artery until it is "wedged." The balloon is then deflated to show pulmonary artery pressure. Pulmonary capillary wedge pressure was about 8 mm Hg, and mean pulmonary artery pressure was about 17 mm Hg.

trace as a Swan-Ganz catheter is advanced through the right atrium, the right ventricle, the main pulmonary artery, and into a branch of the pulmonary artery until it is "wedged." The balloon is then deflated to show pulmonary artery pressure.

Determination of Regional Pulmonary Blood Flow

Regional pulmonary blood flow can be determined by pulmonary angiography, by lung scans after injection of macroaggregates of albumin labeled with radioactive iodine (^{131}I) or technetium (^{99m}TC), and by lung scans after the infusion of dissolved radiolabeled gases such as ^{133}Xe.

PULMONARY ANGIOGRAPHY

A radiopaque substance is injected into the pulmonary artery, and its movement through the lung is monitored during fluoroscopy. Unperfused areas secondary to vascular obstruction by emboli or from other causes are evident because none of the radiopaque substance enters these areas.

MACROAGGREGATES OF ALBUMIN

Macroaggregates of albumin labeled with ^{131}I or ^{99m}TC in the size range of 10 to 50 μm are injected in small quantities into a peripheral vein. Most of these become trapped in small pulmonary vessels as they enter the lung. Lung scans for radioactivity demonstrate the perfused areas of the lung. The aggregates fragment and are removed from the lung within a day or so.

^{133}Xe

^{133}Xe is dissolved in saline and injected intravenously. Xenon is not particularly soluble in saline or blood, and so it comes out of solution in the lung and enters the alveoli. If the ^{133}Xe is well mixed in the blood as it enters the pulmonary artery, then the amount of radioactivity coming into a region of the lung is proportional to the amount of blood flow to that area. By making corrections for regional lung volume, the blood flow *per unit volume* of a region of the lung can be determined.

The Regional Distribution of Pulmonary Blood Flow

If ^{133}Xe is used to determine regional pulmonary blood flow in a person seated upright or standing up, a pattern like that shown in Figure 4–8 is seen. There is greater blood flow per unit volume ("per alveolus") to lower regions of the lung than to upper regions of the lung. Note that the test was made with the subject at the total lung capacity.

If the subject lies down, this pattern of regional perfusion is altered so that perfusion to the *anatomically* upper and lower portions of the lung is roughly evenly distributed, but blood flow per unit volume is still greater in the more gravity-dependent regions of the lung. For example, if the subject were to lie down on his or her left side, the left lung would receive more blood flow per unit volume than would the right lung. Exercise, which increases the cardiac output, increases the

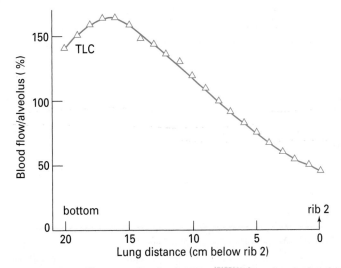

Figure 4–8. Relative blood flow per alveolus (100% = perfusion of each alveolus if all were perfused equally) versus distance from the bottom of the lung in a human seated upright. Measurement of regional blood flow was determined using an intravenous injection of ^{133}Xe. TLC = total lung capacity. (Redrawn from Hughes, 1968, with permission.)

blood flow per unit volume to all regions of the lung, but the perfusion gradient persists so that there is still relatively greater blood flow per unit volume in more gravity-dependent regions of the lung.

The reason for this gradient of regional perfusion of the lung is obviously gravity. As already discussed, the pressure at the bottom of a column of a liquid is proportional to the height of the column times the density of the liquid times gravity. Thus, the intravascular pressures in more gravity-dependent portions of the lung are greater than those in upper regions. Because the pressures are greater in the more gravity-dependent regions of the lung, the *resistance to blood flow is lower* in lower regions of the lung owing to more *recruitment* or *distention* of vessels in these regions. It is therefore not only gravity but also the peculiar characteristics of the pulmonary circulation that cause the increased blood flow to more gravity-dependent regions of the lung. After all, the same hydrostatic effects occur to an even greater extent in the left side of the circulation, but the thick walls of the systemic arteries are not affected.

Recent studies have also demonstrated that blood travels through the more gravity-dependent regions of the lung at a faster rate. That is, the mean *capillary transit time* is less in the lower regions of the lung.

There is also considerable heterogeneity in pulmonary blood flow at any vertical distance up the lung. That is, there may be significant variations in pulmonary blood flow *within* a given horizontal plane of the lung. These variations are caused by local factors and mechanical stresses.

The Interaction of Gravity & Extravascular Pressure: The Zones of the Lung

Experiments done on excised, perfused, upright animal lungs have demonstrated the same gradient of increased perfusion per unit volume from the top of the lung to the bottom. When the experiments were done at low pump outputs so that the pulmonary artery pressure was low, the uppermost regions of the lung received no blood flow. Perfusion of the lung ceased at the point at which alveolar pressure (PA) was just equal to pulmonary arterial pressure (Pa). Above this point, there was no perfusion because alveolar pressure exceeded pulmonary artery pressure, and so the transmural pressure across capillary walls was negative. Below this point, perfusion per unit volume increased steadily with increased distance down the lung.

 Thus, under circumstances in which alveolar pressure is higher than pulmonary artery pressure in the upper parts of the lung, no blood flow occurs in that region, and the region is referred to as being in zone 1, as shown in Figure 4–9. (Note that in this figure blood flow is on the *x* axis and that distance up the lung is on the *y* axis.) Any zone 1, then, is ventilated but not perfused. It is *alveolar dead space*. Fortunately, during normal, quiet breathing in a person with a normal cardiac output, pulmonary artery pressure, even in the uppermost regions of the lung, is greater than alveolar pressure, and so there is no zone 1. Some experiments have also demonstrated perfusion of the corner vessels under zone 1 conditions.

The lower portion of the lung in Figure 4–9 is said to be in zone 3. In this region, the pulmonary artery pressure and the pulmonary vein pressure (Pv) are both greater than alveolar pressure. The driving pressure for blood flow through the lung in this region is simply pulmonary artery pressure minus pulmonary vein pressure. Note that this driving pressure stays constant as one moves further down the lung in zone 3 because the hydrostatic pressure effects are the same for both the arteries and the veins.

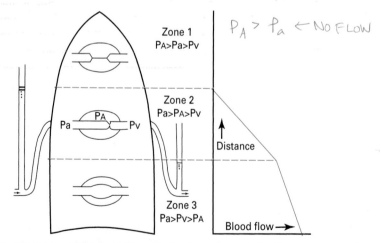

Figure 4–9. The zones of the lung. The effects of gravity and alveolar pressure on the perfusion of the lung. Described in text. (Redrawn from West, 1964, with permission.)

The middle portion of the lung in Figure 4–9 is in zone 2. In zone 2, pulmonary artery pressure is greater than alveolar pressure, and so blood flow does occur. Nevertheless, because alveolar pressure is greater than pulmonary vein pressure, the *effective* driving pressure for blood flow is pulmonary artery pressure minus alveolar pressure in zone 2. (This is analogous to the situation described in Chapter 2: During a forced expiration the driving pressure for airflow is equal to alveolar pressure minus intrapleural pressure.) Notice that in zone 2 (at right in Figure 4–9) the increase in blood flow per distance down the lung is greater than it is in zone 3. This is because the upstream driving pressure, the pulmonary artery pressure, increases according to the hydrostatic pressure increase, but the effective downstream pressure, alveolar pressure, is constant throughout the lung at any instant.

To summarize then: In *zone 1,*

$$P_A > P_a > P_v$$

and there is no blood flow (except perhaps in "corner vessels," which are not exposed to alveolar pressure); in *zone 2,*

$$P_a > P_A > P_v$$

and the effective driving pressure for blood flow is $P_a - P_A$; in *zone 3,*

$$P_a > P_v > P_A$$

and the driving pressure for blood flow is $P_a - P_v$.

It is important to realize that the boundaries between the zones are dependent on physiologic conditions—they are not fixed anatomic landmarks. Alveolar pressure changes during the course of each breath. During eupneic breathing these changes are only a few centimeters of water, but they may be much greater during speech, exercise, and other conditions. A patient on a positive-pressure ventilator with PEEP may have substantial amounts of zone 1 because alveolar pressure is always high. Similarly, after a hemorrhage or during general anesthesia, pulmonary blood flow and pulmonary artery pressure are low and zone 1 conditions are also likely. During exercise, cardiac output and pulmonary artery pressure increase and any existing zone 1 will be recruited to zone 2. The boundary between zones 2 and 3 will move upward as well. Pulmonary artery pressure is highly pulsatile, and so the borders between the zones probably even move up a bit with each contraction of the right ventricle.

Changes in lung volume also affect the regional distribution of pulmonary blood flow and will therefore affect the boundaries between zones. Finally, changes in body position alter the orientation of the zones with respect to the anatomic locations in the lung, but the same relationships exist with respect to gravity and alveolar pressure.

HYPOXIC PULMONARY VASOCONSTRICTION

Alveolar hypoxia or atelectasis causes an active vasoconstriction in the pulmonary circulation. The site of vascular smooth muscle constriction appears to be in the arterial (precapillary) vessels very close to the alveoli.

Mechanism of Hypoxic Pulmonary Vasoconstriction

The mechanism of hypoxic pulmonary vasoconstriction is not completely understood. The response occurs locally, that is, only in the area of the alveolar hypoxia. Connections to the central nervous system are not necessary: An isolated, excised lung, perfused with blood by a mechanical pump with a constant output, exhibits an increased perfusion pressure when ventilated with hypoxic gas mixtures. This indicates that the increase in PVR can occur without the influence of extrinsic nerves. Thus, it is not surprising that hypoxic pulmonary vasoconstriction was recently demonstrated to persist in human patients who had received heart-lung transplants. Hypoxia may cause the release of a vasoactive substance from the pulmonary parenchyma or mast cells in the area. Histamine, serotonin, catecholamines, and prostaglandins have all been suggested as the mediator substance, but none appears to completely mimic the response. *Decreased* release of a vasodilator such as nitric oxide may also be involved in hypoxic pulmonary vasoconstriction. Possibly several mediators act together. Recent studies have strongly indicated that hypoxia acts *directly* on pulmonary vascular smooth muscle to produce hypoxic pulmonary vasoconstriction. Hypoxia inhibits an outward potassium current, which causes pulmonary vascular smooth muscle cells to depolarize, allowing calcium to enter the cells. This, in turn, causes them to contract. The potassium channel appears to be open when it is oxidized and closed when it is reduced.

The hypoxic pulmonary vasoconstriction response is graded—constriction begins to occur at alveolar P_{O_2}s in the range of 100 to 150 mm Hg and increases until $P_{A_{O_2}}$ falls to about 20 to 30 mm Hg.

Physiologic Function of Hypoxic Pulmonary Vasoconstriction

The function of hypoxic pulmonary vasoconstriction in localized hypoxia is fairly obvious. If an area of the lung becomes hypoxic because of airway obstruction or if localized atelectasis occurs, any mixed venous blood flowing to that area will undergo little or no gas exchange (Figure 4–10B) and will mix with blood draining well-ventilated areas of the lung as it enters the left atrium. This mixing will lower the overall arterial P_{O_2} and may even increase the arterial P_{CO_2} (see Chapter 5). The hypoxic pulmonary vasoconstriction diverts mixed venous blood flow away from poorly ventilated areas of the lung by locally increasing vascular resistance, as shown in Figure 4–10C. Therefore, mixed venous blood is sent to better-ventilated areas of the lung (Figure 4–10D). The problem with hypoxic pulmonary vasoconstriction is that it is not a very strong response because there is so little smooth muscle in the pulmonary vasculature. Very high pulmonary artery pressures can interfere with hypoxic pulmonary vasoconstriction, as can other physiologic disturbances, such as alkalosis.

In hypoxia of the whole lung, such as might be encountered at high altitude (see Chapter 11) or in hypoventilation, hypoxic pulmonary vasoconstriction occurs throughout the lung. Even this may be useful in increasing gas exchange because greatly increasing the pulmonary artery pressure recruits many previously unperfused pulmonary capillaries. This increases the surface area available for gas diffusion (see Chapter 6) and improves the matching of ventilation and perfusion,

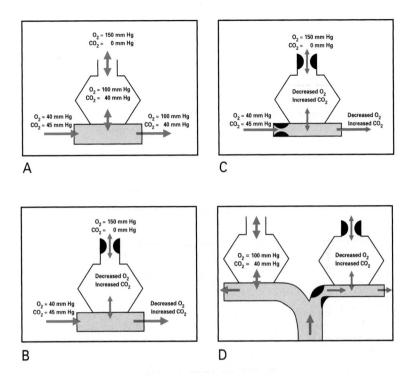

Figure 4–10. Illustration of the physiologic function of hypoxic pulmonary vasoconstriction (HPV). **A:** Normal alveolar-capillary unit. **B:** Perfusion of a hypoventilated alveolus results in blood with a decreased P_{O_2} and an increased P_{CO_2} entering the left atrium. **C:** HPV increases the resistance to blood flow to the hypoventilated alveolus. **D:** This diverts blood flow away from the hypoventilated alveolus to better-ventilated alveoli, thus helping to maintain $\dot{V}/\dot{Q}$ matching. HPV = hypoxic pulmonary vasoconstriction; $\dot{V}/\dot{Q}$ = ventilation-perfusion.

as will be discussed in the next chapter. On the other hand, such a whole-lung hypoxic pulmonary vasoconstriction greatly increases the workload on the right ventricle, and the high pulmonary artery pressure may overwhelm hypoxic pulmonary vasoconstriction in some parts of the lung, increase the capillary hydrostatic pressure in those vessels, and lead to pulmonary edema (see the next section of this chapter).

The mechanism of hypoxic pulmonary vasoconstriction has been controversial, but as noted above many researchers currently believe that inhibition of oxygen-sensitive voltage-gated potassium ion channels depolarizes smooth muscle cells in small branches of the pulmonary artery. This activates voltage-gated calcium ion channels in the smooth muscle cells, allowing influx of calcium ions, which causes the smooth muscle to contract and the vessels to constrict.

Alveolar hypercapnia (high carbon dioxide) also causes pulmonary vasoconstriction. It is not clear whether this occurs by the same mechanism as that of hypoxic pulmonary vasoconstriction.

PULMONARY EDEMA

Pulmonary edema is the extravascular accumulation of fluid in the lung. This pathologic condition may be caused by one or more physiologic abnormalities, but the result is inevitably impaired gas transfer. As the edema fluid builds up, first in the interstitium and later in alveoli, diffusion of gases—particularly oxygen—decreases (see Chapter 6).

The capillary endothelium is much more permeable to water and solutes than is the alveolar epithelium. Edema fluid therefore accumulates in the interstitium before it accumulates in the alveoli.

The Factors Influencing Liquid Movement in the Pulmonary Capillaries

The Starling equation describes the movement of liquid across the capillary endothelium:

$$\dot{Q}_f = K_f[(P_c - P_{is}) - \sigma(\pi_{pl} - \pi_{is})]$$

where $\dot{Q}_f$ = net flow of fluid

K_f = capillary filtration coefficient; this describes the permeability characteristics of the membrane to fluids

P_c = capillary hydrostatic pressure

P_{is} = hydrostatic pressure of the interstitial fluid

σ = reflection coefficient; this describes the ability of the membrane to prevent extravasation of solute particles

π_{pl} = colloid osmotic (oncotic) pressure of the plasma

π_{is} = colloid osmotic pressure of the interstitial fluid

The equation is shown schematically in Figure 4–11. The Starling equation is very useful in understanding the potential causes of pulmonary edema, even though only the plasma colloid osmotic pressure (π_{pl}) can be measured clinically.

Lymphatic Drainage of the Lung

Any fluid that makes its way into the pulmonary interstitium must be removed by the lymphatic drainage of the lung. The volume of lymph flow from the human lung is now believed to be as great as that from other organs under normal circumstances, and it is capable of increasing as much as 10-fold under pathologic conditions. It is only when this large safety factor is overwhelmed that pulmonary edema occurs.

Conditions That May Lead to Pulmonary Edema

The Starling equation provides a useful method of categorizing most of the potential causes of pulmonary edema (Table 4–3).

PERMEABILITY

Infections, circulating or inhaled toxins, oxygen toxicity, and other factors that destroy the integrity of the capillary endothelium lead to localized or generalized pulmonary edema.

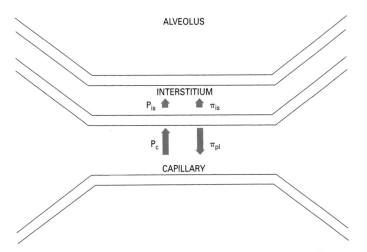

ALVEOLUS

INTERSTITIUM
P_{is} ⬆   ⬆ π_{is}

P_c ⬆   ⬇ π_{pl}

CAPILLARY

Figure 4–11. Illustration of the factors affecting liquid movement from the pulmonary capillaries. P_c = capillary hydrostatic pressure; P_{is} = interstitial hydrostatic pressures; π_{pl} = plasma colloid osmotic pressure; π_{is} = interstitial colloid osmotic pressure. (P_{is} is assumed to be negative, so the arrow points outward instead of inward.)

CAPILLARY HYDROSTATIC PRESSURE

The capillary hydrostatic pressure is estimated to be about 10 mm Hg under normal conditions. If the capillary hydrostatic pressure increases dramatically, the filtration of fluid across the capillary endothelium will increase greatly, and enough fluid may leave the capillaries to exceed the lymphatic drainage. The pulmonary capillary hydrostatic pressure often increases secondary to problems in the left side of the circulation, such as infarction of the left ventricle, left ventricular failure, or mitral stenosis. As left atrial pressure and pulmonary venous pressure rise because of accumulating blood, the pulmonary capillary hydrostatic pressure also increases. Other causes of elevated pulmonary capillary hydrostatic pressure include overzealous administration of intravenous fluids by the physician and diseases that occlude the pulmonary veins.

INTERSTITIAL HYDROSTATIC PRESSURE

Some investigators believe the interstitial hydrostatic pressure of the lung to be slightly positive, whereas others have shown evidence that it may be in the range of −5 to −7 mm Hg. Conditions that would decrease the interstitial pressure would increase the tendency for pulmonary edema to develop. These appear to be limited mainly to potential actions of the physician, such as rapid evacuation of chest fluids or reduction of pneumothorax. Situations that increase alveolar surface tension, for example, when decreased amounts of pulmonary surfactant are present, could also make the interstitial hydrostatic pressure more negative and increase the tendency for the formation of pulmonary edema. Note that as fluid accumulates in the interstitium, the interstitial hydrostatic pressure increases, which helps limit further fluid extravasation.

Table 4–3. Factors Predisposing to Pulmonary Edema

Factor in Starling Equation	Clinical Problems
Increased capillary permeability (K_f, σ)	Acute respiratory distress syndrome
	Oxygen toxicity
	Inhaled or circulating toxins
Increased capillary hydrostatic pressure (P_c)	Increased left atrial pressure resulting from left ventricular infarction or mitral stenosis
	Overadministration of intravenous fluids
Decreased interstitial hydrostatic pressure (P_{is})	Too rapid evacuation of pneumothorax or hemothorax
Decreased colloid osmotic pressure (π_{pl})	Protein starvation
	Dilution of blood proteins by intravenous solutions
	Renal problems resulting in urinary protein loss (proteinuria)

Other Etiologies	Clinical Problems
Insufficient pulmonary lymphatic drainage	Tumors
	Interstitial fibrosing diseases
Unknown etiology	High-altitude pulmonary edema
	Pulmonary edema after head injury (neurogenic pulmonary edema)
	Drug overdose

Reproduced with permission from Levitzky MG, Cairo JM, Hall SM. Introduction to *Respiratory Care*. Philadelphia, PA: Saunders WB and Company; 1990.

THE REFLECTION COEFFICIENT

Any situation that permits more solute to leave the capillaries will lead to more fluid movement out of the vascular space.

PLASMA COLLOID OSMOTIC PRESSURE

Decreases in the colloid osmotic pressure of the plasma, which helps retain fluid in the capillaries, may lead to pulmonary edema. Plasma colloid osmotic pressure, normally in the range of 25 to 28 mm Hg, falls in hypoproteinemia or overadministration of intravenous solutions.

INTERSTITIAL COLLOID OSMOTIC PRESSURE

Increased concentration of solute in the interstitium will pull fluid from the capillaries.

LYMPHATIC INSUFFICIENCY

Conditions that block the lymphatic drainage of the lung, such as tumors or scars, may predispose patients to pulmonary edema.

OTHER CONDITIONS ASSOCIATED WITH PULMONARY EDEMA

Pulmonary edema is often seen associated with head injury, heroin overdose, and high altitude. The causes of the edema formation in these conditions are not known, although high-altitude pulmonary edema may be caused by high pulmonary artery pressures secondary to the hypoxic pulmonary vasoconstriction.

KEY CONCEPTS

 Compared with the systemic arteries, the pulmonary arteries have much less vascular smooth muscle and therefore offer much less resistance to blood flow. Pulmonary arteries are more distensible and because their intravascular pressures are lower, more compressible than systemic arteries. The vascular **transmural pressure gradient** is therefore an important determinant of pulmonary vascular resistance (PVR).

 Although pulmonary vascular smooth muscle can actively contract or relax in response to neural and humoral influences, **"passive" factors** play a more important role in determining PVR than they do in determining systemic vascular resistance.

 PVR is usually lowest at the functional residual capacity and increases at higher and at lower lung volumes.

 PVR usually decreases with increases in pulmonary blood flow, pulmonary artery pressure, left atrial pressure, or pulmonary capillary blood volume because of **distention** of already open blood vessels, **recruitment** of previously unopened vessels, or both.

 There is more blood flow in lower regions of the lung than in upper regions. The effects of pulmonary artery pressure, pulmonary vein pressure, and alveolar pressure on pulmonary blood flow are described as the **"zones of the lung."**

 Alveolar hypoxia (or hypercapnia) can cause constriction of precapillary pulmonary vessels, diverting blood flow away from poorly ventilated or unventilated alveoli.

 CLINICAL PROBLEMS

4–1. A patient's mean arterial blood pressure is 100 mm Hg and his right atrial pressure is 2 mm Hg. His mean pulmonary artery pressure and pulmonary capillary wedge pressure ($\approx$ left atrial pressure) determined using a Swan-Ganz catheter, are 15 and 5 mm Hg, respectively. If his cardiac output is 5 L/min, calculate his pulmonary vascular resistance and systemic vascular resistance.

4–2. Which of the following situations would be expected to decrease pulmonary vascular resistance?

a. Ascent to 15,000 ft above sea level

b. Inspiration to the total lung capacity

   c. *Expiration to the residual volume*

   d. *Moderate exercise*

   e. *Blood loss secondary to trauma*

4–3. Which of the following situations would be expected to lead to an increase *in the amount of the lung under zone 1 conditions?*

   a. *Ascent to 15,000 ft above sea level*

   b. *Blood loss secondary to trauma*

   c. *Moderate exercise*

   d. *Positive-pressure ventilation with positive end-expiratory pressure (PEEP)*

   e. *Changing from the standing to the supine position*

4–4. Which of the following circumstances might be expected to contribute to the formation *of pulmonary edema?*

   a. *Overtransfusion with saline*

   b. *Occlusion of the lymphatic drainage of an area of the lung*

   c. *Left ventricular failure*

   d. *Low concentration of plasma proteins*

   e. *Destruction of portions of the pulmonary capillary endothelium by toxins*

   f. *All of the above*

SUGGESTED READINGS

Aaronson PI, Robertson TP, Knock GA, Becker S, Lewis TH, Snetkov V, Ward JPT. Hypoxic pulmonary vasoconstriction: mechanisms and controversies. *J Physiol.* 2006;570:53–58.

Borst HG, McGregor M, Whittenberger JL, Berglund E. Influence of pulmonary arterial and left atrial pressure on pulmonary vascular resistance. *Circ Res.* 1956;4:393–399.

Deffebach ME, Charan NB, Lakshminarayan S, Butler J. The bronchial circulation: Small, but a vital attribute of the lung. *Am Rev Respir Dis.* 1987;135:463–481.

Dumas JP, Bardou M, Goirand F, Dumas M. Hypoxic pulmonary vasoconstriction. *General Pharm.* 1999;33:289–297.

Hughes JMB, Glazier JB, Maloney JE, West JB. Effect of lung volume on the distribution of pulmonary blood flow in man. *Respir Physiol.* 1968;4:58–72.

Hughes JM, Glazier JB, Maloney JE, West JB. Effect of extraalveolar vessels on distribution of blood flow in the dog lung. *J Appl Physiol.* 1968;25:701–712.

Levitzky MG, Cairo JM, Hall SM. *Introduction to Respiratory Care.* Philadelphia Pa: WB Saunders and Company; 1990.

Moudgil R, Michelakis ED, Archer, SL. Hypoxic pulmonary vasoconstriction. *J Appl Physiol.* 2005;98:390–403.

Murray JF. *The Normal Lung.* Philadelphia, Pa: WB Saunders and Company; 1976:131.

Murray JF. *The Normal Lung.* 2nd ed. Philadelphia, Pa: WB Saunders and Company; 1986:35–43, 139–162.

Schuster DP. Pulmonary edema. In: Fishman AP, ed. *Pulmonary Diseases and Disorders.* 3rd ed. New York, NY: McGraw-Hill; 1998:1331–1356.

Ward JPT, Aaronson PI. Mechanisms of hypoxic pulmonary vasoconstriction: can anyone be right? *Respir Physiol.* 1999;115:261–271.

West JB. *Ventilation/Blood Flow and Gas Exchange.* 5th ed. Oxford: Blackwell; 1990:15–25.

West JB, Dollery CT, Naimark A. Distribution of blood flow in isolated lung: Relation to vascular and alveolar pressures. *J Appl Physiol.* 1964;19:713–724.

Ventilation-Perfusion Relationships

5

OBJECTIVES

The reader understands the importance of the matching of ventilation and perfusion in the lung.

▶ *Predicts the consequences of mismatched ventilation and perfusion.*

▶ *Describes the methods used to assess the matching of ventilation and perfusion.*

▶ *Describes the methods used to determine the uniformity of the distribution of the inspired gas and pulmonary blood flow.*

▶ *Explains the regional differences in the matching of ventilation and perfusion of the normal upright lung.*

▶ *Predicts the consequences of the regional differences in the ventilation and perfusion of the normal upright lung.*

Gas exchange between the alveoli and the pulmonary capillary blood occurs by diffusion, as will be discussed in the next chapter. Diffusion of oxygen and carbon dioxide occurs passively, according to their concentration gradients across the alveolar-capillary barrier. These concentration gradients must be maintained by ventilation of the alveoli and perfusion of the pulmonary capillaries.

THE CONCEPT OF MATCHING VENTILATION & PERFUSION

Alveolar ventilation brings oxygen into the lung and removes carbon dioxide from it. Similarly, the mixed venous blood brings carbon dioxide into the lung and takes up alveolar oxygen. The alveolar P_{O_2} and P_{CO_2} are thus determined by the relationship between alveolar ventilation and perfusion. Alterations in the ratio of ventilation to perfusion, called the $\dot{V}_A/\dot{Q}_c$, will result in changes in the alveolar P_{O_2} and P_{CO_2}, as well as in gas delivery to or removal from the lung.

Alveolar ventilation is normally about 4 to 6 L/min and pulmonary blood flow (which is equal to cardiac output) has a similar range, and so the $\dot{V}/\dot{Q}$ for the whole lung is in the range of 0.8 to 1.2. However, ventilation and perfusion must be matched on the *alveolar-capillary level,* and the $\dot{V}/\dot{Q}$ for the whole lung is really of interest only as an approximation of the situation in all the alveolar-capillary units of the lung. For instance, suppose that all 5 L/min of the cardiac output went to the left lung and all 5 L/min of alveolar ventilation went to the right lung. The whole lung $\dot{V}/\dot{Q}$ would be 1.0, but there would be no gas exchange because there could be no gas diffusion between the ventilated alveoli and the perfused pulmonary capillaries.

CONSEQUENCES OF HIGH & LOW $\dot{V}/\dot{Q}$

Oxygen is delivered to the alveolus by alveolar ventilation, is removed from the alveolus as it diffuses into the pulmonary capillary blood, and is carried away by blood flow. Similarly, carbon dioxide is delivered to the alveolus in the mixed venous blood and diffuses into the alveolus in the pulmonary capillary. The carbon dioxide is removed from the alveolus by alveolar ventilation. As will be discussed in Chapter 6, at resting cardiac outputs the diffusion of both oxygen and carbon dioxide is normally limited by pulmonary perfusion. Thus, the alveolar partial pressures of both oxygen and carbon dioxide are determined by the $\dot{V}/\dot{Q}$. If the $\dot{V}/\dot{Q}$ in an alveolar-capillary unit *increases,* the delivery of oxygen relative to its removal will increase, as will the removal of carbon dioxide relative to its delivery. Alveolar P_{O_2} will therefore rise, and alveolar P_{CO_2} will fall. If the $\dot{V}/\dot{Q}$ in an alveolar-capillary unit *decreases,* the removal of oxygen relative to its delivery will increase and the delivery of carbon dioxide relative to its removal will increase. Alveolar P_{O_2} will therefore fall, and alveolar P_{CO_2} will rise.

Figure 5–1 shows the consequences of alterations in the relationship of ventilation and perfusion on hypothetical alveolar-capillary units. Unit A has a normal $\dot{V}/\dot{Q}$. Inspired air enters the alveolus with a P_{O_2} of about 150 mm Hg and a P_{CO_2} of nearly 0 mm Hg. Mixed venous blood enters the pulmonary capillary with a P_{O_2} of about 40 mm Hg and a P_{CO_2} of about 45 mm Hg. This results in an alveolar P_{O_2} of about 100 mm Hg and an alveolar P_{CO_2} of 40 mm Hg (see Chapter 3). The partial pressure gradient for oxygen diffusion from alveolus to pulmonary capillary is thus about $100 - 40$ mm Hg, or 60 mm Hg; the partial pressure gradient for CO_2 diffusion from pulmonary capillary to alveolus is about $45 - 40$, or 5 mm Hg.

The airway supplying unit B has become completely occluded. Its $\dot{V}/\dot{Q}$ is zero. As time goes on, the air trapped in the alveolus equilibrates by diffusion with the gas dissolved in the mixed venous blood entering the alveolar-capillary unit. (If the occlusion persists, the alveolus is likely to collapse.) No gas exchange can occur, and any blood perfusing this alveolus will leave it exactly as it entered it. Unit B is therefore acting as a right-to-left shunt.

The blood flow to unit C is blocked by a pulmonary embolus, and unit C is therefore completely unperfused. It has an infinite $\dot{V}/\dot{Q}$. Because no oxygen can diffuse from the alveolus into pulmonary capillary blood and because no carbon dioxide can enter the alveolus from the blood, the P_{O_2} of the alveolus is approximately 150 mm Hg and its P_{CO_2} is approximately zero. That is, the gas composition of this unperfused alveolus is the same as that of inspired air. Unit C is alveolar dead space. If unit C were unperfused because its alveolar pressure exceeded its precapillary pressure (rather than because of an embolus), then it would also correspond to part of zone 1.

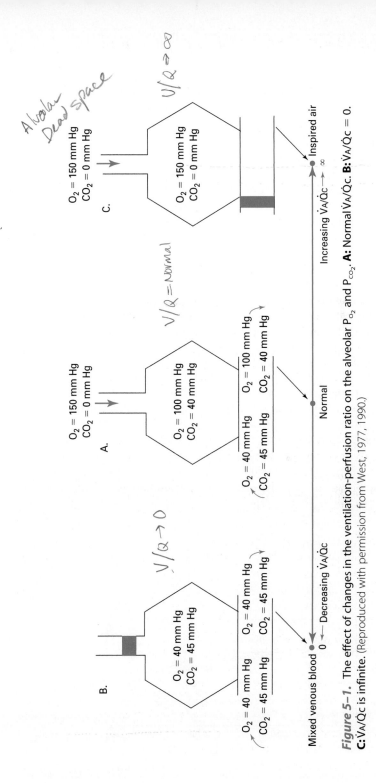

Figure 5–1. The effect of changes in the ventilation-perfusion ratio on the alveolar P_{O_2} and P_{CO_2}. **A:** Normal $\dot{V}_A/\dot{Q}_C$. **B:** $\dot{V}_A/\dot{Q}_C = 0$. **C:** $\dot{V}_A/\dot{Q}_C$ is infinite. (Reproduced with permission from West, 1977, 1990.)

115

Units B and C represent the two extremes of a *continuum* of ventilation-perfusion ratios. The $\dot{V}/\dot{Q}$ ratio of a particular alveolar-capillary unit can fall anywhere along this continuum, as shown at the bottom of Figure 5–1. The alveolar P_{O_2} and P_{CO_2} of such units will therefore fall between the two extremes shown in the figure: Units with *low* $\dot{V}/\dot{Q}$ ratios will have relatively low P_{O_2}s and high P_{CO_2}s; units with *high* $\dot{V}/\dot{Q}$ ratios will have relatively high P_{O_2}s and low P_{CO_2}s. This is demonstrated graphically in an O_2-CO_2 diagram such as that seen in Figure 5–2. The diagram shows the results of mathematical calculations of alveolar P_{O_2}s and P_{CO_2}s for $\dot{V}/\dot{Q}$ ratios between zero (for mixed venous blood) and infinity (for inspired air). The resulting curve is known as the *ventilation-perfusion ratio line*. This simple O_2-CO_2 diagram can be modified to include correction lines for other factors, such as the respiratory exchange ratios of the alveoli and the blood or the dead space. The position of the $\dot{V}/\dot{Q}$ ratio line is altered if the partial pressures of the inspired gas or mixed venous blood are altered.

TESTING FOR NONUNIFORM DISTRIBUTION OF INSPIRED GAS & PULMONARY BLOOD FLOW

Nonuniform ventilation of the alveoli can be caused by uneven *resistance* to airflow or nonuniform *compliance* in different parts of the lung. Uneven resistance to airflow may be a result of collapse of airways, as seen in emphysema; bronchoconstriction, as in asthma; decreased lumen diameter due to inflammation, as in bronchitis; obstruction by mucus, as in asthma or chronic bronchitis; or compression by tumors or edema. Uneven compliance may be a result of fibrosis, regional variations in surfactant production, pulmonary vascular congestion or edema, emphysema, diffuse or regional atelectasis, pneumothorax, or compression by tumors or cysts.

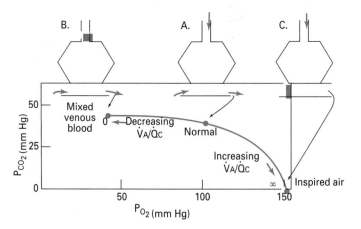

Figure 5–2. The ventilation-perfusion ratio line on an O_2-CO_2 diagram. Unit with a $\dot{V}A/\dot{Q}c$ of zero has the P_{O_2} and P_{CO_2} of mixed venous blood; a unit with an infinite $\dot{V}A/\dot{Q}c$ has the P_{O_2} and P_{CO_2} of inspired air. (Reproduced with permission from West 1977, 1990.)

Nonuniform perfusion of the lung can be caused by embolization or thrombosis; compression of pulmonary vessels by high alveolar pressures, tumors, exudates, edema, pneumothorax, or hydrothorax; destruction or occlusion of pulmonary vessels by various disease processes; pulmonary vascular hypotension; or collapse or overexpansion of alveoli.

As already noted in Chapters 3 and 4, gravity, local factors, and regional differences in intrapleural pressure cause a degree of nonuniformity in the distribution of ventilation and perfusion in normal lungs. This will be discussed in detail later in this chapter.

The methods used for testing for nonuniform ventilation, nonuniform perfusion, and ventilation-perfusion mismatch are summarized in Table 5–1.

Testing for Nonuniform Distribution of Inspired Gas

Several methods can be used to demonstrate an abnormal distribution of ventilation in a patient.

SINGLE-BREATH-OF-OXYGEN TEST

A rising expired nitrogen concentration in phase III (the "alveolar plateau") of the single-breath-of-oxygen test shown in Figure 3–14 indicates the possibility of a maldistribution of ventilation (see "The Closing Volume" section of Chapter 3).

Table 5–1. Testing for $\dot{V}/\dot{Q}$ Mismatch

I. Nonuniform gas distribution
  A. Alveolar plateau of closing volume test
  B. Nitrogen washout
  C. Trapped gas
  D. Single breath of ^{133}Xe
  E. ^{99m}Tc-labeled DTPA (diethylene triamine pentaacetic acid)
II. Nonuniform pulmonary blood flow
  A. Pulmonary angiogram
  B. Lung scans:
    1. ^{131}I-labeled MAA
    2. ^{99m}Tc-labeled MAA
    3. ^{133}Xe
III. Mismatched $\dot{V}/\dot{Q}$
  A. Physiologic shunts: shunt equation
    1. Anatomic
    2. Intrapulmonary
      a. Absolute
      b. Shuntlike states (low $\dot{V}/\dot{Q}$)
  B. Physiologic dead space: Bohr equation
    1. Anatomic
    2. Alveolar: $(a\text{-}A)D_{CO_2}$
  C. $(A\text{-}a)D_{O_2}$
  D. Lung scans after inhaled and infused markers
  E. Multiple inert gas technique

$\dot{V}/\dot{Q}$ = ventilation-perfusion; $(A\text{-}a)D_{O_2}$ = alveolar-arterial oxygen difference.

NITROGEN-WASHOUT TEST

The same equipment used in the single-breath-of-oxygen test mentioned above can be used in another test for nonuniform ventilation of the lungs. In this test, the subject breathes normally from a bag of 100% oxygen, and the expired nitrogen concentration is monitored over a number of breaths. With each successive inspiration of 100% oxygen and subsequent expiration, the expired end-tidal nitrogen concentration falls as nitrogen is washed out of the lung (Figure 5–3).

The rate of decrease of the expired end-tidal nitrogen concentration depends on several factors. A high functional residual capacity (FRC), a low tidal volume, a large dead space, or a low breathing frequency could each contribute to a slower washout of alveolar nitrogen. Nonetheless, subjects with a normal distribution of airways resistance will reduce their expired end-tidal nitrogen concentration to less than 2.5% within 7 minutes. Subjects breathing normally who take more than 7 minutes to reach an alveolar nitrogen concentration of less than 2.5% have high-resistance pathways, or "slow alveoli" (see section "Dynamic Compliance" in Chapter 2).

If the logarithms of the end-tidal nitrogen concentrations are plotted against the number of breaths taken (for a subject breathing regularly), a straight line results (Figure 5–4A). (Many nitrogen meters have a log [N₂] output.) On the other hand, the log [N₂] plotted for a patient with a maldistribution of airways resistance, such as that produced experimentally by inhaling a histamine aerosol (Figure 5–4B), displays a more complex curve. After a short period of relatively rapid nitrogen washout, a long period of extremely slow nitrogen washout occurs, indicating a population of poorly ventilated "slow alveoli."

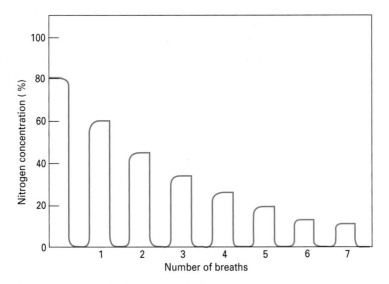

Figure 5–3. Illustration of a nitrogen-washout curve.

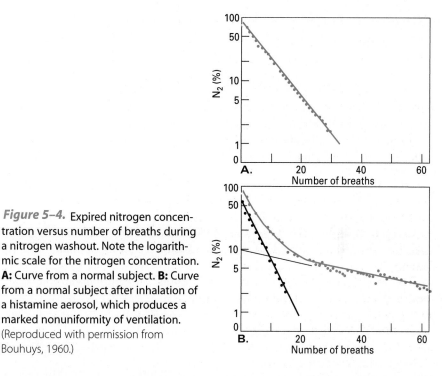

Figure 5–4. Expired nitrogen concentration versus number of breaths during a nitrogen washout. Note the logarithmic scale for the nitrogen concentration. **A:** Curve from a normal subject. **B:** Curve from a normal subject after inhalation of a histamine aerosol, which produces a marked nonuniformity of ventilation. (Reproduced with permission from Bouhuys, 1960.)

TRAPPED GAS

Differences between the FRC determined by the helium-dilution technique and the FRC determined using a body plethysmograph may indicate gas trapped in the alveoli because of airway closure (see Chapter 3). In fact, if a number of high-resistance pathways are present in the lung of the patient being tested, it may take an exceptionally long time for the patient's expired end-tidal helium concentration to equilibrate with the helium concentration in the spirometer. The closing volume determination, discussed at the end of Chapter 3, can also demonstrate airway closure in the lung.

RADIOACTIVE MARKERS

The methods described thus far can indicate the presence of poorly ventilated regions of the lung but not their location. Pictures of the whole lung taken with a scintillation counter, after the subject has taken a breath of a radioactive gas mixture such as ^{133}Xe or ^{99m}Tc DTPA (technetium-labeled diethylene triamine pentaacetic acid) and oxygen, can indicate which regions of the lung are poorly ventilated.

Testing for Nonuniform Distribution of Pulmonary Blood Flow

These methods were all discussed briefly in Chapter 4. They include *angiograms,* lung scans after intravenous injection of radiolabeled (with radioactive iodine or

technetium) *macroaggregates of albumin,* and lung scans after intravenous administration of dissolved ^{133}Xe. Each of these methods can indicate the locations of relatively large regions of poor perfusion.

Testing for Mismatched Ventilation & Perfusion

Several methods can demonstrate the presence or location of areas of the lung
with mismatched ventilation and perfusion. These methods include calculations
of the physiologic shunt, the physiologic dead space, differences between the alveolar and arterial P_{O_2}s and P_{CO_2}s, and lung scans after inhaled and intravenously
administered ^{133}Xe or ^{99m}Tc.

PHYSIOLOGIC SHUNTS AND THE SHUNT EQUATION

A right-to-left shunt is the mixing of venous blood that has not been oxygenated
(or not fully oxygenated) into the arterial blood. The *physiologic shunt,* which corresponds to the physiologic dead space, consists of the anatomic shunts plus the
intrapulmonary shunts. The intrapulmonary shunts can be *absolute shunts,* or they
can be *"shuntlike states,"* that is, areas of low ventilation-perfusion ratios in which
alveoli are underventilated and/or overperfused.

Physiologic shunt = Anatomic shunt + Intrapulmonary shunt

Absolute shunts   "Shunt-like states"

Anatomic Shunts— Anatomic shunts consist of systemic venous blood entering
the left ventricle without having entered the pulmonary vasculature. In a normal
healthy adult, about 2–5% of the cardiac output, including venous blood from the
bronchial veins, the thebesian veins, and the pleural veins, enters the left side of the
circulation directly without passing through the pulmonary capillaries. (This normal anatomic shunt is also occasionally referred to as the *physiologic shunt* because
it does not represent a pathologic condition.) Pathologic anatomic shunts such as
right-to-left intracardiac shunts can also occur, as in tetralogy of Fallot.

Absolute Intrapulmonary Shunts— Mixed venous blood perfusing pulmonary
capillaries associated with totally unventilated or collapsed alveoli constitutes an
absolute shunt (like the anatomic shunts) because no gas exchange occurs as the
blood passes through the lung. Absolute shunts are sometimes also referred to as
true shunts.

Shuntlike States— Alveolar-capillary units with low $\dot{V}A/\dot{Q}$cs also act to lower the
arterial oxygen content because blood draining these units has a lower P_{O_2} than
blood from units with well-matched ventilation and perfusion.

The Shunt Equation— The shunt equation *conceptually* divides all alveolar-
capillary units into two groups: those with well-matched ventilation and perfusion
and those with ventilation-perfusion ratios of zero. Thus, the shunt equation combines
the areas of absolute shunt (including the anatomic shunts) and the shuntlike areas

into a single conceptual group. The resulting ratio of shunt flow to the cardiac output, often referred to as the *venous admixture,* is the part of the cardiac output that would have to be perfusing *absolutely unventilated alveoli* to cause the systemic arterial oxygen content obtained from a patient. A much larger portion of the cardiac output could be *overperfusing* poorly ventilated alveoli and yield the same ratio.

The shunt equation can be derived as follows: Let $\dot{Q}t$ represent the total pulmonary blood flow per minute (i.e., the cardiac output), and let $\dot{Q}s$ represent the amount of blood flow per minute entering the systemic arterial blood without receiving any oxygen (the "shunt flow"). The volume of blood per minute that perfuses alveolar-capillary units with well-matched ventilation and perfusion then equals $\dot{Q}t - \dot{Q}s$.

The total volume of oxygen per time entering the systemic arteries is therefore

$$\dot{Q}t \times Ca_{O_2}$$

where Ca_{O_2} equals oxygen *content* of arterial blood in milliliters of oxygen per 100 mL of blood. This total amount of oxygen per time entering the systemic arteries is composed of the oxygen coming from the well-ventilated and well-perfused alveolar-capillary units:

$$(\dot{Q}t - \dot{Q}s) \times Cc'_{O_2}$$

where Cc'_{O_2} equals the oxygen content of the blood at the end of the ventilated and perfused pulmonary capillaries, *plus* the oxygen in the unaltered mixed venous blood coming from the shunt, $\dot{Q}s \times C\bar{v}_{O_2}$ (where $C\bar{v}_{O_2}$ is equal to the oxygen content of the mixed venous blood).

That is,

$$\dot{Q}t \times Ca_{O_2} = (\dot{Q}t - \dot{Q}s) \times Cc'_{O_2} + \dot{Q}s \times C\bar{v}_{O_2}$$

Oxygen delivery	Oxygen coming	Oxygen from
to systemic arteries	from normal	shunted blood
	$\dot{V}a/\dot{Q}c$ units	flow

$$\dot{Q}t \times Ca_{O_2} = \dot{Q}t \times Cc'_{O_2} - \dot{Q}s \times Cc'_{O_2} + \dot{Q}s \times C\bar{v}_{O_2}$$

$$\dot{Q}s \times (Cc'_{O_2} - C\bar{v}_{O_2}) = \dot{Q}t \times (Cc'_{O_2} - Ca_{O_2})$$

$$\frac{\dot{Q}s}{\dot{Q}t} = \frac{Cc'_{O_2} - Ca_{O_2}}{Cc'_{O_2} - C\bar{v}_{O_2}}$$

The shunt fraction $\dot{Q}s/\dot{Q}t$ is usually multiplied by 100% so that the shunt flow is expressed as a percentage of the cardiac output.

The arterial and mixed venous oxygen contents can be determined if blood samples are obtained from a systemic artery and from the pulmonary artery (for mixed venous blood), but the oxygen content of the blood at the end of the pulmonary capillaries with well-matched ventilation and perfusion is, of course, impossible to measure directly. This must be calculated from the *alveolar air equation,* discussed in Chapter 3, and the patient's hemoglobin concentration, which will be discussed in Chapter 7.

The relative contributions of the true intrapulmonary shunts and the shuntlike states to the calculated shunt flow can be estimated by repeating the measurements and calculations with the patient on a normal or slightly elevated inspired concentration of oxygen and then on a very high inspired oxygen concentration ($F_{I_{O_2}}$ of 0.95 to 1.00). At the lower inspired oxygen concentrations, the calculated $\dot{Q}s/\dot{Q}t$ will include both the true shunts and the alveolar-capillary units with low $\dot{V}/\dot{Q}$ ratios. After a patient has inspired nearly 100% oxygen for 20 to 30 minutes, even alveoli with very low $\dot{V}/\dot{Q}s$ will have high enough alveolar $P_{O_2}s$ to completely saturate the hemoglobin in the blood perfusing them. These units will therefore no longer contribute to the calculated $\dot{Q}s/\dot{Q}t$, and the new calculated shunt should include only areas of absolute shunt. Unfortunately, very high inspired oxygen concentrations may lead to absorption atelectasis of very poorly ventilated alveoli that remain perfused, and so this test may alter what it is trying to measure when high levels of $F_{I_{O_2}}$ are used.

PHYSIOLOGIC DEAD SPACE

The use of the Bohr equation to determine the physiologic dead space was discussed in detail in Chapter 3. If the anatomic dead space is subtracted from the physiologic dead space, the result (if there is a difference) is *alveolar dead space,* or areas of infinite $\dot{V}/\dot{Q}s$. Alveolar dead space also results in an *arterial-alveolar CO_2 difference;* that is, the end-tidal P_{CO_2} is normally equal to the arterial P_{CO_2}. An arterial P_{CO_2} greater than the end-tidal P_{CO_2} usually indicates the presence of alveolar dead space.

ALVEOLAR-ARTERIAL OXYGEN DIFFERENCE

Throughout most of this book, the alveolar and arterial $P_{O_2}s$ are treated as though they are equal. However, the arterial P_{O_2} is normally a few mm Hg less than the alveolar P_{O_2}. This normal *alveolar-arterial oxygen difference,* the $(A-a)D_{O_2}$, is caused by the normal anatomic shunt, some degree of ventilation-perfusion mismatch (see later in this chapter), and diffusion limitation in some parts of the lung. Of these, $\dot{V}/\dot{Q}$ mismatch is usually the most important, with a small contribution from shunts and very little from diffusion limitation. Larger-than-normal differences between the alveolar and arterial P_{O_2} may indicate significant ventilation-perfusion mismatch; however, increased alveolar-arterial oxygen differences (Table 5–2) can also be caused by anatomic or intrapulmonary shunts, diffusion block, low mixed venous $P_{O_2}s$, breathing higher than normal oxygen concentrations, or shifts of the oxyhemoglobin dissociation curve (also see Table 8–6).

The alveolar-arterial P_{O_2} difference is normally about 5 to 15 mm Hg in a young healthy person breathing room air at sea level. It increases with age because of the progressive decrease in arterial P_{O_2} that occurs with aging for the reasons discussed at the end of Chapter 3. The normal alveolar-arterial P_{O_2} difference increases by about 20 mm Hg between the ages of 20 and 70.

Table 5–2. Causes of Increased Alveolar-Arterial Oxygen Difference

Increased right-to-left shunt
  Anatomic
  Intrapulmonary
Increased ventilation-perfusion mismatch
Impaired diffusion
Increased inspired partial pressure of oxygen
Decreased mixed venous partial pressure of oxygen
Shift of oxyhemoglobin dissociation curve

Reproduced with permission from Marshall and Wyche, 1972.

Note that the "alveolar" P_{O_2} used in determining the alveolar-arterial oxygen difference is the $P_{A_{O_2}}$ calculated using the alveolar air equation. As noted in Chapter 3, it is an idealized average alveolar P_{O_2} that represents what alveolar P_{O_2} should be, not necessarily what it is.

Another useful clinical index in addition to the alveolar-arterial oxygen difference is the ratio of arterial P_{O_2} to the fractional concentration of oxygen in the inspired air. The $P_{A_{O_2}}/F_{I_{O_2}}$ should be greater than or equal to 200; a $P_{A_{O_2}}/F_{I_{O_2}}$ less than 200 is seen in acute respiratory distress syndrome.

SINGLE-BREATH CARBON DIOXIDE TEST

The expired concentration of carbon dioxide can be monitored by a rapid-response carbon dioxide meter in a manner similar to that used in the single-breath tests utilizing a nitrogen meter, as described in Chapter 3 (see Figure 3–9). The alveolar plateau phase of the expired carbon dioxide concentration *may* show signs of poorly matched ventilation and perfusion if such regions empty asynchronously with other regions of the lung.

LUNG SCANS AFTER INHALED AND INFUSED MARKERS

Lung scans after both inhaled and injected markers can be used to inspect the location and amount of ventilation and perfusion to the various regions of the lung (see Chapters 3 and 4).

MULTIPLE INERT GAS ELIMINATION TECHNIQUE

A more specific graphic method for assessing ventilation-perfusion relationships in human subjects is called *the multiple inert gas elimination technique.* This technique uses the concept that the elimination via the lungs of different gases dissolved in the mixed venous blood is affected differently by variations in the ventilation-perfusion ratios of alveolar-capillary units, according to the solubility of each gas in the blood. At a ventilation-perfusion ratio of 1.0, a greater volume of a relatively soluble gas would be retained in the blood than would be the case with a relatively insoluble gas. Thus, the retention of any particular gas by a single alveolar-capillary unit is dependent on the blood-gas partition coefficient of the gas and the ventilation-perfusion ratio of the unit. Gases with very low solubilities in the blood would be retained in the blood only by units with very low (or zero) $\dot{V}/\dot{Q}s$. Gases with very high solubilities in the blood would be eliminated mainly in the expired air of units with very high $\dot{V}/\dot{Q}s$.

In the standard multiple inert gas elimination technique for assessing $\dot{V}/\dot{Q}$ relationships, a mixture of six gases dissolved in saline is infused into a peripheral arm vein at a constant rate of 2 to 5 mL/min until a steady state of gas exchange is established. This usually takes about 20 minutes. The six gases—sulfur hexafluoride, ethane, cyclopropane, halothane, diethyl ether, and acetone—were chosen to represent a wide range of solubilities in blood, with acetone the most soluble and sulfur hexafluoride the least soluble. Samples of expired air and arterial blood are analyzed by gas chromatography to determine the concentrations of each of the six gases. Other data usually obtained include cardiac output by indicator dilution, minute ventilation, and arterial and mixed venous blood gases.

Graphs plotting the blood-gas partition coefficients for each of the six gases versus their retentions and excretions are constructed. A computer is then used to convert these data into graphs like the one shown in Figure 5–5A. The graph, which shows the distribution of ventilation-perfusion ratios in a young healthy male subject, can be read as a frequency histogram. The x axis is the spectrum of ventilation-perfusion ratios from 0 to 100, displayed as a logarithmic scale. The y axis shows the amount of ventilation or blood flow going to alveolar-capillary units with the $\dot{V}/\dot{Q}$ ratio on the x axis. The figure demonstrates that in this young, healthy subject almost all the blood flow and ventilation go to alveolar-capillary units with $\dot{V}/\dot{Q}$ ratios near 1. There is no ventilation or perfusion of units with ratios below 0.3 or above 3.0. Figure 5–5B shows the distribution of ventilation and perfusion in a healthy middle-aged subject. Note the wider dispersion of ventilation and perfusion, with more perfusion going to units with ratios above 3.0 and much more going to units with ratios below 0.3.

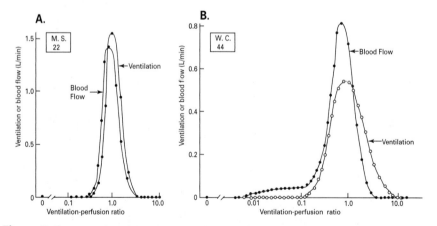

Figure 5–5. Examples of distributions of ventilation-perfusion ratios in normal subjects. **A:** The results in a young subject. **B:** The results in an older man. (Reproduced from Wagner PD, Laravuso RB, Uhl RR, West JB: The Journal of Clinical Investigation, 1974, 54:54–68 by copyright permission of The American Society for Clinical Investigation.)

Similarly, the ventilation is also more widely distributed. Note that there was no true intrapulmonary shunt in either subject, that is, no blood flow to alveolar-capillary units with $\dot{V}/\dot{Q}s$ of zero.

REGIONAL $\dot{V}/\dot{Q}$ DIFFERENCES & THEIR CONSEQUENCES IN THE LUNG

The regional variations in ventilation in the normal upright lung were discussed in Chapter 3. As summarized on the left side of Figure 5–6, gravity-dependent regions of the lung receive more ventilation per unit volume than do upper regions of the lung when one is breathing near the FRC. The reason for this regional difference in ventilation is that there is a gradient of pleural surface pressure, which is probably caused by gravity and the mechanical interaction of the lung and the chest wall. The pleural surface pressure is more negative in nondependent regions of the lung, and so the alveoli in these areas are subjected to greater transpulmonary pressures. As a result, these alveoli have larger volumes than do alveoli in more dependent regions of the lung and are therefore on a less steep portion of their pressure-volume curves. These less-compliant alveoli change their volume less with each breath than do those in more dependent regions.

The right side of Figure 5–6 shows that the more gravity-dependent regions of the lung also receive more blood flow per unit volume than do the upper regions

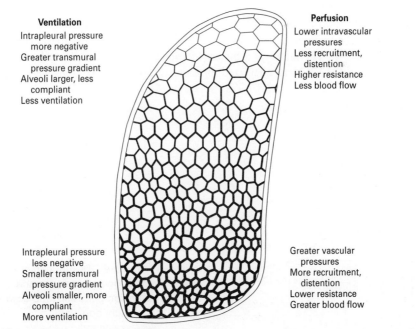

Ventilation

Intrapleural pressure
   more negative
Greater transmural
   pressure gradient
Alveoli larger, less
   compliant
Less ventilation

Perfusion

Lower intravascular
   pressures
Less recruitment,
   distention
Higher resistance
Less blood flow

Intrapleural pressure
   less negative
Smaller transmural
   pressure gradient
Alveoli smaller, more
   compliant
More ventilation

Greater vascular
   pressures
More recruitment,
   distention
Lower resistance
Greater blood flow

Figure 5–6. Summary of regional differences in ventilation (left) and perfusion (right) in the normal upright lung.

of the lung, as discussed in Chapter 4. The reason for this is that the intravascular pressure in the lower regions of the lung is greater because of hydrostatic effects. Blood vessels in more dependent regions of the lung are therefore more distended, or more vessels are perfused because of recruitment.

Regional Differences in the Ventilation-Perfusion Ratios in the Upright Lung

Simplified graphs of the gradients of ventilation and perfusion from the bottom to the top of normal upright dog lungs are shown plotted on the same axes in Figure 5–7. The ventilation-perfusion ratio was then calculated for several locations.

Figure 5–7 shows that the gradient of perfusion from the bottom of the lung to the top is greater than the gradient of ventilation. Because of this, the ventilation-perfusion ratio is relatively low in more gravity-dependent regions of the lung and higher in upper regions of the lung. In fact, if pulmonary perfusion pressure is low, for example, because of hemorrhage, or if alveolar pressure is high, because of positive-pressure ventilation with positive end-expiratory pressure, or if both factors are present, then there may be areas of zone 1 with infinite ventilation-perfusion ratios in the upper parts of the lung.

The Consequences of Regional Ventilation-Perfusion Differences in the Normal Upright Lung

The effects of the regional differences in $\dot{V}/\dot{Q}$ on the alveolar P_{O_2} and P_{CO_2} can be seen in Figure 5–8. The lung was arbitrarily divided into nine imaginary horizontal sections, and the $\dot{V}/\dot{Q}$ was calculated for each section. These sections were then

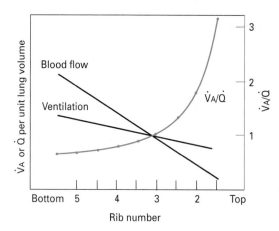

Figure 5–7. Distribution of ventilation and perfusion and ventilation-perfusion ratio down the upright dog lung. (Reproduced with permission from West, 1977, 1990.)

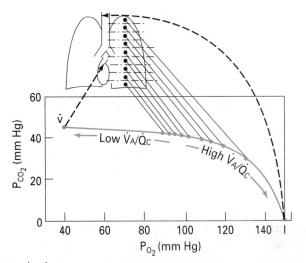

Figure 5–8. The V̇A/Q̇c for each of nine imaginary sections of a vertical lung on the ventilation-perfusion line of an O_2-CO_2 diagram. Upper sections have higher V̇A/Q̇c with higher P_{O_2} and lower P_{CO_2}, and lower sections have lower V̇A/Q̇c with lower P_{O_2} and higher P_{CO_2}. (Reproduced with permission from West JB. Respiratory Physiology. 4th ed. Philadelphia, Pa: Lippincott Williams & Wilkins; 1990.)

positioned on the ventilation-perfusion line of the O_2-CO_2 diagram, and the P_{O_2} and P_{CO_2} of the alveoli in each section could be estimated. Under normal circumstances the blood in the pulmonary capillaries equilibrates with the alveolar P_{O_2} and P_{CO_2} as it travels through the lung, and so the effects of regional differences in V̇/Q̇ on the regional gas exchange could be predicted. As can be seen from the figure, the upper sections have relatively high P_{O_2} and low P_{CO_2}; the lower sections have relatively low P_{O_2} and high P_{CO_2}.

Figures 5–7 and 5–8 demonstrate that the lower regions of the lung receive both better ventilation and better perfusion than do the upper portions of the lung. However, the perfusion gradient is much steeper than the ventilation gradient, and so the ventilation-perfusion ratio is higher in the apical regions than it is in the basal regions. As a result, the alveolar P_{O_2} is higher and the alveolar P_{CO_2} is lower in upper portions of the lung than they are in lower regions. This means that the oxygen *content* of the blood draining the upper regions is higher and the carbon dioxide *content* is lower than that of the blood draining the lower regions. However, these contents are based on *milliliters of blood* (see Chapter 7), and there is much less *blood flow* to the uppermost sections than there is to the bottom sections. Therefore, even though the uppermost sections have the highest V̇/Q̇ and P_{O_2} and the lowest P_{CO_2}, there is more *gas exchange* in the more basal sections.

KEY CONCEPTS

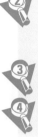

(1) Ventilation and perfusion must be matched on the alveolar-capillary level for optimal gas exchange.

(2) Ventilation-perfusion ratios close to 1.0 result in alveolar P_{O_2}s of approximately 100 mm Hg and P_{CO_2}s close to 40 mm Hg; ventilation-perfusion ratios greater than 1.0 increase the P_{O_2} and decrease the P_{CO_2}; ventilation-perfusion ratios less than 1.0 decrease the P_{O_2} and increase the P_{CO_2}.

(3) **Alveolar dead space** and **intrapulmonary shunt** represent the two extremes of ventilation-perfusion ratios, infinite and zero, respectively.

(4) The ventilation-perfusion ratios in lower regions of the normal upright lung are lower than 1.0, resulting in lower P_{O_2}s and higher P_{CO_2}s; the ventilation-perfusion ratios in upper parts of the lung are greater than 1.0, resulting in higher P_{O_2}s and lower P_{CO_2}s; nonetheless, there is normally more gas exchange in lower regions of the lung because they receive more blood flow.

CLINICAL PROBLEMS

5–1. An otherwise normal person is brought to the emergency department after having accidentally aspirated a foreign body into the right main-stem bronchus, partially occluding it. Which of the following is/are likely to occur?

   a. The right lung's $P_{A_{O_2}}$ will be lower and its $P_{A_{CO_2}}$ will be higher than those of the left lung.

   b. The calculated shunt fraction, $\dot{Q}s/\dot{Q}t$, will increase.

   c. Blood flow to the right lung will decrease.

   d. The arterial P_{O_2} will fall.

   e. All of the above are correct.

5–2. A normal person lies down on her right side and breathes normally. Her right lung, in comparison to her left lung, will be expected to have a

   a. Lower $P_{A_{O_2}}$ and a higher $P_{A_{CO_2}}$

   b. Higher blood flow per unit volume

   c. Greater ventilation per unit volume

   d. Higher ventilation-perfusion ratio

   e. Larger alveoli

SUGGESTED READINGS

Bouhuys A, Jonsson R, Lichtneckert S, et al. Effects of histamine on pulmonary ventilation in man. *Clin Sci.* 1960;19:79–94.

Comroe JH. *Physiology of Respiration.* 2nd ed. Chicago, Ill: Year Book; 1974:168–182.

Marshall BE, Wyche MQ Jr. Hypoxemia during and after anesthesia. *Anesthesiology.* 1972;37:178–209.

Nunn JF. *Nunn's Applied Respiratory Physiology.* 4th ed. Oxford: Butterworth-Heinemann; 1993:156–197.

Roca J, Wagner PD. Principles and information content of the multiple inert gas elimination technique. *Thorax.* 1993;49:815–824.

Wagner PD, Laravuso RB, Uhl RR, West JB. Continuous distributions of ventilation-perfusion ratios in normal subjects breathing air and 100% O_2. *J Clin Invest.* 1974;54:54–58.

West JB. *Ventilation/Blood Flow and Gas Exchange.* 3rd ed. Oxford: Blackwell; 1977:33–52.

West JB. *Ventilation/Blood Flow and Gas Exchange.* 5th ed. Oxford: Blackwell; 1990:29–49, 80–109.

West JB. *Respiratory Physiology—The Essentials.* 5th ed. Baltimore, Md: Lippincott Williams & Wilkins; 1995:51–69.

Diffusion of Gases

6

OBJECTIVES

The reader understands the diffusion of gases in the lung.

▶ *Defines diffusion, and distinguishes it from "bulk flow."*

▶ *States Fick's law for diffusion.*

▶ *Distinguishes between perfusion limitation and diffusion limitation of gas transfer in the lung.*

▶ *Describes the diffusion of oxygen from the alveoli into the blood.*

▶ *Describes the diffusion of carbon dioxide from the blood to the alveoli.*

▶ *Defines the diffusing capacity and discusses its measurement.*

Diffusion of a gas occurs when there is a net movement of molecules from an area in which *that particular gas* exerts a high partial pressure to an area in which it exerts a lower partial pressure. Movement of a gas by diffusion is therefore different from the movement of gases through the conducting airways, which occurs by "bulk flow" (mass movement or convection). During bulk flow, gas movement results from differences in *total* pressure, and molecules of different gases move together along the total pressure gradient. During diffusion, different gases each move according to their own individual partial pressure gradients. Gas transfer during diffusion occurs by random molecular movement. It is therefore dependent on temperature because molecular movement increases at higher temperatures. Gases move in both directions during diffusion, but the area of higher partial pressure, because of its greater number of molecules per unit volume, has proportionately more random "departures." Thus, the *net* movement of gas is dependent on the partial pressure difference between the two areas. In a static situation, diffusion continues until no partial pressure differences exist for any gases in the two areas; in the lungs, oxygen and carbon dioxide continuously enter and leave the alveoli, and so such an equilibrium does not take place.

FICK'S LAW FOR DIFFUSION

Oxygen is brought into the alveoli by bulk flow through the conducting airways. When air flows through the conducting airways during inspiration, the linear velocity of the bulk flow decreases as the air approaches the alveoli. This is because the total cross-sectional area increases dramatically in the distal portions of the tracheobronchial tree, as was seen in Figure 1–5. By the time the air reaches the alveoli, bulk flow probably ceases, and further gas movement occurs by diffusion. Oxygen then moves through the gas phase in the alveoli according to its own partial pressure gradient. The distance from the alveolar duct to the alveolar-capillary interface is usually less than 1 mm. Diffusion in the alveolar gas phase is believed to be greatly assisted by the pulsations of the heart and blood flow, which are transmitted to the alveoli and increase molecular motion.

Oxygen then diffuses through the alveolar-capillary interface. It must first, therefore, move from the gas phase to the liquid phase, according to *Henry's law*, which states that the amount of a gas absorbed by a liquid with which it does not combine chemically is directly proportional to the partial pressure of the gas to which the liquid is exposed and the solubility of the gas in the liquid. Oxygen must dissolve in and diffuse through the thin layer of pulmonary surfactant, the alveolar epithelium, the interstitium, and the capillary endothelium, as was shown in Figure 1–4 (step 2, near the arrow). It must then diffuse through the plasma (step 3), where some remains dissolved and the majority enters the erythrocyte and combines with hemoglobin (step 4). The blood then carries the oxygen out of the lung by bulk flow and distributes it to the other tissues of the body, as was shown in Figure 1–1. At the tissues, oxygen diffuses from the erythrocyte through the plasma, capillary endothelium, interstitium, tissue cell membrane, and cell interior and into the mitochondrial membrane. The process is almost entirely reversed for carbon dioxide, as shown in Figure 1–1.

The factors that determine the rate of diffusion of gas through the alveolar-capillary barrier are described by *Fick's law for diffusion*, shown here in a simplified form:

$$\dot{V}_{gas} = \frac{A \times D \times (P_1 - P_2)}{T}$$

where $\dot{V}_{gas}$ = volume of gas diffusing through the tissue barrier per time, mL/min

A = surface area of the barrier available for diffusion

D = diffusion coefficient, or diffusivity, of the particular gas in the barrier

T = thickness of the barrier or the diffusion distance

$P_1 - P_2$ = partial pressure difference of the gas across the barrier

That is, the volume of gas per unit of time moving across the alveolar-capillary barrier is directly proportional to the area of the barrier, the diffusivity, and the difference in concentration between the two sides, but is inversely proportional to the barrier thickness.

The surface area of the blood-gas barrier is believed to be at least 70 m^2 in a healthy average-sized adult at rest. That is, about 70 m^2 of the *potential* surface area is both ventilated and perfused at rest. If more capillaries are recruited, as in exercise, the surface area available for diffusion increases; if venous return falls, for example, because of hemorrhage, or if alveolar pressure is raised by positive-pressure ventilation, then capillaries may be derecruited and the surface area available for diffusion may decrease.

The thickness of the alveolar-capillary diffusion barrier is only about 0.2 to 0.5 μm. This barrier thickness can increase in interstitial fibrosis or interstitial edema, thus interfering with diffusion. Diffusion probably increases at higher lung volumes because as alveoli are stretched, the diffusion distance decreases slightly (and also because small airways subject to closure may be open at higher lung volumes).

The diffusivity, or diffusion constant, for a gas is directly proportional to the solubility of the gas in the diffusion barrier and is inversely proportional to the square root of the molecular weight (MW) of the gas:

$$D \propto \frac{\text{solubility}}{\sqrt{MW}}$$

The relationship between solubility and diffusion through the barrier has already been discussed. The diffusivity is inversely proportional to the square root of the molecular weight of the gas because different gases with equal numbers of molecules in equal volumes have the same molecular energy if they are at the same temperature. Therefore, light molecules travel faster, have more frequent collisions, and diffuse more rapidly. Thus, *Graham's law* states that the relative rates of diffusion of two gases are inversely proportional to the square roots of their molecular weights, if all else is equal.

For the two gases of greatest interest in the lung,

$$\frac{\sqrt{MW \text{ of } O_2}}{\sqrt{MW \text{ of } CO_2}} = 0.85$$

Because the relative diffusion rates are *inversely* proportional to the ratio of the square roots of their molecular weights,

$$\frac{\text{Diffusion rate for } O_2}{\text{Diffusion rate for } CO_2} \propto \frac{1}{0.85} = 1.17$$

That is, because oxygen is less dense than carbon dioxide, it should diffuse 1.2 times as fast as carbon dioxide (which it does as it moves through the alveoli). In the alveolar-capillary barrier, however, the relative solubilities of oxygen and carbon dioxide must also be considered. The solubility of carbon dioxide in the liquid phase is about 24 times that of oxygen, and so carbon dioxide diffuses about 0.85 × 24, or about *20 times,* more rapidly through the alveolar-capillary barrier than does oxygen. For this reason, patients develop problems in oxygen diffusion through the alveolar-capillary barrier before carbon dioxide retention due to diffusion impairment occurs.

LIMITATIONS OF GAS TRANSFER

The factors that limit the movement of a gas through the alveolar-capillary barrier, as described by Fick's law for diffusion, can be arbitrarily divided into three components: the diffusion coefficient, the surface area and thickness of the alveolar-capillary membrane, and the partial pressure gradient across the barrier for each particular gas. The diffusion coefficient, as discussed in the previous section, is dependent on the physical properties of the gases and the alveolar-capillary membrane. The surface area and thickness of the membrane are physical properties of the barrier, but they can be altered by changes in the pulmonary capillary blood volume, the cardiac output or the pulmonary artery pressure, or by changes in lung volume. The partial pressure gradient of a gas (across the barrier) is the final major determinant of its rate of diffusion. The partial pressure of a gas in the *mixed venous blood* and in the *pulmonary capillaries* is just as important a factor as its *alveolar* partial pressure in determining its rate of diffusion. This will be demonstrated in the next section.

Diffusion Limitation

An erythrocyte and its attendant plasma spend an average of about 0.75 to 1.2 seconds inside the pulmonary capillaries at resting cardiac outputs. This time can be estimated by dividing the pulmonary capillary blood volume by the pulmonary blood flow (expressed in milliliters per second). Some erythrocytes may take less time to traverse the pulmonary capillaries; others may take longer. Figure 6–1 shows schematically the calculated change with time in the partial pressures in the blood of three gases: oxygen, carbon monoxide, and nitrous oxide. These are shown in comparison to the alveolar partial pressures for each gas, as indicated by the dotted line. This alveolar partial pressure is different for each of the three gases, and it depends on its concentration in the inspired gas mixture and on how rapidly it is removed by the pulmonary capillary blood. The schematic is drawn as though all three gases were administered simultaneously, but this is not necessarily the case. Consider each gas as though it were acting independently of the others.

The partial pressure of carbon monoxide in the pulmonary capillary blood rises very slowly compared with that of the other two gases in the figure. (Obviously, a low inspired concentration of carbon monoxide must be used for a very short time in such an experiment.) Nevertheless, if the *content* of carbon monoxide (in milliliters of carbon monoxide per milliliter of blood) were measured simultaneously, it would be rising very rapidly. The reason for this rapid rise is that carbon monoxide combines chemically with the hemoglobin in the erythrocytes. Indeed, the affinity of carbon monoxide for hemoglobin is about 210 times that of oxygen for hemoglobin. The carbon monoxide that is chemically combined with hemoglobin does not contribute to the partial pressure of carbon monoxide in the blood because it is no longer *physically dissolved* in it. Therefore, the partial pressure of

carbon monoxide in the pulmonary capillary blood does not come close to the partial pressure of carbon monoxide in the alveoli during the time that the blood is exposed to the alveolar carbon monoxide. The partial pressure

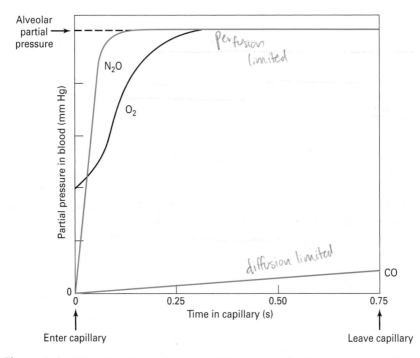

Figure 6–1. Calculated changes in the partial pressures of carbon monoxide, nitrous oxide, and oxygen in the blood as it passes through a functional pulmonary capillary. There are no units on the ordinate because the scale is different for each of the three gases, depending on the alveolar partial pressure of each gas. The abscissa is in seconds, indicating the time the blood has spent in the capillary. At resting cardiac outputs, blood spends an average of 0.75 of a second in a pulmonary capillary. The alveolar partial pressure of each gas is indicated by the dotted line. Note that the partial pressures of nitrous oxide and oxygen equilibrate rapidly with their alveolar partial pressure. (Reproduced with permission from Comroe, 1962.)

gradient across the alveolar-capillary barrier for carbon monoxide is thus well maintained for the entire time the blood spends in the pulmonary capillary, and the diffusion of carbon monoxide is limited only by its diffusivity in the barrier and by the surface area and thickness of the barrier. Carbon monoxide transfer from the alveolus to the pulmonary capillary blood is referred to as *diffusion-limited* rather than *perfusion-limited*.

Perfusion Limitation

The partial pressure of nitrous oxide in the pulmonary capillary blood equilibrates very rapidly with the partial pressure of nitrous oxide in the alveolus because nitrous oxide moves through the alveolar-capillary barrier very easily and because it does not combine chemically with the hemoglobin in the erythrocytes. After only about 0.1 of a second of exposure of the pulmonary capillary blood to the alveolar nitrous oxide, the partial pressure gradient across the alveolar-capillary barrier has been abolished. From this point on, no further nitrous oxide transfer occurs from the alveolus to that portion of the blood in the capillary that has already equilibrated with the alveolar nitrous oxide partial pressure; during the last 0.6 to 0.7 of a second, no net diffusion occurs between the alveolus and the blood as it travels through the pulmonary capillary. Of course, blood just entering the capillary at the arterial end will not be equilibrated with the alveolar partial pressure of nitrous oxide, and so nitrous oxide can diffuse into the blood at the arterial end. The transfer of nitrous oxide is therefore *perfusion-limited.* Nitrous oxide transfer from a particular alveolus to one of its pulmonary capillaries can be increased by increasing the cardiac output and thus reducing the amount of time the blood stays in the pulmonary capillary after equilibration with the alveolar partial pressure of nitrous oxide has occurred. (Because increasing the cardiac output may recruit previously unperfused capillaries, the *total* diffusion of both carbon monoxide and nitrous oxide may increase as the surface area for diffusion increases.)

DIFFUSION OF OXYGEN

As can be seen in Figure 6–1, the time course for oxygen transfer falls between those for carbon monoxide and nitrous oxide. The partial pressure of oxygen rises fairly rapidly (note that it starts at the P_{O_2} of the mixed venous blood, about 40 mm Hg, rather than at zero), and equilibration with the alveolar P_{O_2} of about 100 mm Hg occurs within about 0.25 of a second, or about one third of the time the blood is in the pulmonary capillary at normal resting cardiac outputs. Oxygen moves easily through the alveolar-capillary barrier and into the erythrocytes, where it combines chemically with hemoglobin. The partial pressure of oxygen rises more rapidly than the partial pressure of carbon monoxide. Nonetheless, the oxygen chemically bound to hemoglobin (and therefore no longer physically dissolved) exerts no partial pressure, and so the partial pressure gradient across the alveolar-capillary membrane is initially well maintained and oxygen transfer occurs. The chemical combination of oxygen and hemoglobin, however, occurs rapidly (within hundredths of a second), and at the normal alveolar partial pressure of oxygen, the hemoglobin becomes nearly saturated with oxygen very quickly, as will be discussed in the next chapter. As this happens, the partial pressure of oxygen in the blood rises rapidly to that in the alveolus, and from that point, no further oxygen transfer from the alveolus to the equilibrated blood can occur. Therefore, under the conditions of normal alveolar P_{O_2} and a normal resting cardiac output, oxygen transfer from alveolus to pulmonary capillary is *perfusion-limited.*

Figure 6–2A shows similar graphs of calculated changes in the partial pressure of oxygen in the blood as it moves through a pulmonary capillary. The alveolar P_{O_2}

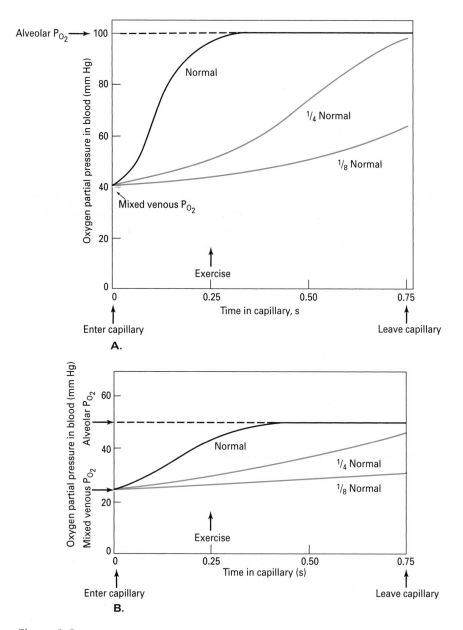

Figure 6–2. Calculated changes in the partial pressure of oxygen as blood passes through a pulmonary capillary. Upper panel shows the patterns with a normal alveolar P_{O_2} of about 100 mm Hg and normal and abnormal diffusion through the alveolar-capillary barrier. Lower panel shows the patterns with low alveolar P_{O_2} and normal and abnormal diffusion through the alveolar-capillary barrier. Alveolar P_{O_2} is indicated by the dotted line. (Reproduced with permission from Wagner, 1972, and West JB, Respiratory Physiology—The Essentials, 4th ed. Philadelphia, Pa: Lippincott Williams & Wilkins; 1990.)

is normal. During exercise, blood moves through the pulmonary capillary much more rapidly than it does at resting cardiac outputs. In fact, the blood may stay in the "functional" pulmonary capillary an average of only about 0.25 of a second during severe exercise, as indicated on the graph. Oxygen transfer into the blood per time will be greatly increased because there is little or no perfusion limitation of oxygen transfer. (Indeed, that part of the blood that stays in the capillary *less* than the average may be subjected to diffusion limitation of oxygen transfer.) Of course, *total* oxygen transfer is also increased during exercise because of recruitment of previously unperfused capillaries, which increases the surface area for diffusion, and because of better matching of ventilation and perfusion. A person with an abnormal alveolar-capillary barrier due to a fibrotic thickening or interstitial edema may approach diffusion limitation of oxygen transfer at rest and may have a serious diffusion limitation of oxygen transfer during strenuous exercise, as can be seen in the middle curve in Figure 6–2A. A person with an extremely abnormal alveolar-capillary barrier might have diffusion limitation of oxygen transfer even at rest, as seen at right in the figure.

The effect of a low alveolar partial pressure of oxygen on oxygen transfer from the alveolus to the capillary is seen in Figure 6–2B. The low alveolar P_{O_2} sets the upper limit for the end-capillary blood P_{O_2}. Because the oxygen content of the arterial blood is decreased, the mixed venous P_{O_2} is also depressed. The even greater decrease in the alveolar partial pressure of oxygen, however, causes a decreased alveolar-capillary partial pressure gradient, and the blood P_{O_2} takes longer to equilibrate with the alveolar P_{O_2}. For this reason, a normal person exerting himself or herself at high altitude might be subject to diffusion limitation of oxygen transfer.

DIFFUSION OF CARBON DIOXIDE

The time course of carbon dioxide transfer from the pulmonary capillary blood to the alveolus is shown in Figure 6–3. In a normal person with a mixed venous partial pressure of carbon dioxide of 45 mm Hg and an alveolar partial pressure of carbon dioxide of 40 mm Hg, an equilibrium is reached in about 0.25 of a second, or about the same time as that for oxygen. This fact may seem surprising, considering that the diffusivity of carbon dioxide is about 20 times that of oxygen, but the partial pressure gradient is normally only about 5 mm Hg for carbon dioxide, whereas it is about 60 mm Hg for oxygen. Carbon dioxide transfer is therefore normally *perfusion-limited*, although it may be diffusion-limited in a person with an abnormal alveolar-capillary barrier, as shown in the figure.

MEASUREMENT OF DIFFUSING CAPACITY

It is often useful to determine the diffusion characteristics of a patient's lungs during their assessment in the pulmonary function laboratory. It may be particularly

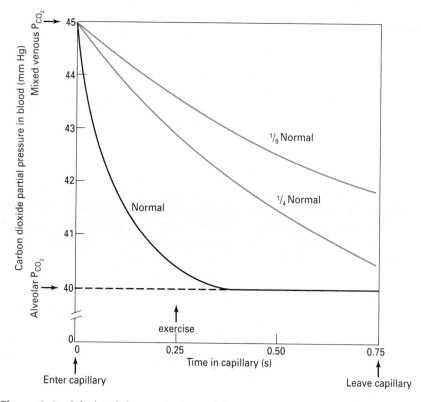

Figure 6–3. Calculated changes in the partial pressure of carbon dioxide as blood passes through a pulmonary capillary. The mixed venous P_{CO_2} is about 45 mm Hg. The alveolar P_{CO_2} is indicated by the dotted line. Patterns for normal and abnormal diffusion through the alveolar-capillary barrier are shown. Note that the partial pressure of CO_2 in the pulmonary capillary blood normally equilibrates rapidly with the alveolar P_{CO_2}. (Reproduced with permission from Wagner, 1972.)

important to determine whether an apparent impairment in diffusion is a result of *perfusion limitation* or *diffusion limitation*.

The *diffusing capacity* (or *transfer factor*) is the rate at which oxygen or carbon monoxide is absorbed from the alveolar gas into the pulmonary capillaries (in milliliters per minute) per unit of partial pressure gradient (in millimeters of mercury). The diffusing capacity of the lung (for gas x), D_{L_x}, is therefore equal to the uptake of gas x, $\dot{V}_x$, divided by the difference between the alveolar partial pressure of gas x, PA_x, and the mean capillary partial pressure of gas x, $P\bar{c}_x$:

$$D_{L_x} = \frac{\dot{V}_x}{PA_x - P\bar{c}_x} \text{ mL/min/mm Hg}$$

This is really just a rearrangement of the Fick equation given at the beginning of this chapter. The terms for area, diffusivity, and thickness have been combined into D_{L_x} and the equation has been rearranged:

$$\dot{V}_x = \frac{A \times D \times (P_1 - P_2)}{T}$$

$$\frac{\dot{V}_x}{P_1 - P_2} = \frac{A \times D}{T}$$

$$D_{L_x} = \frac{\dot{V}_x}{P_1 - P_2}$$

The mean partial pressure of oxygen or carbon monoxide is, as already discussed, affected by their chemical reactions with hemoglobin, as well as by their transfer through the alveolar-capillary barrier. For this reason, the diffusing capacity of the lung is determined by both the diffusing capacity of the membrane, D_M, and the reaction with hemoglobin, expressed as $\theta \times V_C$, where θ is the volume of gas in milliliters per minute taken up by the erythrocytes in 1 mL of blood per millimeter of mercury partial pressure gradient between the plasma and the erythrocyte and V_C is the capillary blood volume in milliliters. (The units of $\theta \times V_C$ are therefore mL/min/mm Hg.) The diffusing capacity of the lung, D_L, can be shown to be related to D_M and $\theta \times V_C$ as follows:

$$\frac{1}{D_L} = \frac{1}{D_M} + \frac{1}{\theta \times V_C} \left(+ \frac{1}{D_A} \right)$$

D_A, or diffusion through the alveolus, is normally very rapid and usually can be disregarded.

Carbon monoxide is most frequently used in determinations of the diffusing capacity because the mean pulmonary capillary partial pressure of carbon monoxide is virtually zero when nonlethal alveolar partial pressures of carbon monoxide are used:

$$D_{L_{CO}} = \frac{\dot{V}_{CO}}{P_{A_{CO}} - P\bar{c}_{CO}}$$

$$\text{but } P\bar{c}_{CO} \simeq 0$$

$$\text{and so } D_{L_{CO}} = \frac{\dot{V}_{CO}}{P_{A_{CO}}}$$

Several different methods are used clinically to measure the carbon monoxide diffusing capacity and involve both single-breath and steady-state techniques, sometimes during exercise. The $D_{L_{CO}}$ is decreased in diseases associated with interstitial or alveolar fibrosis, such as sarcoidosis, scleroderma, and asbestosis, or with conditions causing interstitial or alveolar pulmonary edema, as indicated in

Table 6–1. It is also decreased in conditions causing a decrease in the surface area available for diffusion, such as emphysema, tumors, a low cardiac output, or a low pulmonary capillary blood volume, as well as in conditions leading to ventilation-perfusion mismatch, which effectively decreases the surface area available for diffusion.

Table 6–1. Conditions That Decrease the Diffusing Capacity

Thickening of the barrier
  Interstitial or alveolar edema
  Interstitial or alveolar fibrosis
    Sarcoidosis
    Scleroderma
Decreased surface area
  Emphysema
  Tumors
  Low cardiac output
  Low pulmonary capillary blood volume
Decreased uptake by erythrocytes
  Anemia
  Low pulmonary capillary blood volume
Ventilation-perfusion mismatch

KEY CONCEPTS

The volume of gas per unit of time moving across the alveolar-capillary barrier is directly proportional to the area of the barrier, the diffusivity of the gas in the barrier, and the difference in concentration of the gas between the two sides of the barrier, but is inversely proportional to the barrier thickness.

*If the partial pressure of a gas in the plasma equilibrates with the alveolar partial pressure of the gas within the amount of time the blood is in the pulmonary capillary, its transfer is **perfusion limited**; if equilibration does not occur within the time the blood is in the capillary, its transfer is **diffusion limited**.*

CLINICAL PROBLEMS

6–1. *How would each of the following conditions or circumstances be expected to affect the diffusing capacity (D_L) of the lungs? Explain your answers.*

    a. Changing from the supine to the upright position

    b. Exercise

    c. Valsalva maneuver

    d. Anemia

e. Low cardiac output due to blood loss

f. Diffuse interstitial fibrosis of the lungs

g. Emphysema

6–2. If the pulmonary capillary partial pressure of a gas equilibrates with that in the alveolus before the blood leaves the capillary (assume the gas is diffusing from the alveolus to the pulmonary capillary):

a. its transfer is said to be perfusion limited.

b. its transfer is said to be diffusion limited.

c. increasing the cardiac output will not increase the amount of the gas diffusing across the alveolar-capillary barrier.

d. increasing the alveolar partial pressure of the gas will not increase the amount of the gas diffusing across the alveolar-capillary barrier.

e. recruiting additional pulmonary capillaries will not increase the amount of the gas diffusing across the alveolar capillary barrier.

SUGGESTED READINGS

Comroe JH, Forster RE II, DuBois AB, Briscoe WA, Carlsen E. *The Lung*. 2nd ed. Chicago, Ill: Year Book; 1962:111–139.

Forster RE II, Dubois AB, Briscoe WA, Fisher AB. *The Lung: Physiologic Basis of Pulmonary Function Tests*. 3rd ed. Chicago, Ill: Year Book; 1986:190–222.

Maeda N, Shiga T. Velocity of oxygen transfer and erythrocyte rheology. *News Physiol Sci*. 1994;9:22–27.

Wagner PD, West JB. Effects of diffusion impairment on O_2 and CO_2 time courses in pulmonary capillaries. *J Appl Physiol*. 1972;33:62–71.

West JB. *Respiratory Physiology—The Essentials*. 6th ed. Baltimore, Md: Lippincott Williams & Wilkins; 2000:21–28.

The Transport of Oxygen & Carbon Dioxide in the Blood

7

OBJECTIVES

The reader understands how oxygen and carbon dioxide are transported to and from the tissues in the blood.

▶ States the relationship between the partial pressure of oxygen in the blood and the amount of oxygen physically dissolved in the blood.

▶ Describes the chemical combination of oxygen with hemoglobin and the "oxyhemoglobin dissociation curve."

▶ Defines hemoglobin saturation, the oxygen-carrying capacity, and the oxygen content of blood.

▶ States the physiologic consequences of the shape of the oxyhemoglobin dissociation curve.

▶ Lists the physiologic factors that can influence the oxyhemoglobin dissociation curve, and predicts their effects on oxygen transport by the blood.

▶ States the relationship between the partial pressure of carbon dioxide in the blood and the amount of carbon dioxide physically dissolved in the blood.

▶ Describes the transport of carbon dioxide as carbamino compounds with blood proteins.

▶ Explains how most of the carbon dioxide in the blood is transported as bicarbonate.

▶ Describes the carbon dioxide dissociation curve for whole blood.

▶ Explains the Bohr and Haldane effects.

The final step in the exchange of gases between the external environment and the tissues is the transport of oxygen and carbon dioxide to and from the lung by the blood. Oxygen is carried both physically dissolved in the blood and chemically combined to hemoglobin. Carbon dioxide is carried physically dissolved in the blood, chemically combined to blood proteins as carbamino compounds, and as bicarbonate.

TRANSPORT OF OXYGEN BY THE BLOOD

Oxygen is transported both physically dissolved in blood and chemically combined to the hemoglobin in the erythrocytes. Much more oxygen is normally transported combined with hemoglobin than is physically

142

dissolved in the blood. Without hemoglobin, the cardiovascular system could not supply sufficient oxygen to meet tissue demands.

Physically Dissolved

At a temperature of 37°C, 1 mL of plasma contains 0.00003 mL O_2/mm Hg P_{O_2}. This corresponds to Henry's law, as discussed in Chapter 6. Whole blood contains a similar amount of dissolved oxygen per milliliter because oxygen dissolves in the fluid of the erythrocytes in about the same amount. Therefore, normal arterial blood with a P_{O_2} of approximately 100 mm Hg contains only about 0.003 mL O_2/mL of blood, or 0.3 mL O_2/100 mL of blood. (Blood oxygen content is conventionally expressed in milliliters of oxygen per 100 mL of blood, or *volumes percent.*)

A few simple calculations can demonstrate that the oxygen physically dissolved in the blood is not sufficient to fulfill the body's oxygen demand (at normal $F_{I_{O_2}}$ and barometric pressure). The resting oxygen consumption of an adult is approximately 250 to 300 mL O_2/min. If the tissues were able to remove the entire 0.3 mL O_2/100 mL of blood flow they receive, the cardiac output would have to be about 83.3 L/min to meet the tissue demand for oxygen at rest:

$$\frac{250 \text{ mL } O_2}{\text{min}} \div \frac{0.3 \text{ mL } O_2}{100 \text{ mL blood}} = \frac{83.333 \text{ mL}}{\text{min}} = \frac{83.3 \text{ L}}{\text{min}}$$

During severe exercise, the oxygen demand can increase as much as 16-fold to 4 L/min or more. Under such conditions, the cardiac output would have to be greater than 1000 L/min if physically dissolved oxygen were to supply all the oxygen required by the tissues. The maximum cardiac outputs attainable by normal adults during severe exercise are in the range of 25 L/min. Clearly, the *physically dissolved* oxygen in the blood cannot meet the metabolic demand for oxygen, even at rest.

Chemically Combined with Hemoglobin

THE STRUCTURE OF HEMOGLOBIN

Hemoglobin is a complex molecule with a molecular weight of about 64,500. The protein portion (globin) has a tetrameric structure consisting of four linked polypeptide chains, each of which is attached to a protoporphyrin (heme) group. Each heme group consists of four symmetrically arranged pyrroles with a ferrous (Fe^{2+}) iron atom at its center. The iron atom is bound to each of the pyrrole groups and to one of the four polypeptide chains. A sixth binding site on the ferrous iron atom is freely available to bind with oxygen (or carbon monoxide). Therefore *each* of the four polypeptide chains can bind a molecule of oxygen (or carbon monoxide) to the iron atom in its own heme group, and so the tetrameric hemoglobin molecule can combine chemically with four oxygen molecules (or eight oxygen atoms). Both the globin component and the heme component (with its iron atom in the ferrous state), in their proper spatial orientation to each other, are necessary for the chemical reaction with oxygen to take place—neither heme nor globin alone will combine with oxygen. Each of the tetrameric hemoglobin subunits can combine with oxygen by itself (see Figure 7–4C).

Variations in the amino acid sequences of the four globin subunits may have important physiologic consequences. Normal adult hemoglobin (HbA) consists of two alpha (α) chains, each of which has 141 amino acids, and two beta (β) chains, each of which has 146 amino acids. Fetal hemoglobin (HbF), which consists of two α chains and two gamma (γ) chains, has a higher affinity for oxygen than does adult hemoglobin. Synthesis of β chains normally begins about 6 weeks before birth, and HbA usually replaces almost all the HbF by the time an infant is 4 months old. Other, *abnormal* hemoglobin molecules may be produced by genetic substitution of a single amino acid for the normal one in an α or β chain or (rarely) by alterations in the structure of heme groups. These alterations may produce changes in the affinity of the hemoglobin for oxygen, change the physical properties of hemoglobin, or alter the interaction of hemoglobin and other substances that affect its combination with oxygen, such as 2,3-bisphosphoglycerate (2,3-BPG) (discussed later in this chapter). More than 120 abnormal variants of normal adult hemoglobin have been demonstrated in patients. The best known of these, hemoglobin S, is present in sickle cell disease. Hemoglobin S tends to polymerize and crystallize in the cytosol of the erythrocyte when it is not combined with oxygen. This polymerization and crystallization decreases the solubility of hemoglobin S within the erythrocyte and changes the shape of the cell from the normal biconcave disk to a crescent or "sickle" shape. A sickled cell is more fragile than a normal cell. In addition, the cells have a tendency to stick to one another, which increases blood viscosity and also favors thrombosis or blockage of blood vessels.

Chemical Reaction of Oxygen & Hemoglobin

Hemoglobin rapidly combines *reversibly* with oxygen. It is the reversibility of the reaction that allows oxygen to be released to the tissues; if the reaction did not proceed easily in both directions, hemoglobin would be of little use in delivering oxygen to satisfy metabolic needs. The reaction is very fast, with a half-time of 0.01 of a second or less. Each gram of hemoglobin is capable of combining with about 1.39 mL of oxygen under optimal conditions, but under normal circumstances some hemoglobin exists in forms such as methemoglobin (in which the iron atom is in the ferric state) or is combined with carbon monoxide, in which case the hemoglobin cannot bind oxygen. For this reason, the oxygen-carrying *capacity* of hemoglobin is conventionally considered to be 1.34 mL O_2/g Hb. That is, each gram of hemoglobin, when *fully saturated* with oxygen, binds 1.34 mL of oxygen. Therefore, a person with 15 g Hb/100 mL of blood has an oxygen-carrying capacity of 20.1 mL O_2/100 mL of blood:

$$\frac{15 \text{ g Hb}}{100 \text{ mL blood}} \times \frac{1.34 \text{ mL } O_2}{\text{g Hb}} = \frac{20.1 \text{ mL } O_2}{100 \text{ mL blood}}$$

The reaction of hemoglobin and oxygen is conventionally written

$$Hb + O_2 \rightleftharpoons HbO_2$$
Deoxyhemoglobin   Oxyhemoglobin

HEMOGLOBIN & THE PHYSIOLOGIC IMPLICATIONS OF THE OXYHEMOGLOBIN DISSOCIATION CURVE

The equilibrium point of the reversible reaction of hemoglobin and oxygen is, of course, dependent on how much oxygen the hemoglobin in blood is exposed to. This corresponds directly to the partial pressure of oxygen in the plasma under the conditions in the body. Thus, the P_{O_2} of the plasma *determines* the amount of oxygen that binds to the hemoglobin in the erythrocytes.

The Oxyhemoglobin Dissociation Curve

One way to express the proportion of hemoglobin that is bound to oxygen is as *percent saturation.* This is equal to the content of oxygen in the blood (minus that part physically dissolved) divided by the oxygen-carrying capacity of the hemoglobin in the blood times 100%:

$$\% \text{ Hb saturation} = \frac{O_2 \text{ bound to Hb}}{O_2 \text{ capacity of Hb}} \times 100\%$$

Note that the oxygen-carrying *capacity* of an individual depends on the amount of hemoglobin in that person's blood. The blood oxygen *content* also depends on the amount of hemoglobin present (as well as on the P_{O_2}). Both content and capacity are expressed as milliliters of oxygen per 100 mL of blood. On the other hand, the percent hemoglobin saturation expresses only a percentage and not an amount or volume of oxygen. Therefore, "percent saturation" is not interchangeable with "oxygen content." For example, two patients might have the same percent of hemoglobin saturation, but if one has a lower blood hemoglobin concentration because of anemia, he or she will have a lower blood oxygen content.

The relationship between the P_{O_2} of the plasma and the percent of hemoglobin saturation is demonstrated graphically as the *oxyhemoglobin dissociation curve.* An oxyhemoglobin dissociation curve for normal blood is shown in Figure 7–1.

The oxyhemoglobin dissociation curve is really a plot of how the availability of one of the reactants, oxygen (expressed as the P_{O_2} of the plasma), affects the reversible chemical reaction of oxygen and hemoglobin. The product, oxyhemoglobin, is expressed as percent saturation—really a percentage of the maximum for any given amount of hemoglobin.

As can be seen in Figure 7–1, the relationship between P_{O_2} and HbO_2 is not linear; it is an S-shaped curve, steep at the lower P_{O_2}s and nearly flat when the P_{O_2} is above 70 mm Hg. It is this S shape that is responsible for several very important physiologic properties of the reaction of oxygen and hemoglobin. The reason that the curve is S-shaped and not linear is that it is actually a plot of four reactions rather than one. That is, each of the four subunits of hemoglobin

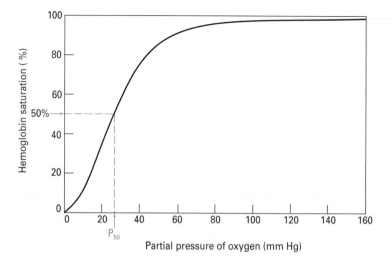

Figure 7–1. A typical "normal" adult oxyhemoglobin dissociation curve for blood at 37°C with a pH of 7.40 and a P_{CO_2} of 40 mm Hg. The P_{50} is the partial pressure of oxygen at which hemoglobin is 50% saturated with oxygen.

can combine with one molecule of oxygen. Indeed, it may be more correct to write the following equation:

$$Hb_4 + 4O_2 \rightleftharpoons Hb_4O_8$$

The reactions of the four subunits of hemoglobin with oxygen do not appear to occur simultaneously. Instead they are believed to occur sequentially in four steps, with an interaction between the subunits occurring in such a way that during the successive combinations of the subunits with oxygen, each combination facilitates the next ("positive cooperativity"). Similarly, dissociation of oxygen from hemoglobin subunits facilitates further dissociations. The dissociation curve for a single monomer of hemoglobin is far different from that for the tetramer (see Figure 7–4C).

As already stated, for hemoglobin to participate in the transport of oxygen from the lungs to the tissues, it must combine with oxygen in the pulmonary capillaries and then release oxygen to the metabolizing tissues in the systemic capillaries. The oxyhemoglobin dissociation curve in Figure 7–1 shows how this is accomplished.

LOADING OXYGEN IN THE LUNG

Mixed venous blood entering the pulmonary capillaries normally has a P_{O_2} of about 40 mm Hg, as discussed in Chapter 5. At a P_{O_2} of 40 mm Hg, hemoglobin is about 75% saturated with oxygen, as seen in Figure 7–1. Assuming a blood hemoglobin concentration of 15 g Hb/100 mL of blood, this corresponds to 15.08 mL O_2/100 mL of blood *bound to hemoglobin* plus an additional 0.12 mL O_2/100 mL of blood *physically dissolved*, or a *total oxygen content* of approximately 15.2 mL O_2/100 mL of blood.

Oxygen-carrying *capacity* is

$$\frac{15 \text{ g Hb}}{100 \text{ mL blood}} \times \frac{1.34 \text{ mL O}_2}{\text{g Hb}} = \frac{20.1 \text{ mL O}_2}{100 \text{ mL blood}}$$

Oxygen *bound to hemoglobin* at a P_{O_2} of 40 mm Hg (37°C, pH 7.4) is

$$\underset{\text{Capacity}}{\frac{20.1 \text{ mL O}_2}{100 \text{ mL blood}}} \times \underset{\text{\% saturation}}{75\%} = \underset{\text{Content}}{\frac{15.08 \text{ mL O}_2}{100 \text{ mL blood}}}$$

Oxygen physically dissolved at a P_{O_2} of 40 mm Hg is

$$\frac{0.003 \text{ mL O}_2}{100 \text{ mL blood} \cdot P_{O_2} \text{ (in mm Hg)}} \times 40 \text{ mm Hg} = \frac{0.12 \text{ mL O}_2}{100 \text{ mL blood}}$$

Total blood oxygen content at a P_{O_2} of 40 mm Hg (37°C, pH 7.4) is

$$\underset{\text{Bound to Hb}}{\frac{15.08 \text{ mL O}_2}{100 \text{ mL blood}}} + \underset{\text{Physically dissolved}}{\frac{0.12 \text{ mL O}_2}{100 \text{ mL blood}}} = \underset{\text{Total}}{\frac{15.2 \text{ mL O}_2}{100 \text{ mL blood}}}$$

As the blood passes through the pulmonary capillaries, it equilibrates with the alveolar P_{O_2} of about 100 mm Hg. At a P_{O_2} of 100 mm Hg, hemoglobin is about 97.4% saturated with oxygen, as seen in Figure 7–1. This corresponds to 19.58 mL O_2/100 mL of *blood bound to hemoglobin* plus 0.3 mL O_2/100 mL of blood *physically dissolved*, or a *total oxygen content* of 19.88 mL O_2/100 mL of blood.

Oxygen *bound to hemoglobin* at a P_{O_2} of 100 mm Hg (37°C, pH 7.4) is

$$\underset{\text{Capacity}}{\frac{20.1 \text{ mL O}_2}{100 \text{ mL blood}}} \times \underset{\text{\% saturation}}{97.4\%} = \underset{\text{Content}}{\frac{19.58 \text{ mL O}_2}{100 \text{ mL blood}}}$$

Oxygen *physically dissolved* at a P_{O_2} of 100 mm Hg is

$$\frac{0.003 \text{ mL O}_2}{100 \text{ mL blood} \cdot P_{O_2} \text{ (in mm Hg)}} \times 100 \text{ mm Hg} = \frac{0.3 \text{ mL O}_2}{100 \text{ mL blood}}$$

Total blood oxygen content at a P_{O_2} of 100 mm Hg (37°C, pH 7.4) is

$$\underset{\text{Bound to Hb}}{\frac{19.58 \text{ mL O}_2}{100 \text{ mL blood}}} + \underset{\text{Physically dissolved}}{\frac{0.3 \text{ mL O}_2}{100 \text{ mL blood}}} = \underset{\text{Total}}{\frac{19.88 \text{ mL O}_2}{100 \text{ mL blood}}}$$

Thus, in passing through the lungs, each 100 mL of blood has loaded (19.88 − 15.20) mL O_2, or 4.68 mL O_2. Assuming a cardiac output of 5 L/min, this means that approximately 234 mL O_2 is loaded into the blood per minute:

$$\frac{5 \text{ L blood}}{\text{min}} \times \frac{46.8 \text{ mL O}_2}{\text{liter blood}} = \frac{234 \text{ mL O}_2}{\text{min}}$$

Note that the oxyhemoglobin dissociation curve is relatively flat when P_{O_2} is greater than approximately 70 mm Hg. This is very important physiologically because it means that there is only a small decrease in the *oxygen content* of blood equilibrated with a P_{O_2} of 70 mm Hg instead of 100 mm Hg. In fact, the curve shows that at a P_{O_2} of 70 mm Hg, hemoglobin is still approximately 94.1% saturated with oxygen. This constitutes an important safety factor because a patient with a relatively low alveolar or arterial P_{O_2} of 70 mm Hg (owing to hypoventilation or intrapulmonary shunting, for example) is still able to load oxygen into the blood with little difficulty. A quick calculation shows that at 70 mm Hg the total blood oxygen content is approximately 19.12 mL O_2/100 mL of blood compared with the 19.88 mL O_2/100 mL of blood at a P_{O_2} of 100 mm Hg. These calculations show that P_{O_2} is often a more sensitive diagnostic indicator of the status of a patient's respiratory system than is the arterial oxygen content. Of course, the oxygen content is more important physiologically to the patient.

It should also be noted that since hemoglobin is approximately 97.4% saturated at a P_{O_2} of 100 mm Hg, raising the alveolar P_{O_2} above 100 mm Hg can combine little additional oxygen with hemoglobin (only about 0.52 mL O_2/100 mL of blood at a hemoglobin concentration of 15 g/100 mL of blood). Hemoglobin is fully saturated with oxygen at a P_{O_2} of about 250 mm Hg.

UNLOADING OXYGEN AT THE TISSUES

As blood passes from the arteries into the systemic capillaries, it is exposed to lower P_{O_2}s, and oxygen is released by the hemoglobin. The P_{O_2} in the capillaries varies from tissue to tissue, being very low in some (e.g., myocardium) and relatively higher in others (e.g., kidney). As can be seen in Figure 7–1, the oxyhemoglobin dissociation curve is very steep in the range of 40 to 10 mm Hg. This means that a small decrease in P_{O_2} can result in a substantial further dissociation of oxygen and hemoglobin, unloading more oxygen for use by the tissues. At a P_{O_2} of 40 mm Hg, hemoglobin is about 75% saturated with oxygen, with a total blood oxygen content of 15.2 mL O_2/100 mL of blood (at 15 g Hb/100 mL of blood). At a P_{O_2} of 20 mm Hg, hemoglobin is only 32% saturated with oxygen. The total blood oxygen content is only 6.49 mL O_2/100 mL of blood, a decrease of 8.71 mL O_2/100 mL of blood for only a 20-mm Hg decrease in P_{O_2}.

The unloading of oxygen at the tissues is also facilitated by other physiologic factors that can *alter the shape and position* of the oxyhemoglobin dissociation curve. These include the pH, P_{CO_2}, temperature of the blood, and concentration of 2,3-BPG in the erythrocytes.

INFLUENCES ON THE OXYHEMOGLOBIN DISSOCIATION CURVE

Figure 7–2 shows the influence of alterations in temperature, pH, P_{CO_2}, and 2,3-BPG on the oxyhemoglobin dissociation curve. High temperature, low pH, high P_{CO_2}, and elevated levels of 2,3-BPG all "shift the oxyhemoglobin dissociation curve to the right." That is, for any particular P_{O_2} there is less oxygen chemically combined with hemoglobin at higher temperatures, lower pHs, higher P_{CO_2}s, and elevated levels of 2,3-BPG.

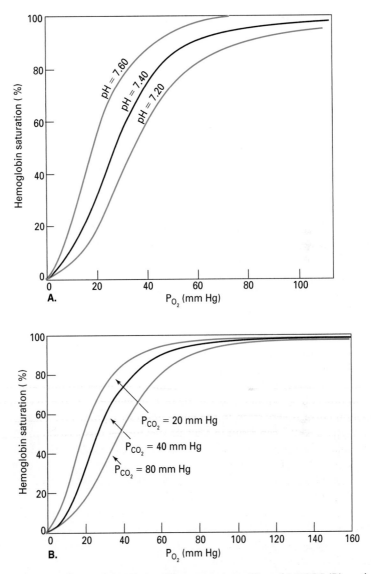

Figure 7–2. The effects of pH (**A**), P_{CO_2} (**B**), temperature (**C**), and 2,3-BPG (**D**) on the oxy-hemoglobin dissociation curve.

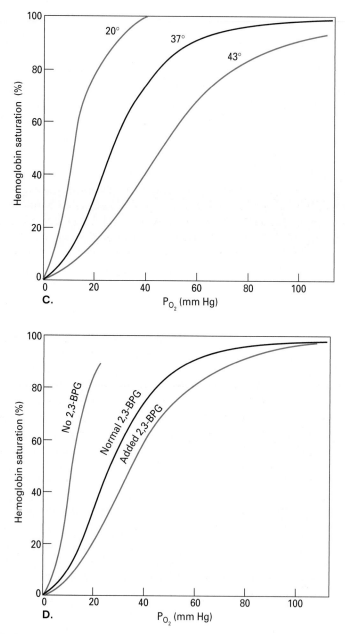

Figure 7–2. (*Continued*)

Effects of pH and P_{CO_2}

The effects of blood pH and P_{CO_2} on the oxyhemoglobin dissociation curve are shown in Figure 7–2A and B. Low pHs and high P_{CO_2}s both shift the curve to the right. High pHs and low P_{CO_2}s both shift the curve to the left. Because high P_{CO_2}s in blood are often associated with low pHs, these two effects often occur together (see below and Chapter 8 for details). The influence of pH (and P_{CO_2}) on the oxyhemoglobin dissociation curve is referred to as the *Bohr effect.* The Bohr effect will be discussed in greater detail at the end of this chapter.

Effects of Temperature

Figure 7–2C shows the effects of blood temperature on the oxyhemoglobin dissociation curve. High temperatures shift the curve to the right; low temperatures shift the curve to the left. At very low blood temperatures, hemoglobin has such a high affinity for oxygen that it does not release the oxygen, even at very low P_{O_2}s. It should also be noted that oxygen is more soluble in water or plasma at lower temperatures than it is at normal body temperature. At 20°C about 50% more oxygen will dissolve in plasma.

Effects of 2,3-BPG

2,3-BPG (also called 2,3-diphosphoglycerate, or 2,3-DPG) is produced by erythrocytes during their normal glycolysis and is present in fairly high concentrations within red blood cells (about 15 mmol/g Hb). 2,3-BPG binds to the hemoglobin in erythrocytes, which decreases the affinity of hemoglobin for oxygen. Higher concentrations of 2,3-BPG therefore shift the oxyhemoglobin dissociation curve to the right, as shown in Figure 7–2D. It has been demonstrated that more 2,3-BPG is produced during chronic hypoxic conditions, thus shifting the dissociation curve to the right and allowing more oxygen to be released from hemoglobin at a particular P_{O_2}. Very low levels of 2,3-BPG shift the curve far to the left, as shown in the figure. This means that blood deficient in 2,3-BPG does not unload much oxygen except at very low P_{O_2}s. It is important to note that blood stored at blood banks for as little as 1 week has been shown to have very low levels of 2,3-BPG. Use of banked blood in patients may result in greatly decreased oxygen unloading to the tissues unless steps are taken to restore the normal levels of 2,3-BPG. In summary, 2,3-BPG is an important regulating mechanism in the release of oxygen by hemoglobin. Without its presence, hemoglobin's high affinity for oxygen would impair the oxygen supply of the tissues.

Physiologic Consequences of the Effects of Temperature, pH, P_{CO_2}, and 2,3-BPG

As blood enters metabolically active tissues, it is exposed to an environment different from that found in the arterial tree. The P_{CO_2} is higher, the pH is lower, and the temperature is also higher than that of the arterial blood. It is evident, then, that in our original discussion of the oxyhemoglobin dissociation curve, shown in Figure 7–1, we were neglecting some important factors. The curve shown in Figure 7–1 is for blood at 37°C, with a pH of 7.4 and a P_{CO_2} of 40 mm Hg. Blood in metabolically active tissues and therefore the venous blood draining them are no longer subject to these conditions because they have been exposed to a different environment. Because low pH, high P_{CO_2}, increased 2,3-BPG, and higher temperature *all shift the oxyhemoglobin dissociation curve to the right,* they all can help unload oxygen from hemoglobin at the tissues. On the other hand, as the venous blood returns to the lung and CO_2 leaves the blood (which increases the pH), the affinity of hemoglobin for oxygen increases as the curve shifts back to the left, as shown in Figure 7–3.

Note that the effects of pH, P_{CO_2}, and temperature shown in Figure 7–2 are all more pronounced at lower P_{O_2}s than at higher P_{O_2}s. That is, they have a more profound effect on enhancing the unloading of oxygen at the tissues than they do interfering with its loading at the lungs.

A convenient way to discuss shifts in the oxyhemoglobin dissociation curve is the P_{50}, shown in Figures 7–1 and 7–3. The P_{50} is the P_{O_2} at which 50% of the hemoglobin present in the blood is in the deoxyhemoglobin state and 50% is in the oxyhemoglobin state. At a temperature of 37°C, a pH of 7.4, and a P_{CO_2} of 40 mm Hg, normal human blood has a P_{50} of 26 or 27 mm Hg. If the oxyhemoglobin dissociation curve is shifted to the right, the P_{50} increases. If it is shifted to the left, the P_{50} decreases.

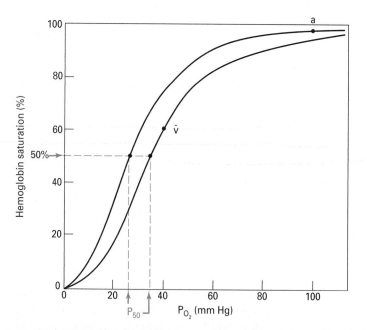

Figure 7–3. Oxyhemoglobin dissociation curves for arterial and venous blood. The venous curve is shifted to the right because the pH is lower and the P_{CO_2} (and possibly the temperature) is higher. The rightward shift results in a higher P_{50} for venous blood. a = arterial point (P_{O_2} = 100 mm Hg); $\bar{v}$ = mixed venous point (P_{O_2} = 40 mm Hg).

Other Factors Affecting Oxygen Transport

ANEMIA

Most forms of anemia do not affect the oxyhemoglobin dissociation curve if the association of oxygen and hemoglobin is expressed as percent saturation. For example, anemia secondary to blood loss does not affect the combination of oxygen and hemoglobin for the remaining erythrocytes. It is the *amount* of hemoglobin that decreases, not the percent saturation or even the arterial P_{O_2}. The arterial *content* of oxygen, however, in milliliters of oxygen per 100 mL of blood, is reduced, as shown in Figure 7–4A, because the decreased amount of hemoglobin per 100 mL of blood decreases the oxygen-carrying *capacity* of the blood.

CARBON MONOXIDE

Carbon monoxide has a much greater affinity for hemoglobin than does oxygen, as discussed in Chapter 6. It can therefore effectively block the combination of oxygen with hemoglobin because oxygen cannot be bound to iron atoms already combined with carbon monoxide. Carbon monoxide has a second deleterious effect: It shifts the oxyhemoglobin dissociation curve to the left. Thus, carbon monoxide can prevent the loading of oxygen into the blood in the lungs and can also interfere with the unloading of oxygen at the tissues. This can be seen in Figure 7–4A.

Carbon monoxide is particularly dangerous for several reasons. A person breathing very low concentrations of carbon monoxide can slowly reach life-threatening levels of carboxyhemoglobin (COHb) in the blood because carbon monoxide has such a high affinity for hemoglobin. The effect is cumulative. What is worse is that a person breathing carbon monoxide is not aware of doing so—the gas is colorless, odorless, and tasteless and does not elicit any reflex coughing or sneezing, increase in ventilation, or feeling of difficulty in breathing.

Smoking and living in urban areas cause small amounts of carboxyhemoglobin to be present in the blood of healthy adults. A nonsmoker who lives in a rural area may have only about 1% carboxyhemoglobin; a smoker who lives in an urban area may have 5–8% carboxyhemoglobin in the blood.

NITRIC OXIDE

Hemoglobin within erythrocytes can rapidly scavenge nitric oxide (NO). NO can react with oxyhemoglobin to form methemoglobin and nitrate or react with deoxyhemoglobin to form a hemoglobin–nitric oxide complex. In addition, hemoglobin may act as a carrier for nitric oxide, in the form of S-nitrosothiol, on the cysteine residues on the β-globin chain. This is called s-nitrosohemoglobin (SNO-Hb). When hemoglobin binds oxygen, the formation of this S-nitrosothiol is enhanced; when hemoglobin releases oxygen, nitric oxide could be released. Thus, in regions where the P_{O_2} is low, nitric oxide—a potent vasodilator—could be released. Some researchers have proposed that this mechanism plays an important role in hypoxia-induced vasodilation or that nitric oxide scavenging by hemoglobin plays a role in hypoxic pulmonary vasoconstriction, but this has not yet been established.

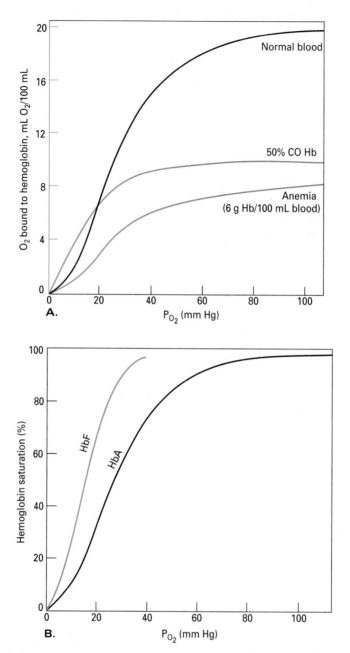

Figure 7–4. **A:** The effects of carbon monoxide and anemia on the carriage of oxygen by hemoglobin. Note that the ordinate is expressed as the *volume* of oxygen bound to hemoglobin in milliliters of oxygen per 100 mL of blood. **B:** A comparison of the oxyhemoglobin dissociation curves for normal adult hemoglobin (HbA) and fetal hemoglobin (HbF). **C:** Dissociation curves for normal HbA, a single monomeric subunit of hemoglobin (Hb subunit), and myoglobin (Mb).

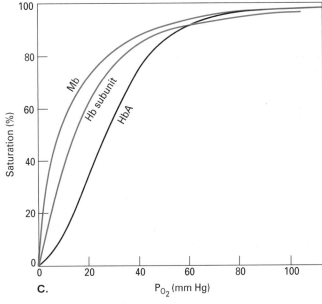

Figure 7–4. (Continued)

METHEMOGLOBIN

Methemoglobin is hemoglobin with iron in the ferric (Fe^{3+}) state. It can be caused by nitrite poisoning or by toxic reactions to oxidant drugs, or it can be found congenitally in patients with hemoglobin M. Iron atoms in the Fe^{3+} state will not combine with oxygen.

HEMOGLOBINS OTHER THAN HBA

As already discussed in this chapter, variants of the normal adult hemoglobin A (HbA) may have different affinities for oxygen. Fetal hemoglobin (HbF) in red blood cells has a dissociation curve to the left of that for HbA, as shown in Figure 7–4B. This is perfectly reasonable because fetal P_{O_2}s are much lower than those of an adult. The curve is located properly for its operating range. Furthermore, fetal hemoglobin's greater affinity for oxygen relative to the maternal hemoglobin promotes transport of oxygen across the placenta by maintaining the diffusion gradient. The shape of the HbF curve in blood appears to be a result of the fact that 2,3-BPG has little effect on the affinity of HbF for oxygen. Indeed, the curve is similar to that of HbA without 2,3-BPG (Figure 7–2D). Abnormal hemoglobins may have either increased or decreased affinities for oxygen. For example, Hb Seattle and Hb Kansas have lower affinities for oxygen than does HbA; Hb Rainier has a higher affinity for oxygen.

MYOGLOBIN

Myoglobin (Mb), a heme protein that occurs naturally in muscle cells, consists of a single polypeptide chain attached to a heme group. It can therefore combine chemically with a single molecule of oxygen and is similar structurally to a single subunit of hemoglobin.

As can be seen in Figure 7–4C, the hyperbolic dissociation curve of myoglobin (which is similar to that of a single hemoglobin subunit) is far to the left of that of normal adult hemoglobin. That is, at lower P_{O_2}s, much more oxygen remains bound to myoglobin. Myoglobin can therefore act to transport and store oxygen in skeletal muscle. As blood passes through the muscle, oxygen leaves hemoglobin and binds to myoglobin. It can be released from the myoglobin when conditions cause lower P_{O_2}s.

ARTIFICIAL BLOOD

Oxygen can bind reversibly to emulsions of *fluorocarbons.* Although these fluorocarbon emulsions do not have nearly as much oxygen-carrying capacity as does hemoglobin at normal P_{O_2}s, they can carry significantly more oxygen than plasma can. At very high P_{O_2}s (e.g., around 660 mm Hg, which would be attained in the pulmonary capillaries of alveoli ventilated with 100% O_2), these fluorocarbon emulsions can carry nearly as much oxygen as hemoglobin can. Fluorocarbons may become useful as emergency blood substitutes, for transfusions, and to augment blood transport in anemic patients or during surgery. They are already used for oxygenating the myocardium during coronary angioplasty procedures.

CYANOSIS

Cyanosis is not really an influence on the transport of oxygen but rather is a sign of poor transport of oxygen. Cyanosis occurs when more than 5 g Hb/100 mL of arterial blood is in the deoxy state. It is a bluish purple discoloration of the skin, nail beds, and mucous membranes, and its presence is indicative of an abnormally high concentration of deoxyhemoglobin in the arterial blood. Its absence, however, does not exclude hypoxemia because an anemic patient with hypoxemia may not have sufficient hemoglobin to appear cyanotic. Patients with abnormally high levels of hemoglobin in their arterial blood, such as those with polycythemia, may appear cyanotic without being hypoxemic.

TRANSPORT OF CARBON DIOXIDE BY THE BLOOD

Carbon dioxide is carried in the blood in physical solution, chemically combined to amino acids in blood proteins, and as bicarbonate ions. About 200 to 250 mL of carbon dioxide is produced by the tissue metabolism each minute in a resting 70-kg person and must be carried by the venous blood to the lung for removal from the body. At a cardiac output of 5 L/min, each 100 mL of blood passing through the lungs must therefore unload 4 to 5 mL of carbon dioxide.

Physically Dissolved

Carbon dioxide is about 20 times as soluble in the plasma (and inside the erythrocytes) as is oxygen. About 5% to 10% of the total carbon dioxide transported by the blood is carried in physical solution.

About 0.0006 mL CO_2/mm Hg P_{CO_2} will dissolve in 1 mL of plasma at 37°C. One hundred milliliters of plasma or whole blood at a P_{CO_2} of 40 mm Hg, therefore, contains about 2.4 mL CO_2 in physical solution. Figure 7–5 shows that the

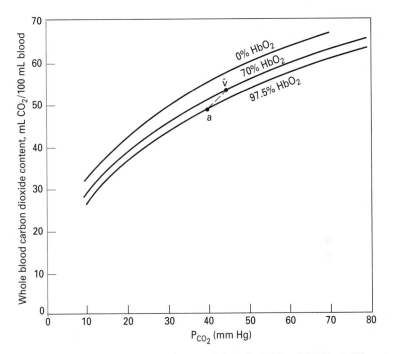

Figure 7–5. Carbon dioxide dissociation curves for whole blood (37°C) at different oxyhemoglobin saturations. Note that the ordinate is whole blood CO_2 content in milliliters of CO_2 per 100 mL of blood. a = arterial point; v = mixed venous point.

total CO_2 content of whole blood is about 48 mL $CO_2/100$ mL of blood at 40 mm Hg, and so approximately 5% of the carbon dioxide carried in the arterial blood is in *physical solution*. Similarly, multiplying 0.06 mL $CO_2/100$ mL of blood/mm Hg P_{CO_2} times a venous P_{CO_2} of 45 mm Hg shows that about 2.7 mL CO_2 is physically dissolved in the mixed venous blood. The total carbon dioxide content of venous blood is about 52.5 mL $CO_2/100$ mL of blood; a little more than 5% of the total carbon dioxide content of venous blood is in physical solution.

Carbamino Compounds

Carbon dioxide can combine chemically with the terminal amine groups in blood proteins, forming *carbamino compounds*.

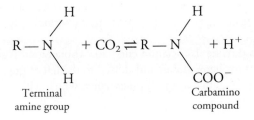

The reaction occurs rapidly; no enzymes are necessary. Note that a hydrogen ion is released when a carbamino compound is formed.

Because the protein found in greatest concentration in the blood is the globin of hemoglobin, most of the carbon dioxide transported in this manner is bound to amino acids of hemoglobin ("carbaminohemoglobin"). Deoxyhemoglobin can bind more carbon dioxide as carbamino groups than can oxyhemoglobin. Therefore, as the hemoglobin in the venous blood enters the lung and combines with oxygen, it releases carbon dioxide from its terminal amine groups. About 5% to 10% of the total carbon dioxide content of blood is in the form of carbamino compounds.

Bicarbonate

The remaining 80% to 90% of the carbon dioxide transported by the blood is carried as bicarbonate ions. This is made possible by the following reaction:

$$CO_2 + H_2O \overset{\text{carbonic}}{\underset{\text{anhydrase}}{\rightleftharpoons}} H_2CO_3 \rightleftharpoons H^+ + HCO_3^-$$

Carbon dioxide can combine with water to form carbonic acid, which then dissociates into a hydrogen ion and a bicarbonate ion.

Very little carbonic acid is formed by the association of water and carbon dioxide without the presence of the enzyme carbonic anhydrase because the reaction occurs so slowly. Carbonic anhydrase, which is present in high concentration in erythrocytes (but not in plasma), makes the reaction proceed about 13,000 times faster. Hemoglobin also plays an integral role in the transport of carbon dioxide because it can accept the hydrogen ion liberated by the dissociation of carbonic acid, thus allowing the reaction to continue. This will be discussed in detail in the last section of this chapter.

THE CARBON DIOXIDE DISSOCIATION CURVE

The carbon dioxide dissociation curve for whole blood is shown in Figure 7–5. Within the normal physiologic range of P_{CO_2}s, the curve is nearly a straight line, with no steep or flat portions. If it is plotted on axes similar to those for oxygen, the carbon dioxide dissociation curve for whole blood is steeper than the oxygen dissociation curve for whole blood. That is, there is a greater change in CO_2 content per mm Hg change in P_{CO_2} than there is in oxygen content per mm Hg change in P_{O_2}.

The carbon dioxide dissociation curve for whole blood is shifted to the right at greater levels of oxyhemoglobin and shifted to the left at greater levels of deoxyhemoglobin. This is known as the *Haldane effect,* which will be explained in the next section. The Haldane effect allows the blood to load more carbon dioxide at the tissues, where there is more deoxyhemoglobin, and unload more carbon dioxide in the lungs, where there is more oxyhemoglobin.

THE BOHR & HALDANE EFFECTS EXPLAINED

The Bohr and Haldane effects are both explained by the fact that *deoxyhemoglobin is a weaker acid than oxyhemoglobin.* That is, deoxyhemoglobin more readily accepts the hydrogen ion liberated by the dissociation of carbonic acid, thus permitting more carbon dioxide to be transported in the form of bicarbonate ion. This is referred to as the *isohydric shift.* Conversely, the association of hydrogen ions with the amino acids of hemoglobin lowers the affinity of hemoglobin for oxygen, thus shifting the oxyhemoglobin dissociation curve to the right at low pHs or high P_{CO_2}s. The following "equation" can therefore be written

$$H^+ Hb + O_2 \rightleftharpoons H^+ + HbO_2$$

These effects can be seen in the schematic diagrams of oxygen and carbon dioxide transport shown in Figure 7–6.

At the tissues, the P_{O_2} is low and the P_{CO_2} is high. Carbon dioxide dissolves in the plasma, and some diffuses into the erythrocyte. Some of this carbon dioxide dissolves in the cytosol, some forms carbamino compounds with hemoglobin, and some is hydrated by carbonic anhydrase to form carbonic acid. At low P_{O_2}s, there are substantial amounts of deoxyhemoglobin in the erythrocytes and the deoxyhemoglobin is able to accept the hydrogen ions liberated by the dissociation of carbonic acid and the formation of carbamino compounds. The hydrogen ions released by the dissociation of carbonic acid and the formation of carbamino compounds bind to specific amino acid residues on the globin chains and facilitate the release of oxygen from hemoglobin (the Bohr effect). Bicarbonate ions diffuse out of the erythrocyte through the cell membrane much more readily than do hydrogen ions. Because more bicarbonate ions than hydrogen ions leave the erythrocyte, electrical neutrality is maintained by the exchange of chloride ions for bicarbonate ions by the bicarbonate-chloride carrier protein. This is the "chloride shift." Small amounts of water also move into the cell to maintain the osmotic equilibrium.

At the lung, the P_{O_2} is high and the P_{CO_2} is low. As oxygen combines with hemoglobin, the hydrogen ions that were taken up when it was in the deoxyhemoglobin state are released. They combine with bicarbonate ions, forming carbonic acid. This breaks down into carbon dioxide and water. At the same time, carbon dioxide is also released from the carbamino compounds. Carbon dioxide then diffuses out of the red blood cells and plasma and into the alveoli. A chloride shift opposite in direction to that in the tissues also occurs to maintain electrical neutrality.

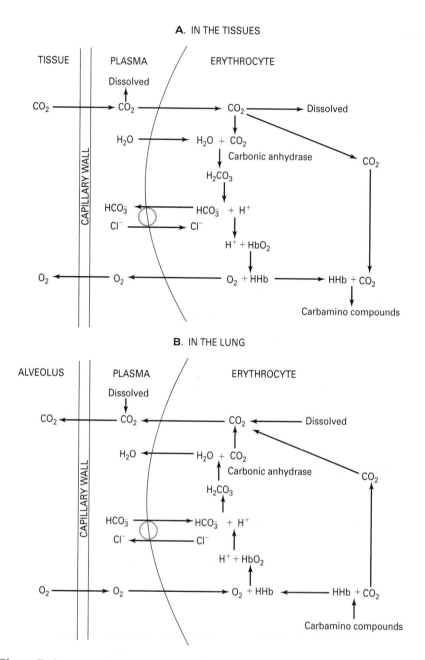

A. IN THE TISSUES

B. IN THE LUNG

Figure 7–6. Schematic representation of uptake and release of carbon dioxide and oxygen at the tissues (**A**) and in the lung (**B**). Note that small amounts of carbon dioxide can form carbamino compounds with blood proteins other than hemoglobin and may also be hydrated in trivial amounts in the plasma to form carbonic acid and then bicarbonate (not shown in diagram). The circles represent the bicarbonate-chloride exchange carrier protein.

KEY CONCEPTS

Blood normally carries a small amount of oxygen physically dissolved in the plasma and a large amount chemically combined to hemoglobin: only the physically dissolved oxygen contributes to the partial pressure, but the partial pressure of oxygen determines how much combines chemically with hemoglobin.

*The oxyhemoglobin dissociation curve describes the **reversible** reaction of oxygen and hemoglobin to form oxyhemoglobin; it is relatively flat at a P_{O_2} above approximately 70 mm Hg and is very steep at a P_{O_2} in the range of 20 to 40 mm Hg.*

Decreased pH, increased P_{CO_2}, increased temperature, and increased 2,3-BPG concentration of the blood all shift the oxyhemoglobin dissociation curve to the right.

*Blood normally carries small amounts of carbon dioxide physically dissolved in the plasma and chemically combined to blood proteins as **carbamino compounds** and a large amount in the form of bicarbonate ions.*

Deoxyhemoglobin favors the formation of carbamino compounds, and it promotes the transport of carbon dioxide as bicarbonate ions by buffering hydrogen ions formed by the dissociation of carbonic acid.

CLINICAL PROBLEMS

7–1. An otherwise normal person has lost enough blood to decrease his body's hemoglobin concentration from 15 g/100 mL blood to 12 g/100 mL blood. Which of the following would be expected to decrease?

   a. Arterial P_{O_2}

   b. Blood oxygen-carrying capacity

   c. Arterial hemoglobin saturation

   d. Arterial oxygen content

7–2. Results of tests on a patient's blood show the hemoglobin concentration to be 10 g/100 mL of blood. The blood is 97.4% saturated with oxygen at a Pa_{O_2} of 100 mm Hg. What is the patient's arterial oxygen content, including physically dissolved oxygen (37°C, pH 7.40, P_{CO_2} of 40 mm Hg)?

7–3. What is the approximate hemoglobin oxygen saturation (S_{O_2}) of a blood sample that contains 10 g Hb/100 mL blood and has an oxygen content of 10 mL O_2/100 mL blood (ignore physically dissolved O_2)?

7–4. *Which of the following should increase the P_{50} of the oxyhemoglobin dissociation curve?*

a. *Hypercapnia*

b. *Acidosis*

c. *Increased blood levels of 2,3-BPG*

d. *Increased body temperature*

e. *All of the above*

SUGGESTED READINGS

Comroe JH. *Physiology of Respiration.* 2nd ed. Chicago, Ill: Year Book; 1974:183–196.

Hsia CCW. Respiratory function of hemoglobin. *N Engl J Med.* 1998;338:239–247.

Robinson JM, Lancaster JR. Hemoglobin-mediated hypoxia-induced vasodilation via nitric oxide. *Am J Respir Cell Mol Biol.* 2005;32:257–261.

Roughton FJW. Transport of oxygen and carbon dioxide. In: Fenn WO, Rahn H, eds. *Handbook of Physiology,* sec 3: Respiration. Washington, DC: American Physiological Society; 1964;1:767–825.

Veeramachaneni NK, Harken AH, Cairns CB. Clinical implications of hemoglobin as a nitric oxide carrier. *Arch Surg.* 1999;134:434–437.

The Regulation of Acid-Base Status

8

OBJECTIVES

The reader understands the basic concepts of the regulation of the acid-base status of the body.

▶ *Defines acids, bases, and buffers.*

▶ *Lists the buffer systems available in the human body.*

▶ *Describes the interrelationships of the pH, the P_{CO_2} of the blood, and the plasma bicarbonate concentration, and states the Henderson-Hasselbalch equation.*

▶ *States the normal ranges of arterial pH, P_{CO_2}, and bicarbonate concentration, and defines alkalosis and acidosis.*

▶ *Lists the potential causes of respiratory acidosis and alkalosis and metabolic acidosis and alkalosis.*

▶ *Discusses the respiratory and renal mechanisms that help compensate for acidosis and alkalosis.*

▶ *Evaluates blood gas data to determine a subject's acid-base status.*

▶ *Classifies and explains the causes of tissue hypoxia.*

The maintenance of a relatively constant internal environment is one of the major physiologic functions of the organ systems of the body. Body temperature, fluid volume and osmolarity, and electrolytes—including acids and bases—are normally carefully regulated. A thorough knowledge of the mechanisms that control these variables is essential to clinical practice.

The respiratory system is intimately involved in the maintenance of the balance of acids and bases in the body. This chapter will introduce the major concepts of acid-base balance, particularly with respect to the respiratory system; a more detailed study of this important subject is strongly encouraged.

THE CHEMISTRY OF ACIDS, BASES, & BUFFERS

Although there are several ways to define acids and bases, the most useful physiologically is to define an *acid* as a substance that can donate a hydrogen ion (a proton) to another substance and a *base* as a substance that can accept a hydrogen ion from another substance. A *strong acid* is a substance that is completely or almost completely dissociated into a hydrogen ion and its corresponding or *conjugate* base in dilute aqueous solution; a *weak acid* is only slightly ionized in aqueous solution. In general, a strong acid has a weak conjugate base and a weak acid has a strong conjugate base. The strength of an acid or a base should not be confused with its concentration.

A *buffer* is a mixture of substances in aqueous solution (usually a combination of a weak acid and its conjugate base) that can resist changes in hydrogen ion concentration when strong acids or bases are added. That is, the changes in hydrogen ion concentration that occur when a strong acid or base is added to a buffer system are much smaller than those that would occur if the same amount of acid or base were added to pure water or another nonbuffer solution.

The Quantification of Acidity

The acidity of a solution is determined by the *activity* of the hydrogen ions in the solution. The hydrogen ion activity, which is denoted by the symbol $\alpha_H{}^+$, is closely related to the concentration of hydrogen ions ($[H^+]$) in a solution. In extremely dilute solutions, the hydrogen ion activity is equal to the hydrogen ion concentration; in highly concentrated solutions, the activity is less than the concentration. The hydrogen ion concentration of the blood is low enough that the hydrogen ion activity may be considered to be equal to the hydrogen ion concentration.

The hydrogen ion activity of pure water is about 1.0×10^{-7} mol/L. By convention, solutions with hydrogen ion activities above 10^{-7} mol/L are considered to be acid; those with hydrogen ion activities below 10^{-7} are considered to be alkaline. The range of hydrogen ion concentrations or activities *in the body* is normally from about 10^{-1} for gastric acid to about 10^{-8} for the most alkaline pancreatic secretion. This wide range of hydrogen ion activities necessitates the use of the more convenient *pH scale*. The pH of a solution is the negative logarithm of its hydrogen ion activity. With the exception of the highly concentrated gastric acid, in most instances in the body the hydrogen ion activity is about equal to the hydrogen ion concentration. Therefore,

$$pH = -\log(\alpha_H+)$$
$$\text{or } pH = -\log[H^+]$$

Thus, the pH of gastric acid is on the order of 1; the pH of the alkaline pancreatic secretion may be as high as 8.

The pH of *arterial blood* is normally close to 7.40, with a normal range considered to be about 7.35 to 7.45. An arterial pH less than 7.35 is considered *acidemia;* an arterial pH greater than 7.45 is considered *alkalemia.* The underlying condition characterized by hydrogen ion retention or by loss of bicarbonate or other bases is referred to as *acidosis;* the underlying condition characterized by hydrogen ion loss or retention of base is referred to as *alkalosis.* Under pathologic conditions the extremes of arterial blood pH have been noted to range as high as 7.8 and as low as 6.9. These correspond to hydrogen ion concentrations as follows [hydrogen ion concentrations are expressed as *nanomoles* (10^{-9} mol/L) for convenience]:

pH	Concentration (nmol/Liter)
6.90	126
7.00	100
7.10	79
7.20	63
7.30	50
7.40	40
7.50	32
7.60	25
7.70	20
7.80	16

Note that the pH scale is "inverted" by the negative sign and is also logarithmic as it is defined. Therefore, an *increase* in pH from 7.40 to 7.70 represents a *decrease* in hydrogen ion concentration. In fact, the increase of only 0.3 pH units indicates that hydrogen ion concentration was cut *in half.*

The Importance of Body pH Regulation

Hydrogen ions are the most reactive cations in body fluids, and they interact with negatively charged regions of other molecules, such as those of body proteins. Interactions of hydrogen ions with negatively charged functional groups of proteins can lead to marked changes in protein structural conformations with resulting alterations in the behavior of the proteins. An example of this was already seen in Chapter 7, where hemoglobin was noted to combine with less oxygen at a lower pH (the Bohr effect). Alterations in the structural conformations and charges of protein enzymes will obviously affect their activities, with resulting alterations in the functions of body tissues. The absorption and efficacy of drugs administered by the physician may also be affected by the pH. Extreme changes in the hydrogen ion concentration of the body can result in loss of organ system function and structural integrity; under acute conditions, arterial pHs above approximately 7.80 or below 6.9 are not compatible with life.

Sources of Acids in the Body

Under normal circumstances, cellular metabolism is the main source of acids in the body. These acids are the waste products of substances ingested as foodstuffs. The greatest source of hydrogen ions is the carbon dioxide produced as one of the end products of the oxidation of glucose and fatty acids during aerobic metabolism. The hydration of carbon dioxide results in the formation of carbonic acid, which then can dissociate into a hydrogen ion and a bicarbonate ion, as discussed in

Chapter 7. This process is reversed in the pulmonary capillaries, and CO_2 then diffuses through the alveolar-capillary barrier into the alveoli, from which it is removed by alveolar ventilation. Carbonic acid is therefore said to be a *volatile acid* because it can be converted into a gas and then removed from an open system like the body. Very great amounts of carbon dioxide can be removed from the lungs by alveolar ventilation: Under normal circumstances, about 15,000 to 25,000 mmol of carbon dioxide is removed via the lungs daily.

A much smaller quantity of *fixed* or *nonvolatile* acids is also normally produced during the course of the metabolism of foodstuffs. The fixed acids produced by the body include sulfuric acid, which originates from the oxidation of sulfur-containing amino acids such as cysteine; phosphoric acid from the oxidation of phospholipids and phosphoproteins; hydrochloric acid, which is produced during the conversion of ingested ammonium chloride to urea and by other reactions; and lactic acid from the anaerobic metabolism of glucose. Of course, lactic acid is sometimes converted to carbon dioxide, and so it is not always a fixed acid. Other fixed acids may be ingested accidentally or formed in abnormally large quantities by disease processes, such as the acetoacetic and butyric acid formed during diabetic ketoacidosis. About 70 mEq of fixed acids is normally removed from the body each day (about 1 mEq/kg/body weight/day); the range is 50 to 100 mEq. A vegetarian diet may produce significantly less fixed acid and may even result in no net production of fixed acids. The removal of fixed acids is accomplished mainly by the kidneys, as will be discussed later in this chapter. Some may also be removed via the gastrointestinal tract. Fixed acids normally represent only about 0.2% of the total body acid production.

BUFFER SYSTEMS OF THE HUMAN BODY

The body contains a variety of substances that can act as buffers in the physiologic pH range. These include bicarbonate, phosphate, and proteins in the blood, the interstitial fluid, and inside cells. One way to express the ability of a substance to act as a buffer is its *buffer value*. The buffer value of a solution is the amount of hydrogen ions in milliequivalents per liter that can be added to or removed from the solution with a resultant change of one pH unit. Another way is to determine the substance's titration curve. The pK of the acid is another important consideration.

An acid, HA, can dissociate into a hydrogen ion, H^+, and its base, A^-:

$$HA \rightleftharpoons H^+ + A^-$$

According to the *law of mass action,* the relationship between the undissociated acid and the proton and the base at equilibrium can be expressed as the following ratio:

$$\frac{[H^+][A^-]}{[HA]} = K$$

That is, the product of the concentrations of hydrogen ion and base divided by the concentration of the acid is equal to a constant K, the *dissociation constant*. This can be rearranged to

$$[H^+] = K \frac{[HA]}{[A^-]}$$

After taking the logarithm of both sides,

$$\log [H^+] = \log K + \log \frac{[HA]}{[A^-]}$$

After multiplying both sides by -1,

$$-\log [H^+] = -\log K + \log \frac{[A^-]}{[HA]}$$

$$\text{or pH} = pK + \log \frac{[A^-]}{[HA]}$$

This is the general form of the *Henderson-Hasselbalch equation.*

The buffer value or buffering capacity of a buffer pair is greatest at or near the pK of the weak acid. Note that when the concentrations of HA and A^- are equal, the pH of a solution is equal to its pK.

As already stated, the human body contains a number of buffers and buffer pairs. The *isohydric principle* states that all the buffer pairs in a homogeneous solution are in equilibrium with the same hydrogen ion concentration. For this reason, all the buffer pairs in the *plasma* behave similarly, with the relative concentrations of their undissociated acids and their bases determined by their respective pKs:

$$pH = pK_1 + \log \frac{[A_1^-]}{[HA_1]} = pK_2 + \log \frac{[A_2^-]}{[HA_2]} = pK_3 + \log \frac{[A_3^-]}{[HA_3]}$$

An implication of the isohydric principle is that the detailed analysis of a single buffer pair, like the bicarbonate buffer system, can reveal a great deal about the chemistry of all the plasma buffers.

Buffers of the Blood

The main buffers of the blood are bicarbonate, phosphate, and proteins.

Bicarbonate

The bicarbonate buffer system consists of the buffer pair of the weak acid, carbonic acid, and its conjugate base, bicarbonate. As already stated, in the body:

$$CO_2 \rightleftharpoons \underset{\substack{\text{Dissolved} \\ \text{in the} \\ \text{aqueous phase}}}{CO_2} + H_2O \underset{\substack{\text{carbonic} \\ \text{anhydrase}}}{\rightleftharpoons} H_2CO_3 \rightleftharpoons H^+ + HCO_3^-$$

Gas phase

The ability of the bicarbonate system to function as a buffer of fixed acids in the body is largely due to the ability of the lungs to remove carbon dioxide from the body. In a closed system bicarbonate would not be nearly as effective.

At a temperature of 37°C about 0.03 mmol of carbon dioxide per mm Hg of P_{CO_2} will dissolve in a liter of plasma. (Note that the solubility of CO_2 was expressed as *milliliters of CO₂* per *100 mL* of plasma in Chapter 7.) Therefore, the carbon dioxide *dissolved* in the plasma, expressed as millimoles per liter, is equal to $0.03 \times P_{CO_2}$. At body temperature in the plasma, the equilibrium of the second part of the series of equations given above is far to the left so that there is roughly 1000 times as much carbon dioxide present physically dissolved in the plasma as there is in the form of carbonic acid. The dissolved carbon dioxide is in *equilibrium* with the carbonic acid, though, and so *both* the dissolved carbon dioxide and the carbonic acid are considered as the undissociated HA in the Henderson-Hasselbalch equation for the bicarbonate system:

$$pH = pK + \log \frac{[HCO_3^-]p}{[CO_2 + H_2CO_3]}$$

where $[HCO_3^-]p$ stands for plasma bicarbonate concentration. The concentration of carbonic acid is negligible, and so

$$pH = pK' + \log \frac{[HCO_3^-]p}{0.03 \times P_{CO_2}}$$

where pK' is the pK of the HCO_3^--CO_2 system in blood.

The pK' of this system at physiologic pHs and at 37°C is 6.1. Therefore, at an arterial pH of 7.40 and an arterial P_{CO_2} of 40 mm Hg,

$$7.40 = 6.1 + \log \frac{[HCO_3^-]p}{1.2 \text{ mmol/L}}$$

Therefore, the arterial plasma bicarbonate concentration is about 24 mmol/L (the normal range is 23 to 28 mmol/L) because the logarithm of 20 is equal to 1.3.

Note that the term *total CO₂* refers to the dissolved carbon dioxide (including carbonic acid) *plus* the carbon dioxide present as bicarbonate.

A useful way to display the interrelationships among the variables of pH, P_{CO_2}, and bicarbonate concentration of the plasma, as expressed by the Henderson-Hasselbalch equation, is the *pH-bicarbonate diagram* shown in Figure 8–1.

As can be seen from Figure 8–1, pH is on the abscissa of the pH-bicarbonate diagram, and the plasma bicarbonate concentration in millimoles per liter is on the ordinate. For each value of pH and bicarbonate ion concentration, there is a single corresponding P_{CO_2} on the graph. Conversely, for any particular pH and P_{CO_2}, only one bicarbonate ion concentration will satisfy the Henderson-Hasselbalch equation. If the P_{CO_2} is held constant, for example, at 40 mm Hg, an *isobar* line can be constructed, connecting the resulting points as the pH is varied. The representative

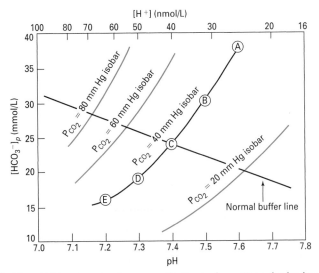

Figure 8–1. The pH-bicarbonate diagram with P_{CO_2} isobars. Note the hydrogen ion concentration in nanomoles per liter at the top of the figure corresponding to the pHs on the abscissa. Points A to E correspond to different pHs and bicarbonate concentrations all falling on the same P_{CO_2} isobar. (Reprinted from Davenport HW, The ABC of Acid-Base Chemistry, 6th ed, 1974, by permission of the University of Chicago Press.)

isobars shown in Figure 8–1 give an indication of the potential alterations of acid-base status when alveolar ventilation is increased or decreased. If everything else remains constant, hypoventilation leads to acidosis; hyperventilation leads to alkalosis.

The buffer value of the bicarbonate system *without the presence of hemoglobin* is about −5.4 mmol/L/pH unit. That is, the bicarbonate concentration increases only 5.4 mmol/L as enough acid in the form of carbon dioxide is added to the bicarbonate system to lower the pH by one unit. The rise in bicarbonate concentration represents the amount of carbonic acid added to the system. The bicarbonate buffer system is therefore a poor buffer for carbonic acid. The presence of hemoglobin makes blood a much better buffer, as can be seen in Figure 8–2.

The figure shows that increasing the hemoglobin concentration in this in vitro experiment makes the buffering curve steeper. That is, the bicarbonate concentration rises more at greater hemoglobin concentrations as carbonic acid (in the form of CO_2) is added to the blood. The increase in bicarbonate concentration is greater with more hemoglobin because as carbon dioxide is added to the blood, the hydrogen ions formed by the dissociation of carbonic acid are buffered by hemoglobin (as will be discussed shortly). Most of the bicarbonate ions formed by this dissociation can therefore move into the plasma. The buffer value of plasma in the presence of hemoglobin is thus four to five times that of plasma separated from erythrocytes. Therefore, the slope of the normal in vivo buffer line shown in Figures 8–1 and 8–3 is mainly determined by the nonbicarbonate buffers present in the body.

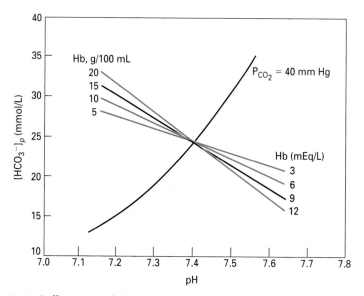

Figure 8–2. Buffer curves of plasma of blood containing 5, 10, 15, or 20 g of hemoglobin per 100 mL of blood. (Reprinted from Davenport HW, The ABC of Acid-Base Chemistry, 6th ed, 1974, by permission of the University of Chicago Press.)

Phosphate

The phosphate buffer system mainly consists of the buffer pair of the dihydrogen phosphate ($H_2PO_4^-$) and the monohydrogen phosphate (HPO_4^{2-}) anions:

$$H_2PO_4^- \rightleftharpoons H^+ + HPO_4^{2-}$$

The pK of the acid form is 6.8, so that in pHs ranging near 7.0, the acid form can readily donate a proton and the base form can accept a proton. Many organic phosphates found in the body also have pKs within ±0.5 pH units of 7.0, and these compounds can also function as buffers under physiologic conditions. These organic phosphates include such compounds as glucose-1-phosphate and adenosine triphosphate.

Proteins

Although several potential buffering groups are found on proteins, only one large group has pKs in the pH range encountered in the blood. These are the imidazole groups in the histidine residues of the peptide chains. The pKs of the various histidine residues on the different *plasma proteins* range from about 5.5 to about 8.5, thus providing a broad spectrum of buffer pairs. The protein present in the greatest quantity in the blood is *hemoglobin*. Thirty-six of the five hundred forty amino acid residues in hemoglobin are histidine, with pKs ranging from 7 to 8; the N-terminal valine residues also have a pK of about 7.8. As already noted, deoxyhemoglobin is a weaker acid than is oxyhemoglobin. That is, the pK of an imidazole group of one of the histidine residues in deoxygenated hemoglobin is greater than it is in the oxyhemoglobin state. Thus, as oxygen leaves hemoglobin in the tissue capillaries, the imidazole group removes hydrogen ions from the erythrocyte interior, allowing more carbon dioxide to be transported as bicarbonate. This process is reversed in the lungs.

Buffers of the Interstitial Fluid

The bicarbonate buffer system is the major buffer found in the interstitial fluid, including the lymph. The phosphate buffer pair is also found in the interstitial fluid. The volume of the interstitial compartment is much larger than that of the plasma, and so the interstitial fluid may play an important role in buffering.

Bone

The extracellular portion of bone contains very large deposits of calcium and phosphate salts, mainly in the form of hydroxyapatite. Although bone growth in a child causes a net production of hydrogen ions, in an otherwise healthy adult, where bone growth and resorption are in a steady state, bone salts can buffer hydrogen ions in chronic acidosis. Chronic buffering of hydrogen ions by the bone salts may therefore lead to demineralization of bone.

Intracellular Buffering

The intracellular proteins and organic phosphates of most cells can function to buffer both fixed acids and carbonic acid. Again, this is largely a function of the histidine groups on the proteins and phosphate groups on such compounds as ATP (adenosine triphosphate) and glucose-1-phosphate. Of course, buffering by the hemoglobin in erythrocytes is intracellular buffering.

ACIDOSIS & ALKALOSIS

Acid-base disorders can be divided into four major categories: respiratory acidosis, respiratory alkalosis, metabolic acidosis, and metabolic alkalosis. These primary acid-base disorders may occur singly ("simple") or in combination ("mixed") or may be altered by compensatory mechanisms.

Respiratory Acidosis

The arterial P_{CO_2} is normally kept at or near 40 mm Hg (normal range is 35 to 45 mm Hg by convention) by the mechanisms that regulate breathing. Sensors exposed to the arterial blood and to the cerebrospinal fluid provide the central controllers of breathing with the information necessary to regulate the arterial P_{CO_2} at or near 40 mm Hg (see Chapter 9). Any short-term alterations (i.e., those which occur without renal compensation) in alveolar ventilation that result in an increase in alveolar and therefore also in arterial P_{CO_2} tend to lower the arterial pH, resulting in respiratory *acidosis*. This can be seen by looking at the P_{CO_2} = 60 mm Hg and P_{CO_2} = 80 mm Hg isobars in Figure 8–1. The exact arterial pH at any Pa_{CO_2} depends on the bicarbonate and other buffers present in the blood. Pure changes in arterial P_{CO_2} caused by changes in ventilation travel along the normal in vivo buffer line (Figures 8–1 and 8–3). This is similar to the in vitro plasma of blood buffer line at 15 g Hb/100 mL of blood seen in Figure 8–2. Pure uncompensated respiratory acidosis would correspond with point C on Figure 8–3 (at the intersection of an elevated P_{CO_2} isobar and the normal buffer line).

In respiratory acidosis, the *ratio* of bicarbonate to CO_2 decreases. Yet, as can be seen at point C in Figure 8–3, in uncompensated primary (simple) respiratory acidosis, the absolute plasma bicarbonate concentration does increase somewhat because of the buffering of some of the hydrogen ions liberated by the dissociation of carbonic acid by nonbicarbonate buffers.

Any impairment of alveolar ventilation can cause respiratory acidosis. As shown in Table 8–1, depression of the respiratory centers in the medulla (see Chapter 9) by anesthetic agents, narcotics, hypoxia, central nervous system disease or trauma, or even greatly elevated Pa_{CO_2} itself results in hypoventilation and respiratory acidosis. Interference with the neural transmission to the respiratory muscles by disease processes, drugs or toxins, or dysfunctions or deformities of the respiratory muscles or the chest wall can result in respiratory acidosis. Restrictive, obstructive, and obliterative diseases of the lungs can also result in respiratory acidosis.

Respiratory Alkalosis

Alveolar ventilation in excess of that needed to keep pace with body carbon dioxide production results in alveolar and arterial P_{CO_2}s below 35 mm Hg. Such hyperventilation

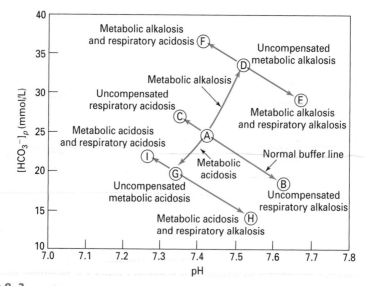

Figure 8–3. Acid-base paths in vivo. (Reprinted from Davenport HW, The ABC of Acid-Base Chemistry, 6th ed, 1974, by permission of the University of Chicago Press.)

Table 8–1. Common Causes of Respiratory Acidosis

Depression of the respiratory control centers
  Anesthetics
  Sedatives
  Opiates
  Brain injury or disease
  Severe hypercapnia, hypoxia
Neuromuscular disorders
  Spinal cord injury
  Phrenic nerve injury
  Poliomyelitis, Guillain-Barré syndrome, etc.
  Botulism, tetanus
  Myasthenia gravis
  Administration of curarelike drugs
  Diseases affecting the respiratory muscles
Chest wall restriction
  Kyphoscoliosis
  Extreme obesity
Lung restriction
  Pulmonary fibrosis
  Sarcoidosis
  Pneumothorax, pleural effusions, etc.
Pulmonary parenchymal diseases
  Pneumonia, etc.
  Pulmonary edema
Airway obstruction
  Chronic obstructive pulmonary disease
  Upper airway obstruction

 leads to respiratory alkalosis. Uncompensated primary respiratory alkalosis results in movement to a lower P_{CO_2} isobar along the normal buffer line, as seen at point B in Figure 8–3. The decreased Pa_{CO_2} shifts the equilibrium of the series of reactions describing carbon dioxide hydration and carbonic acid dissociation to the left. This results in a decreased arterial hydrogen ion concentration, raising the pH, and a decreased plasma bicarbonate concentration. The ratio of bicarbonate to carbon dioxide increases.

The causes of respiratory alkalosis include anything leading to hyperventilation. As shown in Table 8–2, *hyperventilation syndrome,* a psychological dysfunction of unknown cause, results in chronic or recurrent episodes of hyperventilation and respiratory alkalosis. Drugs, hormones (such as progesterone), toxic substances, central nervous system diseases or disorders, bacteremias, fever, overventilation by mechanical ventilators (or the physician), or ascent to high altitude may all result in respiratory alkalosis. Students are often surprised to see acute asthma included in a list of problems that can cause respiratory alkalosis. Asthma is an episodic obstructive disease and it is reasonable to assume that it would cause CO_2 retention and therefore respiratory acidosis during attacks. That is true in *very* severe asthma attacks, but most asthma attacks result in hypocapnia and respiratory alkalosis. As the asthma

Table 8–2. Common Causes of Respiratory Alkalosis

Central nervous system
Anxiety
Hyperventilation syndrome
Inflammation (encephalitis, meningitis)
Cerebrovascular disease
Tumors
Drugs or hormones
Salicylates
Progesterone
Bacteremias, fever
Pulmonary diseases
Acute asthma
Pulmonary vascular diseases (pulmonary embolism)
Overventilation with mechanical ventilators
Hypoxia; high altitude

attack occurs, bronchial smooth muscle spasm and mucus secretion obstruct the ventilation to some alveoli. Although some hypoxic pulmonary vasoconstriction may occur, it is not sufficient to divert all of the mixed venous blood flow away from these poorly ventilated alveoli. That results in a right-to-left shunt or shunt-like state, which would therefore be expected to cause the arterial P_{O_2} to decrease and the arterial P_{CO_2} to increase. However, the P_{CO_2} *decreases* because the patient increases alveolar ventilation if he or she is able to.

Irritant receptors in the airways are stimulated by the mucus and by chemical mediators released during the attack. Hypoxia caused by the shunt stimulates the arterial chemoreceptors; the patient also has the feeling of dyspnea (many asthma attacks have an *emotional* component). All of these things cause *increased* breathing and therefore increased alveolar ventilation.

Increasing ventilation will get more CO_2 out of the blood perfusing ventilated alveoli (and therefore out of the body) but it will not get much oxygen into alveoli supplied by obstructed airways, nor will it get much more oxygen into the blood of the unobstructed alveoli because of the shape of the oxyhemoglobin dissociation curve. Remember that the hemoglobin is already 97.4% saturated with oxygen and not much more will dissolve in the plasma. Therefore, during the attack the patient has *hypoxemia, hypocapnia,* and *respiratory alkalosis.* It is only when the attack is so severe that the patient can't do the additional work of breathing that hypercapnia and respiratory acidosis occur.

Metabolic Acidosis

Metabolic acidosis may be more properly referred to as *nonrespiratory acidosis.* That is, it does not always involve aberrations in metabolism.

Metabolic acidosis can be caused by the ingestion, infusion, or production of a fixed acid; by decreased renal excretion of hydrogen ions; by the movement of

Table 8–3. Common Causes of Metabolic Acidosis

Ingested drugs or toxic substances
  Methanol
  Ethanol
  Salicylates
  Ethylene glycol
  Ammonium chloride
Loss of bicarbonate ions
  Diarrhea
  Pancreatic fistulas
  Renal dysfunction
Lactic acidosis
  Hypoxemia
  Anemia, carbon monoxide
  Shock (hypovolemic, cardiogenic, septic, etc.)
  Severe exercise
  Acute respiratory distress syndrome (ARDS)
Ketoacidosis
  Diabetes mellitus
  Alcoholism
  Starvation
Inability to excrete hydrogen ions
  Renal dysfunction

hydrogen ions from the intracellular to the extracellular compartment; or by the loss of bicarbonate or other bases from the extracellular compartment. As can be seen in Figure 8–3, primary uncompensated metabolic acidosis results in a downward movement along the P_{CO_2} = 40 mm Hg isobar to point G. That is, a net loss of buffer establishes a new blood buffer line lower than and parallel to the normal blood buffer line. P_{CO_2} is unchanged, hydrogen ion concentration is increased, and the ratio of bicarbonate concentration to CO_2 is decreased.

As shown in Table 8–3, ingestion of methyl alcohol or salicylates can cause metabolic acidosis by increasing the fixed acids in the blood. (Salicylate poisoning—e.g., aspirin overdose—causes both metabolic acidosis and later respiratory alkalosis.) Diarrhea can cause very great bicarbonate losses, resulting in metabolic acidosis. Renal dysfunctions can lead to an inability to excrete hydrogen ions, as well as an inability to reabsorb bicarbonate ions, as will be discussed in the next section. True "metabolic" acidosis may be caused by an accumulation of lactic acid in severe hypoxemia or shock and by diabetic ketoacidosis.

Metabolic Alkalosis

 Metabolic, or nonrespiratory, alkalosis occurs when there is an excessive loss of fixed acids from the body, or it may occur as a consequence of the ingestion, infusion, or excessive renal reabsorption of bases such as bicarbonate. Figure 8–3 shows that primary uncompensated metabolic alkalosis results

Table 8–4. Common Causes of Metabolic Alkalosis

Loss of hydrogen ions
   Vomiting
   Gastric fistulas
   Diuretic therapy
   Treatment with or overproduction of steroids (aldosterone or other mineralocorticoids)
Ingestion or administration of excess bicarbonate or other bases
   Intravenous bicarbonate
   Ingestion of bicarbonate or other bases (e.g., antacids)

in an upward movement along the $P_{CO_2} = 40$ mm Hg isobar to point D. That is, a net gain of buffer establishes a new blood buffer line higher than and parallel to the normal blood buffer line. P_{CO_2} is unchanged, hydrogen ion concentration is decreased, and the ratio of bicarbonate concentration to carbon dioxide is increased.

As shown in Table 8–4, loss of gastric juice by vomiting results in a loss of hydrogen ions and may cause metabolic alkalosis. Excessive ingestion of bicarbonate or other bases (e.g., stomach antacids) or over infusion of bicarbonate by the physician may cause metabolic alkalosis. In addition, diuretic therapy, treatment with steroids (or the overproduction of endogenous steroids), and conditions leading to severe potassium depletion may also cause metabolic alkalosis.

RESPIRATORY & RENAL COMPENSATORY MECHANISMS

Uncompensated primary acid-base disturbances, such as those indicated by points B, C, D, and G on Figure 8–3, are seldom seen because respiratory and renal compensatory mechanisms are called into play to offset these disturbances. The two main compensatory mechanisms are functions of the respiratory and renal systems.

Respiratory Compensatory Mechanisms

The respiratory system can compensate for metabolic acidosis or alkalosis by altering alveolar ventilation. As discussed in Chapter 3, if carbon dioxide production is constant, the alveolar P_{CO_2} is roughly inversely proportional to the alveolar ventilation. This can be seen in the upper portion of Figure 3–10. In metabolic acidosis, the elevated blood hydrogen ion concentration stimulates *chemoreceptors,* which, in turn, increase alveolar ventilation, thus decreasing arterial P_{CO_2}. This causes an increase in arterial pHa, returning it toward normal. (The mechanisms by which ventilation is regulated are discussed in detail in Chapter 9.) These events can be better understood by looking at Figure 8–3. Point G represents uncompensated metabolic acidosis. As the respiratory compensation for the metabolic acidosis occurs, in the form of an increase in ventilation, the arterial P_{CO_2} falls. The point representing blood pHa, Pa_{CO_2}, and bicarbonate concentration would then move a short distance along the lower than normal buffer line (from point G toward point H) until a new lower Pa_{CO_2} is attained. This returns the arterial pH *toward* normal; complete compensation does not occur. Of course, the respiratory compensation for metabolic acidosis occurs almost simultaneously with the development of the acidosis.

The blood pH, P_{CO_2}, and bicarbonate concentration point does not really move first from the normal (point A) to point G and *then* move a short distance along line GH; instead the compensation begins to occur as the acidosis develops, and so the point takes an intermediate pathway between the two lines.

The respiratory compensation for metabolic alkalosis is to decrease alveolar ventilation, thus raising Pa_{CO_2}. This decreases arterial pH toward normal, as can be seen on Figure 8–3. Point D represents uncompensated metabolic alkalosis; respiratory compensation would move the blood pHa, Pa_{CO_2}, and bicarbonate concentration point a short distance along the new higher than normal blood buffer line toward point F. Again the compensation occurs as the alkalosis develops, with the point moving along an intermediate course.

Under most circumstances the *cause* of respiratory acidosis or alkalosis is a dysfunction in the ventilatory control mechanism or the breathing apparatus itself. Compensation for acidosis or alkalosis in these conditions must therefore come from outside the respiratory system. The respiratory compensatory mechanism can operate very rapidly (within minutes) to partially correct metabolic acidosis or alkalosis.

Renal Compensatory Mechanisms

The kidneys can compensate for respiratory acidosis and metabolic acidosis of nonrenal origin by excreting fixed acids and by retaining filtered bicarbonate. The kidneys can also compensate for respiratory alkalosis or metabolic alkalosis of nonrenal origin by decreasing hydrogen ion excretion and by decreasing the retention of filtered bicarbonate.

RENAL MECHANISMS IN ACIDOSIS

The renal tubular cells secrete hydrogen ions into the tubular fluid. This is mainly accomplished by the generation of hydrogen ions and bicarbonate ions within the cell by the dissociation of carbonic acid. The carbonic acid is formed by the hydration of carbon dioxide via the carbonic anhydrase reaction. The carbon dioxide may be metabolically produced by the tubular cell itself or may be carried dissolved into the tubular fluid after production elsewhere in the body. The hydrogen ion generated by this process is actively secreted into the tubular lumen, and the new bicarbonate ion is "reabsorbed" into the peritubular capillary. Sodium ions in the tubular fluid are exchanged for the hydrogen ions secreted into the tubular fluid to maintain electrical neutrality. There is also an interrelationship between renal potassium ion secretion and renal hydrogen ion secretion: When the secretion of one of these ions is increased, secretion of the other is decreased because an active hydrogen ion-potassium ion exchange occurs in the cells of the collecting duct. For this reason, disturbances in acid-base balance are usually associated with alterations in potassium ion balance and vice versa. The hydrogen ion secreted into the tubular lumen is buffered by tubular bicarbonate, phosphate, or the small quantities of other buffers found in the tubular fluid.

About 80% of all filtered bicarbonate ions are reabsorbed in the proximal tubule and about 10% in the loop of Henle. The remaining 10% of bicarbonate ions are reabsorbed either by this mechanism in the distal tubules and collecting duct or in the process of titration of tubular phosphate ions, or by the generation of ammonium ions. In each mechanism, bicarbonate ions are returned to the peritubular capillary.

Ammonium (NH_4) is actively formed in the renal cells mainly by the deamination of the amino acid glutamine. Ammonium then diffuses into the tubular lumen.

Normally, the kidneys secrete about 70 mEq of hydrogen ions and reabsorb about 70 mEq of bicarbonate daily. This process can increase during acidosis to the extent that the urine can be acidified to a pH as low as 4.0 to 5.0. This is about 800 times as acidic as normal plasma.

RENAL MECHANISMS IN ALKALOSIS

In alkalotic states, the kidney decreases the secretion of hydrogen ions and decreases bicarbonate reabsorption. The kidney tends to reabsorb almost all the filtered bicarbonate until the plasma bicarbonate concentration reaches about 27 to 28 mEq/L (normally it is about 24 mEq/L). Plasma bicarbonate is excreted above this threshold.

TIME COURSE OF RENAL MECHANISMS

Renal compensatory mechanisms for acid-base disturbances operate much more slowly than respiratory compensatory mechanisms. For example, the renal compensatory responses to sustained respiratory acidosis or alkalosis may take 3 to 6 *days*.

Summary of Renal & Respiratory Contributions to Acid-Base Balance

The kidneys help regulate acid-base balance by altering the excretion of fixed acids and the retention of the filtered bicarbonate; the respiratory system helps regulate body acid-base balance by adjusting alveolar ventilation to alter alveolar P_{CO_2}. For these reasons, some authors suggest that the Henderson-Hasselbalch equation is in effect

$$pH = a\ constant + \frac{kidneys}{lungs}$$

CLINICAL INTERPRETATION OF BLOOD GASES & ACID-BASE STATUS

Samples of arterial blood are usually analyzed clinically to determine the "arterial blood gases": the arterial P_{O_2}, P_{CO_2}, and pH. The plasma bicarbonate can then be calculated from the pH and P_{CO_2} by using the Henderson-Hasselbalch equation. This can be done directly, or by using a nomogram, or by graphical analysis such as the pH-bicarbonate diagram (the "Davenport plot," after its popularizer), the pH-P_{CO_2} diagram (the "Siggaard-Andersen"), or the composite acid-base diagram. Most blood gas analyzers perform these calculations automatically.

Table 8–5 summarizes the changes in pHa, Pa$_{CO_2}$, and plasma bicarbonate concentration seen in simple, mixed, and partially compensated acid-base disturbances. It contains the same information shown in Figure 8–3, depicted

Table 8–5. Acid-Base Disturbances

	pH	P_{CO_2}	HCO_3^-
Uncompensated respiratory acidosis	↓↓	↑↑	↑
Uncompensated respiratory alkalosis	↑↑	↓↓	↓
Uncompensated metabolic acidosis	↓↓	—	↓↓
Uncompensated metabolic alkalosis	↑↑	—	↑↑
Partially compensated respiratory acidosis	↓	↑↑	↑↑
Partially compensated respiratory alkalosis	↑	↓↓	↓↓
Partially compensated metabolic acidosis	↓	↓↓	↓↓
Partially compensated metabolic alkalosis	↑	↑↑	↑↑
Respiratory and metabolic acidosis	↓↓	↑↑	↓
Respiratory and metabolic alkalosis	↑↑	↓↓	↑

differently. A thorough understanding of the patterns shown in Table 8–5 coupled with knowledge of a patient's P_{O_2} and other clinical findings can reveal a great deal about the underlying pathophysiologic processes in progress. This can be seen in the clinical problems at the end of this chapter.

A simple approach to interpreting a blood gas set is to first look at the pH to determine whether the predominant problem is acidosis or alkalosis. (Note that an acidemia could represent more than one cause of acidosis, an acidosis with some compensation, or even an acidosis *and* a separate underlying alkalosis. Similarly, an alkalemia could represent more than one cause of alkalosis, an alkalosis with some compensation, or even an alkalosis *and* a separate underlying acidosis.) After looking at the pH, look at the arterial P_{CO_2} to see if it explains the pH. For example, if the pH is low and the P_{CO_2} is high, then the primary problem is respiratory acidosis. If the pH is low and the P_{CO_2} is near 40 mm Hg, then the primary problem is metabolic acidosis with little or no compensation. If both the pH and the P_{CO_2} are low, there is metabolic acidosis with respiratory compensation. Then look at the bicarbonate concentration to confirm your diagnosis. It should be slightly increased in uncompensated respiratory acidosis, high in partially compensated respiratory acidosis, and low in metabolic acidosis.

If the pH is high and the P_{CO_2} is low, then the primary problem is respiratory alkalosis. If the pH is high and the P_{CO_2} is near 40 mm Hg, then the problem is uncompensated metabolic alkalosis. If both the pH and the P_{CO_2} are high, then there is partially compensated metabolic alkalosis. The bicarbonate should be slightly decreased in respiratory alkalosis, decreased in partially compensated respiratory alkalosis, and increased in metabolic alkalosis.

Base Excess

Calculation of the *base excess* or *base deficit* may be very useful in determining the therapeutic measures to be administered to a patient. The base excess or base deficit is the number of milliequivalents of acid or base needed to titrate 1 L of blood to pH 7.4 at 37°C if the Pa_{CO_2} *were held constant at 40 mm Hg*. It is not, therefore, just the difference between the plasma bicarbonate concentration of the sample in question and the normal plasma bicarbonate concentration because respiratory adjustments also cause a change in bicarbonate concentration: The arterial P_{CO_2} must be considered. Base excess can be determined by actually titrating a sample or by using a nomogram, diagram, or calculator program. Most blood gas analyzers calculate the base excess automatically. The base excess is expressed in milliequivalents per liter above or below the normal buffer-base range—it therefore has a normal value of 0 ± 2 mEq/L. A base deficit is also called a *negative base excess.*

The base deficit can be used to estimate how much sodium bicarbonate (in mEq) should be given to a patient by multiplying the base deficit (in mEq/L) times the patient's estimated extracellular fluid (ECF) space (in liters), which is the distribution space for the bicarbonate. The ECF is usually estimated to be 0.3 times the lean body mass in kilograms.

Anion Gap

Calculation of the *anion gap* can be helpful in determining the cause of a patient's metabolic acidosis. It is determined by subtracting the sum of a patient's plasma chloride and bicarbonate concentrations (in mEq/L) from his or her plasma sodium concentration:

$$\text{Anion gap} = [Na^+] - ([Cl^-] + [HCO_3^-])$$

The anion gap is normally 12 ± 4 mEq/L.

The sum of all of the plasma cations must equal the sum of all of the plasma anions, so the anion gap exists only because all of the plasma cations and anions are not measured when standard blood chemistry is done. Sodium, chloride, and bicarbonate concentrations are almost always reported. The normal anion gap is a result of the presence of more unmeasured anions than unmeasured cations in normal blood.

$$[Na^+] + [\text{unmeasured cations}] = [Cl^-] + [HCO_3^-] + [\text{unmeasured anions}]$$
$$[Na^+] - ([Cl^-] + [HCO_3^-]) = [\text{unmeasured anions}] - [\text{unmeasured cations}]$$

The anion gap is therefore the difference between the unmeasured anions and the unmeasured cations.

The negative charges on the plasma proteins probably make up most of the normal anion gap, because the total charges of the other plasma cations (K^+, Ca^{2+}, Mg^{2+}) are approximately equal to the total charges of the other anions (PO_4^{3-}, SO_4^{2-}, organic anions).

An increased anion gap usually indicates an increased number of unmeasured anions (those other than Cl^- and HCO_3^-) or a decreased number of unmeasured cations (K^+, Ca^{2+}, or Mg^{2+}), or both. This is most likely to happen when the measured anions, [HCO_3^-] or [Cl^-] are lost and replaced by unmeasured anions. For example, the buffering by HCO_3^-s of H^+s from ingested or metabolically produced acids produces an increased anion gap.

Thus, metabolic acidosis with an abnormally great anion gap (i.e., greater than 16 mEq/L) would probably be caused by lactic acidosis or ketoacidosis; ingestion of organic anions such as salicylate, methanol, and ethylene glycol; or renal retention of anions such as sulfate, phosphate, and urate.

THE CAUSES OF HYPOXIA

Thus far only two of the three variables referred to as the arterial blood gases, the arterial P_{CO_2} and pH, have been discussed. Many abnormal conditions or diseases can cause a low arterial P_{O_2}. They are discussed in the following section about the causes of tissue hypoxia in the section on *hypoxic hypoxia*.

 The causes of tissue hypoxia can be classified (in some cases rather arbitrarily) into four or five major groups (Table 8–6). The underlying physiology of most of these types of hypoxia has already been discussed in this or previous chapters.

Hypoxic Hypoxia

Hypoxic hypoxia refers to conditions in which the arterial P_{O_2} is abnormally low. Because the amount of oxygen that will combine with hemoglobin is mainly determined by the P_{O_2}, such conditions may lead to decreased oxygen delivery to the tissues if reflexes or other responses cannot adequately increase the cardiac output or hemoglobin concentration of the blood.

Low Alveolar P_{O_2}

Conditions causing low alveolar P_{O_2}s inevitably lead to low arterial P_{O_2}s and oxygen contents because the alveolar P_{O_2} determines the upper limit of arterial P_{O_2}. *Hypoventilation* leads to both alveolar hypoxia and hypercapnia (high CO_2), as

Table 8–6. A Classification of the Causes of Hypoxia

Classification	$P_{A_{O_2}}$	Pa_{O_2}	Ca_{O_2}	$P\bar{v}_{O_2}$	$C\bar{v}_{O_2}$	Increased $F_{I_{O_2}}$ Helpful?
Hypoxic hypoxia						
Low alveolar P_{O_2}	Low	Low	Low	Low	Low	Yes
Diffusion impairment	N	Low	Low	Low	Low	Yes
Right-to-left shunts	N	Low	Low	Low	Low	No
V̇/Q̇ mismatch	N	Low	Low	Low	Low	Yes
Anemic hypoxia	N	N	Low	Low	Low	No
CO poisoning	N	N	Low	Low	Low	Possibly
Hypoperfusion hypoxia	N	N	N	Low	Low	No
Histotoxic hypoxia	N	N	N	High	High	No

N = Normal.

discussed in Chapter 3. Hypoventilation can be caused by depression or injury of the respiratory centers in the brain (discussed in Chapter 9); interference with the nerves supplying the respiratory muscles, as in spinal cord injury; neuromuscular junction diseases such as myasthenia gravis; and altered mechanics of the lung or chest wall, as in noncompliant lungs due to sarcoidosis, reduced chest wall mobility because of kyphoscoliosis or obesity, and airway obstruction. Ascent to *high altitudes* causes alveolar hypoxia because of the reduced total barometric pressure encountered above sea level. *Reduced $F_{I_{O_2}}s$* (fraction of inspired oxygen) have similar effects. Alveolar carbon dioxide is decreased because of the reflex increase in ventilation caused by hypoxic stimulation, as will be discussed in Chapter 11. Hypoventilation and ascent to high altitudes lead to decreased venous P_{O_2} and oxygen content as oxygen is extracted from the already hypoxic arterial blood. Administration of elevated oxygen concentrations in the inspired gas can alleviate the alveolar and arterial hypoxia in hypoventilation and in ascent to high altitude, but it cannot reverse the hypercapnia of hypoventilation. In fact, administration of elevated $F_{I_{O_2}}s$ to spontaneously breathing patients hypoventilating because of a depressed central response to carbon dioxide (see Chapter 9) can further depress ventilation.

DIFFUSION IMPAIRMENT

Alveolar-capillary diffusion is discussed in greater detail in Chapter 6. Conditions such as interstitial fibrosis and interstitial or alveolar edema can lead to low arterial $P_{O_2}s$ and contents with normal or elevated alveolar $P_{O_2}s$. High $F_{I_{O_2}}s$ that increase the alveolar P_{O_2} to very high levels may raise the arterial P_{O_2} by increasing the partial pressure gradient for oxygen diffusion, as discussed in Chapter 6.

SHUNTS

True right-to-left shunts, such as anatomic shunts and absolute intrapulmonary shunts, can cause decreased arterial $P_{O_2}s$ with normal or even elevated alveolar $P_{O_2}s$. Patients with intrapulmonary shunts have low arterial $P_{O_2}s$, but may not have significantly increased $P_{CO_2}s$ if they are able to increase their alveolar ventilation or if they are mechanically ventilated. This is a result of the different shapes of the oxyhemoglobin dissociation curve (see Figure 7–1) and the carbon dioxide dissociation curve (see Figure 7–5). The carbon dioxide dissociation curve is almost linear in the normal range of arterial $P_{CO_2}s$, and arterial P_{CO_2} is very tightly regulated by the respiratory control system (see Chapter 9). Carbon dioxide retained in the shunted blood stimulates increased alveolar ventilation, and because the carbon dioxide dissociation curve is nearly linear, increased ventilation will allow more carbon dioxide to diffuse from the nonshunted blood into well-ventilated alveoli and be exhaled. On the other hand, increasing alveolar ventilation will not get any more oxygen into the shunted blood and, because of the shape of the oxyhemoglobin dissociation curve, very little more into the unshunted blood. This is because the hemoglobin of well-ventilated and perfused alveoli is nearly saturated with oxygen, and little more will dissolve in the plasma. Similarly, arterial hypoxemia caused by true shunts is not relieved by high $F_{I_{O_2}}s$ because the shunted blood does not come into contact with the high levels of oxygen. The hemoglobin of the *unshunted* blood is nearly completely saturated with oxygen at a normal $F_{I_{O_2}}$ of 0.21, and the small additional volume of oxygen dissolved in the blood at high $F_{I_{O_2}}$s cannot make up for the low hemoglobin saturation of the shunted blood.

VENTILATION-PERFUSION MISMATCH

Alveolar-capillary units with low ventilation-perfusion ($\dot{V}A/\dot{Q}c$) ratios contribute to arterial hypoxia, as already discussed. Units with high $\dot{V}A/\dot{Q}cs$ do not by themselves lead to arterial hypoxia, of course, but large lung areas that are underperfused are usually associated either with overperfusion of other units or with low cardiac outputs (see the section on Hypoperfusion Hypoxia below). Hypoxic pulmonary vasoconstriction (discussed in Chapter 4) and local airway responses (discussed in Chapter 2) normally help minimize $\dot{V}/\dot{Q}$ mismatch.

Note that diffusion impairment, shunts, and $\dot{V}/\dot{Q}$ mismatch increase the alveolar-arterial P_{O_2} difference (see Table 5–2).

Anemic Hypoxia

Anemic hypoxia is caused by a decrease in the amount of functioning hemoglobin, which can be a result of decreased hemoglobin or erythrocyte production, the production of abnormal hemoglobin or red blood cells, pathologic destruction of erythrocytes, or interference with the chemical combination of oxygen and hemoglobin. Carbon monoxide poisoning, for example, results from the greater affinity of hemoglobin for carbon monoxide than for oxygen. Methemoglobinemia is a condition in which the iron in hemoglobin has been altered from the Fe^{2+} to the Fe^{3+} form, which does not combine with oxygen.

Anemic hypoxia results in a decreased oxygen content when both alveolar and arterial P_{O_2} are normal. Standard analysis of arterial blood gases could therefore give normal values unless a *co-oximeter* is also used to determine blood oxygen content. Venous P_{O_2} and oxygen content are both decreased. Administration of high $F_{I_{O_2}}$s is not effective in greatly increasing the arterial oxygen content (except possibly in carbon monoxide poisoning).

Hypoperfusion Hypoxia

Hypoperfusion hypoxia (sometimes called *stagnant hypoxia*) results from low blood flow. This can occur either locally, in a particular vascular bed, or systemically, in the case of a low cardiac output. The alveolar P_{O_2} and the arterial P_{O_2} and oxygen content may be normal, but the reduced oxygen delivery to the tissues may result in tissue hypoxia. Venous P_{O_2} and oxygen content are low. Raising the $F_{I_{O_2}}$ is of little value in hypoperfusion hypoxia (unless it directly increases the perfusion) because the blood flowing to the tissues is already oxygenated normally.

Histotoxic Hypoxia

Histotoxic hypoxia refers to a poisoning of the cellular machinery that uses oxygen to produce energy. Cyanide, for example, binds to cytochrome oxidase in the respiratory chain and effectively blocks oxidative phosphorylation. Alveolar P_{O_2} and arterial P_{O_2} and oxygen content may be normal (or even *elevated*, because low doses of cyanide increase ventilation by stimulating the arterial chemoreceptors). Venous P_{O_2} and oxygen content are elevated because oxygen is not utilized.

Other Causes of Hypoxia

Tissue edema or fibrosis may result in impaired diffusion of oxygen from the blood to the tissues. It is also conceivable that the delivery of oxygen to a tissue is completely normal, but the tissue's metabolic demands still exceed the supply and tissue hypoxia could result. This is known as *overutilization hypoxia.*

The Effects of Hypoxia

Hypoxia can result in reversible tissue injury or even tissue death. The outcome of an hypoxic episode depends on whether the tissue hypoxia is generalized or localized, on how severe the hypoxia is, on the rate of development of the hypoxia (see Chapter 11), and on the duration of the hypoxia. Different cell types have different susceptibilities to hypoxia; unfortunately, brain cells and heart cells are the most susceptible.

KEY CONCEPTS

1. Hypoventilation causes **respiratory acidosis;** the compensation for respiratory acidosis is renal retention of base and excretion of hydrogen ions.

2. Hyperventilation causes **respiratory alkalosis;** the compensation for respiratory alkalosis is renal excretion of base and retention of hydrogen ions.

3. Ingestion, infusion, overproduction, or decreased renal excretion of hydrogen ions, or loss of bicarbonate ions, can cause **metabolic acidosis;** the compensation for metabolic acidosis is increased alveolar ventilation.

4. Ingestion, infusion, or excessive renal reabsorption of bases, or loss of hydrogen ions, can cause **metabolic alkalosis;** the compensation for metabolic alkalosis is decreased alveolar ventilation.

5. Metabolic acidosis with an abnormally elevated **anion gap** indicates an increased plasma concentration of anions other than chloride and bicarbonate or a decreased plasma concentration of potassium, calcium, or magnesium ions.

6. Tissue hypoxia can be a result of low alveolar P_{O_2}, diffusion impairment, right-to-left shunts, or ventilation-perfusion mismatch (**hypoxic hypoxia**); decreased functional hemoglobin (**anemic hypoxia**); low blood flow (**hypoperfusion hypoxia**); or an inability of the mitochondria to use oxygen (**histotoxic hypoxia**).

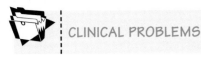

CLINICAL PROBLEMS

8–1 through 8–6: *Match each of the following sets of blood gas data to one of the underlying problems listed below. Assume the body temperature to be 37°C and the hemoglobin concentration to be 15 g Hb/100 mL blood. $F_{I_{O_2}}$ is 0.21 (room air).*

a. *Acute vomiting (10 minutes after vomiting)*

b. *Acute methanol ingestion*

c. *Diarrhea*

d. *Accidental hypoventilation of a patient on a mechanical ventilator for 10 minutes*

e. *Accidental hyperventilation of a patient on a mechanical ventilator for 10 minutes*

f. *Chronic obstructive pulmonary disease*

8–1. *pHa = 7.25*
Pa_{CO_2} = 50 mm Hg
$[HCO_3^-]$ = 26 mEq/L
Pa_{O_2} = 70 mm Hg
Anion gap = 11 mEq/L

8–2. *pHa = 7.47*
Pa_{CO_2} = 46 mm Hg
$[HCO_3^-]$ = 33 mEq/L
Pa_{O_2} = 85 mm Hg
Anion gap = 9 mEq/L

8–3. *pHa = 7.60*
Pa_{CO_2} = 20 mm Hg
$[HCO_3^-]$ = 20 mEq/L
Pa_{O_2} = 110 mm Hg
Anion gap = 12 mEq/L

8–4. *pHa = 7.34*
Pa_{CO_2} = 65 mm Hg
$[HCO_3^-]$ = 40 mEq/L
Pa_{O_2} = 65 mm Hg
Anion gap = 11 mEq/L

8–5. *pHa = 7.25*
Pa_{CO_2} = 30 mm Hg
$[HCO_3^-]$ = 15 mEq/L
Pa_{O_2} = 95 mm Hg
Anion gap = 10 mEq/L

8-6. $pHa = 7.25$
$Pa_{CO_2} = 30\ mm\ Hg$
$[HCO_3^-] = 15\ mEq/L$
$Pa_{O_2} = 95\ mm\ Hg$
Anion gap $= 25\ mEq/L$

Use the Pulmonary Function Test Decision Tree in the Appendix to help answer Questions 8-7 through 8-10.

8-7 and 8-8. A 68-year-old man complains of difficulty breathing. He says he has had the problem for a long time—in fact, he can't remember when it started—and it seems to be getting worse. He coughs frequently and sometimes produces sputum upon arising. He says that he has smoked at least one pack of cigarettes a day since he was 20 years old. He does not appear to be cyanotic.

The results of the patient's pulmonary function tests are shown below.

Lung Volumes (BTPS) (from body plethysmograph)		Pred	Actual	% Pred
VC	Liters	4.48	3.32	74
TLC	Liters	7.03	8.24	117
RV	Liters	2.63	4.91	186
RV/TLC	%	37	59	
FRC	Liters	4.67	7.07	151
ERV	Liters	2.03	2.16	106
IC	Liters	2.35	1.16	49

Dynamic Lung Volumes (BTPS)		Pred	Actual	% Pred
FVC	Liters	4.48	2.67	59
FEV_1	Liters	3.27	0.95	29
FEV_1/FVC	%	73	35	
FEV_3/FVC	%	97	63	
FEF_{25-75}	L/s	2.83	0.43	15
PEF	L/s	8.27	3.04	36

Diffusing Capacity	Pred	Actual	% Pred
D_{LCO} mL/min/mm Hg	25	10	40

8-7. The patient's pulmonary function tests are consistent with
a. Restrictive disease
b. Obstructive disease
c. Both
d. Neither

8–8. *The patient's dynamic lung volumes are not improved after the administration of a bronchodilator. The patient's disease is most likely*

   a. *Asthma*

   b. *Sarcoidosis*

   c. *COPD, primarily emphysema*

   d. *COPD, primarily chronic bronchitis*

   e. *Alveolar fibrosis*

8–9 and 8–10. *A 55-year-old man says he "can't catch his breath" when he jogs or does any physical work. He noticed the problem about 2 years ago, and it seems to be getting worse. He says he coughs a lot, but he doesn't spit anything up. He says he has never smoked, but he has worked in a chemical plant for many years. You note that he has a respiratory rate of 25 breaths per minute, with small tidal volumes. He does not appear to be cyanotic.*

The results of the patient's pulmonary function tests are shown below.

Lung Volumes (BTPS) (from body plethysmograph)		Pred	Actual	% Pred
VC	Liters	4.5	3.0	67
TLC	Liters	6.0	4.0	67
RV	Liters	1.5	1.0	67
RV/TLC	%	25	25	100
FRC	Liters	3.0	2.0	67
ERV	Liters	1.5	1.0	67
IC	Liters	2.5	1.7	68

Dynamic Lung Volumes (BTPS)		Pred	Actual	% Pred
FVC	Liters	4.5	3.0	67
FEV_1	Liters	3.6	2.7	75
FEV_1/FVC	%	80	90	113
FEV_3/FVC	%	97	98	101
FEF_{25-75}	L/s	2.5	2.6	104
PEF	L/s	8	7	88

Diffusing Capacity	Pred	Actual	% Pred
D_{LCO} mL/min/mm Hg	25	8	32

8–9. *The patient's pulmonary function tests are consistent with*

   a. *Restrictive disease*

   b. *Obstructive disease*

   c. *Both*

   d. *Neither*

8–10. *The patient's disease is most likely*

    a. COPD, primarily emphysema

    b. COPD, primarily chronic bronchitis

    c. Interstitial alveolar fibrosis

    d. Arthritis of the rib cage

    e. Respiratory muscle weakness

SUGGESTED READINGS

Davenport HW. *The ABC of Acid-Base Chemistry.* 6th ed. Chicago, Ill: University of Chicago Press; 1974.

Dejours P (translated by Farhi L). *Respiration.* New York, NY: Oxford University Press; 1966:54–56, 201–212.

Koeppen BM. Renal regulation of acid-base balance. *Adv Physiol Educ.* 1998;20:S132–S141.

Rose BD, Post TW. *Clinical Physiology of Acid-Base and Electrolyte Disorders.* 5th ed. New York, NY: McGraw-Hill; 2001.

Siggaard-Anderson O, Ulrich A, Gøthgen IH. Classes of tissue hypoxia. *Acta Anaesthesiol Scand.* 1995;39:S137–S142.

Vander AJ. *Renal Physiology.* 5th ed. New York, NY: McGraw-Hill; 1995:162–189.

The Control of Breathing

OBJECTIVES

The reader understands the organization and function of the respiratory control system.
- Describes the general organization of the respiratory control system.
- Localizes the centers that generate the spontaneous rhythmicity of breathing.
- Describes the groups of neurons that effect inspiration and expiration.
- Describes the other centers in the brainstem that may influence the spontaneous rhythmicity of breathing.
- Lists the cardiopulmonary and other reflexes that influence the breathing pattern.
- States the ability of the brain cortex to override the normal pattern of inspiration and expiration temporarily.
- Describes the effects of alterations in body oxygen, carbon dioxide, and hydrogen ion levels on the control of breathing.
- Describes the sensors of the respiratory system for oxygen, carbon dioxide, and hydrogen ion concentration.

Breathing is spontaneously initiated in the central nervous system. A cycle of inspiration and expiration is *automatically* generated by neurons located in the brainstem; in eupneic states, breathing occurs without a conscious initiation of inspiration and expiration. Normal individuals do not have to worry about forgetting to breathe while they sleep.

This spontaneously generated cycle of inspiration and expiration can be modified, altered, or even temporarily suppressed by a number of mechanisms. As shown in Figure 9–1, these include reflexes arising in the lungs, the airways, and the cardiovascular system; information from receptors in contact with the cerebrospinal fluid; and commands from higher centers of the brain such as the hypothalamus, the centers of speech, or other areas in the cortex. The centers that are responsible for the generation of the spontaneous rhythmicity of inspiration and expiration are, therefore, able to alter their activity to meet the increased metabolic demand on the respiratory system during exercise or may even be temporarily superseded or suppressed during speech or breath holding.

The respiratory control centers in the brainstem affect the automatic rhythmic control of breathing via a "final common pathway" consisting of the spinal cord, the innervation of the muscles of respiration such as the phrenic nerves, and the muscles of respiration themselves. Alveolar ventilation is therefore determined by the *interval* between successive groups of discharges of the respiratory neurons and the innervation of the muscles of respiration, which determines the respiratory *rate* or breathing frequency, and by the *frequency* of neural discharges transmitted by *individual* nerve fibers to their motor units, the *duration* of these discharges, and the *number of motor units activated* during each inspiration or expiration, which determine the *depth* of respiration or the tidal volume. Note that some pathways from the cerebral cortex to the muscles of respiration, such as those involved in voluntary breathing, bypass the medullary respiratory center described below and travel directly to the spinal α motorneurons. These are represented by the dashed line in Figure 9–1.

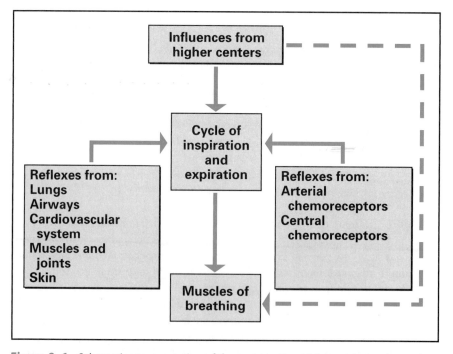

Figure 9–1. Schematic representation of the organization of the respiratory control system. A cycle of inspiration and expiration is automatically established in the medullary respiratory center. Its output represents a final common pathway to the respiratory muscles, except for some voluntary pathways that may go directly from higher centers to the respiratory muscles (dashed line). Reflex responses from chemoreceptors and other sensors may modify the cycle of inspiration and expiration established by the medullary respiratory center.

THE GENERATION OF SPONTANEOUS RHYTHMICITY

The centers that initiate breathing are located in the reticular formation of the medulla, beneath the floor of the fourth ventricle. If the brainstem of an anesthetized animal is sectioned *above* this area, as seen in the transection labeled III in Figure 9–2, a pattern of inspiration and expiration is maintained (although it is somewhat irregular) even if all other afferents to this area, including the vagi, are also severed. If the brainstem is transected *below* this area, as seen in the transection labeled IV in Figure 9–2, breathing ceases. This area, known as the *medullary center* (or medullary respiratory center), was originally believed to consist of two discrete groups of respiratory neurons: the *inspiratory neurons,* which fire during inspiration and the *expiratory neurons,* which fire during expiration.

Activity of the inspiratory neurons is presumably transmitted to the muscles of inspiration, initiating inspiration; activity of the expiratory neurons is presumably transmitted to the muscles of expiration, initiating expiration. It was thought that

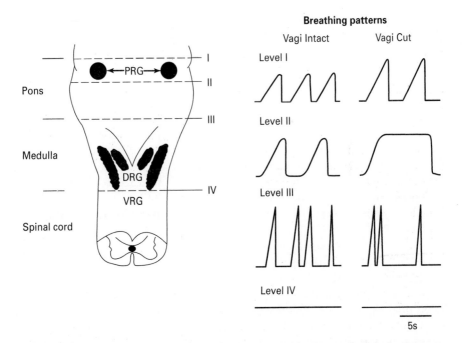

Figure 9–2. The effects of transections at different levels of the brainstem on the ventilatory pattern of anesthetized animals. **Left:** A schematic representation of the dorsal surface of the lower brainstem. **Right:** A schematic representation of the breathing patterns (inspiration is upward) corresponding to the transections with the vagus nerves intact or transected. PRG = pontine respiratory groups; DRG = dorsal respiratory group; VRG = ventral respiratory group. (From *Physiology of Respiration* by Michael P. Hlastala and Albert J. Berger, copyright © 1996 by Oxford University Press, Inc. Used by permission of Oxford University Press, Inc.)

when the inspiratory neurons discharged, their activity was conducted to the expiratory neuron pool via collateral fibers and the activity of the expiratory neurons was inhibited. Similarly, when the expiratory neurons discharged, their activity was conducted to the inspiratory neuron pool via collateral fibers, and the activity of the inspiratory neurons was inhibited. The *reciprocal inhibition* of these two opposing groups of neurons was believed to be the source of the spontaneous respiratory rhythmicity. More recent studies of the medullary center have not entirely supported this early hypothesis. Furthermore, because expiration is passive in normal quiet breathing, the expiratory neurons may not discharge unless expiration is active.

THE MEDULLARY RESPIRATORY CENTER

There are two dense bilateral aggregations of respiratory neurons in the medullary respiratory center known as the *dorsal respiratory groups* (DRG in Figures 9–2 and 9–3) and the *ventral respiratory groups* (VRG in Figures 9–2 and 9–3). Inspiratory and expiratory neurons are anatomically intermingled to a greater or lesser extent within these areas, and the medullary center does not consist of a discrete "inspiratory center" and a discrete "expiratory center."

The Dorsal Respiratory Group

The dorsal respiratory groups are located bilaterally in the *nucleus of the tractus solitarius* (NTS), as shown in Figure 9–3. They consist mainly of *inspiratory neurons*. These inspiratory neurons project primarily to the contralateral spinal cord. They probably serve as the principal initiators of the activity of the phrenic nerves and are therefore responsible for maintaining the activity of the diaphragm. Dorsal respiratory group neurons send many collateral fibers to those in the ventral respiratory group, but the ventral respiratory group sends only a few collateral fibers to the dorsal respiratory group, as will be discussed in the next section. Reciprocal inhibition therefore seems an unlikely explanation of spontaneous inspiratory and expiratory rhythmicity.

The NTS is the primary *projection site* of visceral afferent fibers of the ninth cranial nerve (the glossopharyngeal) and the tenth cranial nerve (the vagus). These nerves carry information about the arterial P_{O_2}, P_{CO_2}, and pH from the carotid and aortic arterial chemoreceptors and information concerning the systemic arterial blood pressure from the carotid and aortic baroreceptors. In addition, the vagus carries information from stretch receptors and other sensors in the lungs that may also exert profound influences on the control of breathing. The effects of information from these sensors on the control of breathing will be discussed in detail later in this chapter. The location of the DRG within the NTS suggests that it may be the site of integration of various inputs that can reflexly alter the spontaneous pattern of inspiration and expiration.

There are two populations of inspiratory neurons in the DRG, as shown in Figure 9–3. One population, called the *I α cells,* increase their activity if lung inflation is withheld; the second population, the *I β cells,* decrease their activity if lung

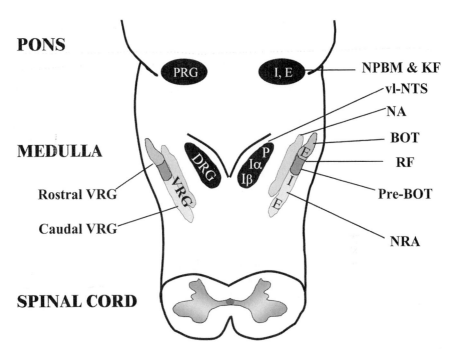

Figure 9–3. Location of pontine and medullary respiratory neuron aggregations (dorsal view of the brainstem). PRG = pontine respiratory group; I = inspiratory; E = expiratory; DRG = dorsal respiratory group; VRG = ventral respiratory group; P = pump cells; NPBM = nucleus parabrachialis medialis; KF = Kölliker-Fuse nucleus; vl-NTS = ventrolateral nucleus of the tractus solitarius; NA = nucleus ambiguus; BOT = Bötzinger complex; RF = retrofacial nucleus; Pre-Bot = pre-Bötzinger complex; NRA = nucleus retroambigualis.

inflation is withheld. These cells may play an important role in the Hering-Breuer reflexes described later in this chapter. A third population of cells, the P-cells (pump cells), appears to be interneurons involved in relaying afferent activity from pulmonary stretch receptors.

In summary, the DRG is probably responsible for driving the diaphragm and is probably the initial integrating site for many cardiopulmonary reflexes that affect the respiratory rhythm.

The Ventral Respiratory Group

The ventral respiratory groups are located bilaterally in the *retrofacial nucleus,* the *nucleus ambiguus,* and the *nucleus retroambigualis,* as shown in Figure 9–3. They consist of both inspiratory and expiratory neurons. The neurons in the nucleus ambiguus are primarily vagal motorneurons that innervate the ipsilateral laryngeal, pharyngeal, and tongue muscles involved in breathing and in maintaining the patency of the upper airway. They are both inspiratory and expiratory neurons. In the nucleus retroambigualis, the inspiratory cells appear to be located more rostrally

and the expiratory cells are located more caudally. There appear to be two populations of inspiratory cells in the nucleus retroambigualis: One group mainly projects
contralaterally to external intercostal muscles, with some fibers also sent to the
phrenic nerves, thus innervating the diaphragm; the second group appears to project only within the medulla to other inspiratory and expiratory cells. The expiratory
neurons in the nucleus retroambigualis project to the contralateral spinal cord to
drive the internal intercostal and abdominal muscles. The retrofacial nucleus,
located most rostrally in the ventral respiratory groups, mainly contains expiratory
neurons in a group of cells called the *Bötzinger complex*. This group of neurons has
been shown to inhibit inspiratory cells in the DRG, as well as some phrenic
motorneurons.

In summary, the VRG neurons consist of both inspiratory and expiratory cells.
Their major function is to drive either spinal respiratory neurons, innervating
mainly the intercostal and abdominal muscles, or the auxiliary muscles of respiration innervated by the vagus nerves. Many expiratory cells may not fire at all during the passive expirations seen in eupneic breathing (see Chapter 2); those that do
discharge do not cause contraction of the expiratory muscles. It now appears that
cells in the *pre-Bötzinger complex* probably act as pacemakers and establish the respiratory rhythm.

The "Apneustic Center"

If the brainstem is transected in the pons at the level denoted by the line labeled II
in Figure 9–2, a breathing pattern called *apneusis* results if the vagus nerves have
also been transected. Apneustic breathing consists of prolonged inspiratory efforts
interrupted by occasional expirations. Afferent information that reaches this so-
called *apneustic center* via the vagus nerves must be important in preventing apneusis because apneusis does not occur if the vagus nerves are intact, as shown
schematically in Figure 9–2.

Apneusis is probably caused by a sustained discharge of medullary inspiratory
neurons. Therefore, the apneustic center may be the site of the normal "inspiratory
cutoff switch"; that is, it is the site of projection and integration of various types of
afferent information that can *terminate inspiration*. Apneusis is a result of the inac-
tivation of the inspiratory cutoff mechanism. The specific group of neurons that
function as the apneustic center has not been identified, but it must be located
somewhere between the lines labeled II and III in Figure 9–2.

THE PONTINE RESPIRATORY GROUPS

If the brainstem is transected immediately caudal to the inferior colliculus, as
denoted by the line labeled I in Figure 9–2, the breathing pattern shows an essen-
tially normal balance between inspiration and expiration, even if the vagus nerves
are transected. As discussed in the previous section, transections made caudal to the
line labeled II in Figure 9–2 lead to apneusis in the absence of the vagus nerves. A
group of respiratory neurons known as the *pontine respiratory groups,* (formerly
called the *pneumotaxic center*) therefore functions to modulate the activity of the

apneustic center. These cells, located in the upper pons in the *nucleus parabrachialis medialis* and the *Kölliker-Fuse nucleus* (shown in Figure 9–3), probably function to "fine-tune" the breathing pattern. Electrical stimulation of these structures can result in synchronization of phrenic nerve activity with the stimulus or premature switching from inspiration to expiration and vice versa. Pulmonary inflation afferent information can inhibit the activity of the pontine respiratory groups, which may in turn act to modulate the threshold for lung inflation inspiratory cutoff. The pontine respiratory groups may also modulate the respiratory control system's response to other stimuli, such as hypercapnia and hypoxia.

SPINAL PATHWAYS

Axons projecting from the DRG, the VRG, the cortex, and other supraspinal sites descend in the spinal white matter to influence the diaphragm and the intercostal and abdominal muscles of respiration, as already discussed. At the level of these spinal respiratory motorneurons, there is integration of descending influences as well as the presence of local spinal reflexes that can affect these motorneurons. Descending axons with inspiratory activity excite phrenic and external intercostal motorneurons and also inhibit internal intercostal motorneurons by exciting spinal inhibitory interneurons. They are actively inhibited during expiratory phases of the respiratory cycle.

Ascending pathways in the spinal cord, carrying information from pain, touch, and temperature receptors, as well as from proprioceptors, can also influence breathing, as will be discussed in the next section. Inspiratory and expiratory fibers appear to be separated in the spinal cord.

REFLEX MECHANISMS OF RESPIRATORY CONTROL

A large number of sensors located in the lungs, the cardiovascular system, the muscles and tendons, and the skin and viscera can elicit reflex alterations in the control of breathing. These are summarized in Table 9–1.

Respiratory Reflexes Arising from Pulmonary Stretch Receptors

Three respiratory reflexes can be elicited by stimulation of the pulmonary stretch receptors: the Hering-Breuer inflation reflex, the Hering-Breuer deflation reflex, and the "paradoxical" reflex of Head.

THE HERING-BREUER INFLATION REFLEX

In 1868, Breuer and Hering reported that a maintained distention of the lungs of anesthetized animals decreased the frequency of the inspiratory effort or caused a transient apnea. The stimulus for this reflex is pulmonary inflation. The sensors are *stretch receptors* located within the smooth muscle of large and small airways. They are sometimes referred to as *slowly adapting pulmonary stretch receptors* because their activity is maintained with sustained stretches. The afferent pathway consists of large myelinated fibers in the vagus; as mentioned previously, these fibers appear to enter the brainstem and project to the DRGs, the apneustic center, and the pontine respiratory groups. The efferent limb of the reflex consists of bronchodilation in addition to the apnea or slowing of the ventilatory frequency (due to an increase in the time spent in expiration) already mentioned. Lung inflation also causes reflex effects in the cardiovascular system: Moderate lung inflations cause an increase in heart rate and may cause a slight vasoconstriction; very large inflations may cause a decrease in heart rate and systemic vascular resistance.

The Hering-Breuer inflation reflex was originally believed to be an important determinant of the rate and depth of ventilation. Vagotomized anesthetized animals breathe much more deeply and less frequently than they did before their vagus nerves were transected. It was therefore assumed that the Hering-Breuer inflation reflex acts tonically to limit the tidal volume and establish the depth and rate of breathing. More recent studies on unanesthetized humans have cast doubt on this conclusion because the central threshold of the reflex is much higher than the normal tidal volume during eupneic breathing. Tidal volumes of 800 to 1500 mL are generally required to elicit this reflex in conscious eupneic adults. The Hering-Breuer inflation reflex may help minimize the work of breathing by inhibiting large tidal volumes (see Chapter 2) as well as to prevent overdistention of the alveoli at large volumes. It may also be important in the control of breathing in babies. Infants have Hering-Breuer inflation reflex thresholds within their normal tidal volume ranges, and the reflex may be an important influence on their tidal volumes and respiratory rates.

THE HERING-BREUER DEFLATION REFLEX

Breuer and Hering also noted that abrupt *deflation* of the lungs increases the ventilatory rate. This could be a result of *decreased* stretch receptor activity or of stimulation of other pulmonary receptors, or rapidly adapting receptors such as the irritant receptors and J receptors, which will be discussed later in this chapter. The afferent pathway is the vagus, and the effect is hyperpnea. This reflex may be responsible for the increased ventilation elicited when the lungs are deflated abnormally, as in pneumothorax, or it may play a role in the periodic spontaneous deep breaths ("sighs") that help prevent atelectasis. These sighs occur occasionally and irregularly during the course of normal, quiet, spontaneous breathing. They consist of a slow deep inspiration (larger than a normal tidal volume) followed by a slow deep expiration. This response appears to be very important because patients maintained on mechanical ventilators must be given large tidal volumes or periodic deep breaths or they develop diffuse atelectasis, which may lead to arterial hypoxemia.

The Hering-Breuer deflation reflex may be very important in helping to *actively* maintain infants' functional residual capacities (FRCs). It is very unlikely that infants' FRCs are determined passively like those of adults because the inward recoil of their lungs is considerably greater than the outward recoil of their very compliant chest walls.

THE PARADOXICAL REFLEX OF HEAD

In 1889, Henry Head performed experiments designed to show the effects of the Hering-Breuer inflation reflex on the control of breathing. Instead of transecting

Table 9–1. Reflex Mechanisms of Respiratory Control

Stimulus	Reflex Name	Receptor	Afferent Pathway	Effects
Lung inflation	Hering-Breuer inflation reflex	Stretch receptors within smooth muscle of large and small airways	Vagus	Respiratory Cessation of inspiratory effort, apnea, or decreased breathing frequency; bronchodilation Cardiovascular Increased heart rate, slight vasoconstriction
Lung deflation	Hering-Breuer deflation reflex	Possibly J receptors, irritant receptors in lungs, or stretch receptors in airways	Vagus	Respiratory Hyperpnea
Lung inflation	Paradoxical reflex of Head	Stretch receptors in lungs	Vagus	Respiratory Inspiration
Negative pressure in the upper airway	Pharyngeal dilator reflex	Receptors in nose, mouth, upper airways	Trigeminal, laryngeal, glossopharyngeal	Respiratory Contraction of pharyngeal dilator muscles
Mechanical or chemical irritation of airways	Cough	Receptors in upper airways, tracheobronchial tree	Vagus	Respiratory Cough; bronchoconstriction
	Sneeze	Receptors in nasal mucosa	Trigeminal, olfactory	Sneeze; bronchoconstriction Cardiovascular Increased blood pressure
Face immersion*	Diving reflex	Receptors in nasal mucosa and face	Trigeminal	Respiratory Apnea Cardiovascular Decreased heart rate; vasoconstriction
Pulmonary embolism		J receptors in pulmonary vessels	Vagus	Respiratory Apnea or tachypnea

(Continued)

Table 9–1. Reflex Mechanisms of Respiratory Control (Continued)

Stimulus	Reflex Name	Receptor	Afferent Pathway	Effects
Pulmonary vascular congestion		J receptors in pulmonary vessels	Vagus	Respiratory Tachypnea, possibly sensation of dyspnea
Specific chemicals in the pulmonary circulation	Pulmonary chemoreflex	J receptors in pulmonary vessels	Vagus	Respiratory Apnea or tachypnea; bronchoconstriction
Low Pa_{O_2}, high Pa_{CO_2}, low pHa	Arterial chemoreceptor reflex	Carotid bodies, aortic bodies	Glossopharyngeal, vagus	Respiratory Hyperpnea; bronchoconstriction, dilation of upper airway Cardiovascular Decreased heart rate (direct effect), vasoconstriction
Increased systemic arterial blood pressure	Arterial baroreceptor reflex	Carotid sinus stretch receptors, aortic arch stretch receptors	Glossopharyngeal, vagus	Respiratory Apnea, bronchodilation Cardiovascular Decreased heart rate, vasodilation etc.
Stretch of muscles, tendons, movement of joints		Muscle spindles, tendon organs, proprioreceptors	Various spinal pathways	Respiratory Provide respiratory controller with feedback about work of breathing, stimulation of proprioreceptors in joints causes hyperpnea
Somatic pain		Pain receptors	Various spinal pathways	Respiratory Hyperpnea Cardiovascular Increased heart rate, vasoconstriction, etc.

*Discussed in Chap. 11.

the vagus nerves, he decided to block their function by cooling them to 0°C. As he rewarmed the vagus nerves, he noted that in the situation of a selective *partial* block of the vagus nerves, lung inflation caused a further inspiration instead of the apnea expected when the vagus nerves were completely functional. The receptors for this paradoxical reflex are located in the lungs, but their precise location is not known. Afferent information travels in the vagus; the effect is very deep inspirations. This reflex may also be involved in the sigh response, or it may be involved in generating the first breath of the newborn baby; very great inspiratory efforts must be generated to inflate the fluid-filled lungs.

Respiratory Reflexes Arising from Receptors in the Airways & the Lungs

THE PHARYNGEAL DILATOR REFLEX

As discussed in Chapter 2, negative pressure in the upper airway causes reflex contraction of the pharyngeal dilator muscles. The receptors appear to be located in the nose, mouth, and upper airways; the afferent pathways appear to be in the trigeminal, laryngeal, and glossopharyngeal nerves.

IRRITANT RECEPTORS

Mechanical or chemical irritation of the airways (and possibly the alveoli) can elicit a reflex cough or sneeze, or it can cause hyperpnea, bronchoconstriction, and increased blood pressure. The receptors are located in the nasal mucosa, upper airways, tracheobronchial tree, and possibly the alveoli themselves. Those in the larger airways of the tracheobronchial tree, which also respond to stretch, are sometimes referred to as *rapidly adapting pulmonary stretch receptors* because their activity decreases rapidly during a sustained stimulus. The afferent pathways are the vagus nerves for all but the receptors located in the nasal mucosa, which send information centrally via the trigeminal and olfactory tracts. The cough and the sneeze reflexes are discussed in greater detail in Chapter 10.

Respiratory Reflexes Arising from Pulmonary Vascular Receptors (J Receptors)

Pulmonary embolism causes apnea or rapid shallow breathing (tachypnea); pulmonary vascular congestion causes tachypnea. Injection of chemicals such as phenyldiguanide and capsaicin into the pulmonary circulation may also elicit apnea or rapid shallow breathing. The receptors responsible for initiating these responses are believed to be located in the walls of the pulmonary capillaries or in the interstitium; therefore, they are called *J* (for juxtapulmonary-capillary) *receptors.* Stimulation of these receptors by pulmonary vascular congestion or an increase in pulmonary interstitial fluid volume leads to tachypnea; decreased stimulation of the receptors caused by pulmonary emboli obstructing vessels *proximal* to the capillaries leads to decreased ventilation. In addition, these receptors might be responsible for the *dyspnea* (a feeling of difficult or labored breathing) encountered during the pulmonary vascular congestion and edema secondary to left ventricular failure or even the dyspnea that healthy people feel at the onset of exercise. The afferent pathway of these reflexes is slow-conducting nonmyelinated vagal fibers. Other possible causes of dyspnea are shown in Table 9–2.

Respiratory Reflexes Arising from the Cardiovascular System

The arterial chemoreceptors, and to a much lesser extent the arterial baroreceptors, can exert a great influence on the respiratory control system. The role of the arterial chemoreceptors in the control of ventilation will be discussed in greater detail in subsequent sections of this chapter and will only be briefly summarized here.

ARTERIAL CHEMORECEPTORS

The arterial chemoreceptors are located bilaterally in the carotid bodies, which are situated near the bifurcations of the common carotid arteries, and in the aortic bodies, which are located in the arch of the aorta. They respond to low arterial P_{O_2}s, high arterial P_{CO_2}s, and low arterial pHs, with the carotid bodies generally capable of a greater response than the aortic bodies. The afferent pathway from the carotid body is Hering's nerve, a branch of the glossopharyngeal nerve;

Table 9–2. Stimuli Postulated to Produce Dyspnea

Stimulus	Receptors	Example of Clinical Disease
Vascular stimuli		
Right atrial pressure	Right atrial stretch receptors	Congestive heart failure
Right ventricular pressure	Right ventricular strain receptors	Congestive heart failure Pulmonary stenosis
Pulmonary artery pressure	Pulmonary artery stretch receptors	Primary pulmonary hypertension
Left atrial pressure	Left atrial stretch receptors	Mitral valve disease
Mechanical stimuli		
Respiratory muscle length-tension inappropriateness	Muscle spindles	Pleural effusion, Pneumothorax
Pulmonary hyperinflation	Stretch receptors (vagal)	Bullous emphysema
Deformation of lung interstitium	J receptors (vagal)	Pulmonary edema Pneumonia
Humoral stimuli		
Hypoxemia	Carotid bodies	Lung diseases
Hypercapnia	Carotid bodies Central chemoreceptors	Chronic obstructive lung disease
Acidosis	Carotid bodies Central chemoreceptors	Cardiovascular
Movement of extremities	Mechanoreceptors Metaboreceptors	None reported
Psychogenic	Cerebral cortex	Psychoneurosis

Reproduced with permission from Wasserman and Casaburi, *Annual Review of Medicine,* vol 39, © 1988 by Annual Reviews, Inc.

the afferent pathway from the aortic body is the vagus. The reflex effects of stimulation of the arterial chemoreceptors are hyperpnea, bronchoconstriction, dilation of the *upper* airway, and increased blood pressure. The *direct* effect of arterial chemoreceptor stimulation is a decrease in heart rate; however, this is usually masked by an increase in heart rate secondary to the increase in lung inflation.

ARTERIAL BARORECEPTORS

The arterial baroreceptors exert a minor influence on the control of ventilation. Baroreceptors are stretch receptors that are responsive to changes in pressure. They are located in the carotid sinuses, which are situated at the origin of the internal carotid arteries near the bifurcation of the common carotid arteries, and in the aortic arch. The afferent pathways are Hering's nerve and the glossopharyngeal nerve for the carotid baroreceptors and the vagus nerve for the aortic baroreceptors. The effects of stimulation of the arterial baroreceptors by elevated blood pressure are a brief apnea and bronchodilation.

Respiratory Reflexes Arising from Muscles & Tendons

Stimulation of receptors located in the muscles, the tendons, and the joints can increase ventilation. Included are receptors in the muscles of respiration (e.g., muscle spindles) and rib cage as well as other skeletal muscles, joints, and tendons. These receptors may play an important role in adjusting the ventilatory effort to elevated workloads and may help minimize the work of breathing. They may also participate in initiating and maintaining the elevated ventilation that occurs during exercise, as will be discussed later in this chapter. Afferent information ascends to the respiratory controller via the spinal cord, as mentioned previously in this chapter.

Reflex Respiratory Responses to Pain

Somatic pain generally causes hyperpnea; visceral pain generally causes apnea or decreased ventilation.

INFLUENCES OF HIGHER CENTERS

The spontaneous rhythmicity generated in the medullary respiratory center can be completely overwhelmed (at least temporarily) by influences from higher brain centers. In fact, the greatest minute ventilations obtainable from healthy conscious human subjects can be attained *voluntarily,* exceeding those obtained with the stimuli of severe exercise, hypercapnia, or hypoxia. This is the underlying concept of the maximum voluntary ventilation (MVV) test often used to assess the respiratory system. Conversely, the respiratory rhythm can be *completely* suppressed for *several minutes* by voluntary breath holding, until the chemical drive to respiration (high P_{CO_2} and low P_{O_2} and pH) overwhelms the voluntary suppression of breathing at the "breakpoint."

During speech, singing, or playing a wind instrument, the normal cycle of inspiration and expiration is automatically modified by higher brain centers.

In certain emotional states, chronic hyperventilation severe enough to cause respiratory alkalosis may occur, as was discussed in Chapter 8.

THE RESPONSE TO CARBON DIOXIDE

The respiratory control system normally reacts very effectively to alterations in the internal "chemical" environment of the body. Changes in the body P_{CO_2}, pH, and P_{O_2} result in alterations in alveolar ventilation designed to return these variables to their normal values. Special neuronal units called *chemoreceptors* alter their activity when their own local chemical environment changes and can therefore supply the central respiratory controller with the afferent information necessary to make the proper adjustments in alveolar ventilation to change the whole-body P_{CO_2}, pH, and P_{O_2}. The respiratory control system therefore functions as a *negative-feedback system.*

The arterial and cerebrospinal fluid partial pressures of carbon dioxide are probably the most important inputs to the ventilatory control system in establishing the breath-to-breath levels of tidal volume and ventilatory frequency. (Of course, changes in carbon dioxide lead to changes in hydrogen ion concentration, and so the effects of these two stimuli can be difficult to separate.) An elevated level of carbon dioxide is a very powerful stimulus to ventilation: Only voluntary hyperventilation and the hyperpnea of exercise can surpass the minute ventilations obtained with hypercapnia. However, the arterial P_{CO_2} is so precisely controlled that it changes little (< 1 mm Hg) during exercise severe enough to increase metabolic carbon dioxide production 10-fold.

Acutely increasing the levels of carbon dioxide in the inspired air (the FI_{CO_2}) increases the minute ventilation. The effect is most pronounced in FI_{CO_2}s in the range of 0.05 to 0.10 (5% to 10% CO_2 in inspired gas), which produces alveolar P_{CO_2}s between about 40 and 70 mm Hg. Above 10% to 15% CO_2 in inspired air, there is little further increase in alveolar ventilation: Very high arterial P_{CO_2}s (> 70 to 80 mm Hg) may directly produce respiratory depression. (Very *low* arterial P_{CO_2}s caused by hyperventilation may temporarily cause apnea because of decreased ventilatory drive. Metabolically produced carbon dioxide will then build up and restore breathing.)

The physiologic response to elevated carbon dioxide is dependent on its concentration. Low concentrations of carbon dioxide in the inspired air are easily tolerated, with an increase in ventilation the main effect. Higher levels cause dyspnea, severe headaches secondary to the cerebral vasodilation caused by the elevated Pa_{CO_2}, restlessness, faintness, and dulling of consciousness, in addition to greatly elevated alveolar ventilation. A loss of consciousness, muscular rigidity, and tremors occur at inspired CO_2 concentrations greater than 15%. With 20% to 30% inspired carbon dioxide, generalized convulsions are produced almost immediately.

The ventilatory response of a normal conscious person to physiologic levels of carbon dioxide is shown in Figure 9–4. Inspired concentrations of carbon dioxide or metabolically produced carbon dioxide producing alveolar (and arterial) P_{CO_2}s in the range of 38 to 50 mm Hg increase alveolar ventilation linearly. The slope of the line is quite steep; it varies from person to person,

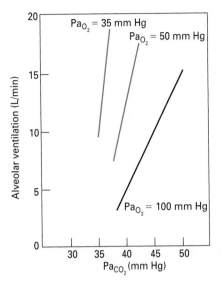

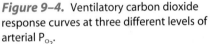

Figure 9–4. Ventilatory carbon dioxide response curves at three different levels of arterial P_{O_2}.

with a mean slope of 2.0 to 2.5 L/min per mm Hg Pa_{CO_2} for younger healthy adults. The slope decreases with age.

Figure 9–4 also shows that *hypoxia* potentiates the ventilatory response to carbon dioxide. At lower arterial P_{O_2}s (e.g., 35 and 50 mm Hg), the response curve is shifted to the left and the slope is steeper. That is, for any particular arterial P_{CO_2}, the ventilatory response is greater at a lower arterial P_{O_2}. This may be caused by the effects of hypoxia at the chemoreceptor itself or at higher integrating sites; changes in the central acid-base status secondary to hypoxia may also contribute to the enhanced response.

Other influences on the carbon dioxide response curve are illustrated in Figure 9–5. Sleep shifts the curve slightly to the right. The arterial P_{CO_2} normally increases during slow-wave sleep, rising as much as 5 to 6 mm Hg during deep sleep. Because of this rightward shift in the CO_2 response curve during non-REM sleep and other evidence, it is possible that there is a "wakefulness" component of respiratory drive. During non-REM sleep, chemoreceptor input would therefore constitute the sole respiratory drive. A depressed response to carbon dioxide during sleep may be involved in central sleep apnea, a condition characterized by abnormally long periods (1 to 2 min) between breaths during sleep. This lack of central respiratory drive is a potentially dangerous condition in both infants and adults. (In *obstructive sleep apnea* the central respiratory controller does issue the command to breathe, but the upper airway is obstructed because the pharyngeal muscles do not contract properly, there is too much fat around the pharynx, or the tongue blocks the airway.) Narcotics and anesthetics may profoundly depress the ventilatory response to carbon dioxide. Indeed, respiratory depression is the most common cause of death in cases of overdose of opiate alkaloids and their derivatives, barbiturates, and most anesthetics. Endorphins also depress the response to carbon dioxide.

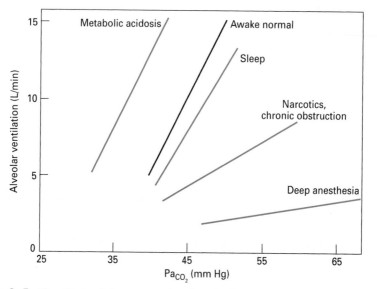

Figure 9–5. The effects of sleep, narcotics, chronic obstructive pulmonary disease, deep anesthesia, and metabolic acidosis on the ventilatory response to carbon dioxide.

Chronic obstructive lung diseases depress the ventilatory response to hypercapnia, in part because of depressed ventilatory drive secondary to central acid-base changes, and because the work of breathing may be so great that ventilation cannot be increased normally. Metabolic acidosis displaces the carbon dioxide response curve to the left, indicating that for any particular Pa_{CO_2}, ventilation is increased during metabolic acidosis.

As already discussed, the respiratory control system constitutes a negative-feedback system. This is exemplified by the response to carbon dioxide. Increased *metabolic production* of carbon dioxide increases the carbon dioxide brought to the lung. If alveolar ventilation stayed constant, the alveolar P_{CO_2} would increase, as would arterial and cerebrospinal P_{CO_2}. This stimulates alveolar ventilation. Increased alveolar ventilation decreases alveolar and arterial P_{CO_2}, as was discussed in Chapter 3 (see Figure 3–10), returning the P_{CO_2} to the original value, as shown in Figure 9–6.

The curve labeled A in Figure 9–6 shows the effect of increasing ventilation (here $\dot{V}_I$, or the inspired minute volume in liters per minute) on the arterial P_{CO_2}. Note that the independent variable for curve A is on the *ordinate* and that the dependent variable is on the abscissa. This graph is really the same as that shown in the upper part of Figure 3–10. Curve B is the steady-state ventilatory response to elevated arterial P_{CO_2}s as obtained by increasing the percentage of inspired carbon dioxide—that is, it is a typical CO_2 response curve (like that seen in Figure 9–4). The point at which the two curves cross is the "set point" for the system, normally a Pa_{CO_2} of 40 mm Hg.

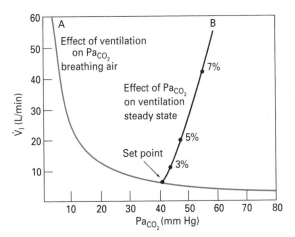

Figure 9–6. *Curve A:* The effect of ventilation on the arterial P_{CO_2}. Note that ventilation is the independent variable and Pa_{CO_2} is the dependent variable. *Curve B:* The steady-state ventilatory response to elevated Pa_{CO_2} as obtained by breathing carbon dioxide mixtures. (From Berger, 1977. Reprinted by permission of the New England Journal of Medicine.)

As can be seen in Figure 9–7, the respiratory control system constitutes a negative-feedback system, with the P_{CO_2}, pH, and P_{O_2} the controlled variables. To act as a negative-feedback system, the respiratory controller must receive information concerning the levels of the controlled variables from sensors in the system. These sensors, or chemoreceptors, are located within the systemic arterial system and within the brain itself. The arterial chemoreceptors, which are often referred to as the *peripheral chemoreceptors,* are located in the carotid and aortic bodies; the *central chemoreceptors* are located bilaterally near the ventrolateral surface of the medulla in the brainstem. Recent studies have suggested that there may be other central chemoreceptor sites in the brainstem (e.g., near the dorsal surface in the vicinities of the NTS and the locus coeruleus). The peripheral chemoreceptors are exposed to arterial blood; the central chemoreceptors are exposed to cerebrospinal fluid. The central chemoreceptors are therefore on the *brain* side of the blood-brain barrier. Both the peripheral and central chemoreceptors respond to elevations in the partial pressure of carbon dioxide, although the response may be related to the local increase in hydrogen ion concentration that occurs with elevated P_{CO_2}. That is, the sensors may be responding to the increased carbon dioxide concentration, the subsequent increase in hydrogen ion concentration, or both.

Peripheral Chemoreceptors

The peripheral chemoreceptors increase their firing rate in response to increased arterial P_{CO_2}, decreased arterial P_{O_2}, or decreased arterial pH. There is considerable impulse traffic in the afferent fibers from the arterial chemoreceptors at normal

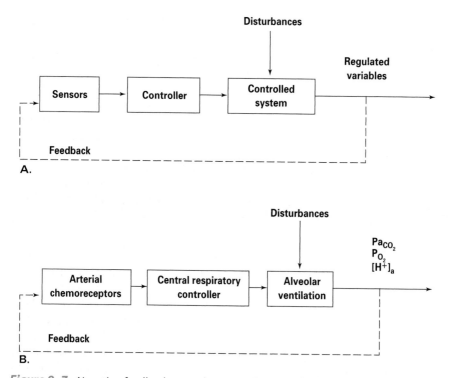

Figure 9–7. Negative-feedback control systems. **A:** General scheme of a negative-feedback control system. **B:** How the respiratory control system works as a negative-feedback control system. Note that the central chemoreceptors also act as sensors for the respiratory control system, with the P_{CO_2} and pH of the cerebrospinal fluid the regulated variables that feed back to the sensors.

levels of arterial P_{O_2}, P_{CO_2}, and pH. The response of the receptors is both rapid enough and sensitive enough that they can relay information concerning breath-to-breath alterations in the composition of the arterial blood to the medullary respiratory center. Recordings made of afferent fiber activity have demonstrated increased impulse traffic in a single fiber to increased P_{CO_2} and decreased pH and P_{O_2}, although the sensors themselves may not react to all three stimuli. The carotid bodies appear to exert a much greater influence on the respiratory controller than do the aortic bodies, especially with respect to decreased P_{O_2} and pH; the aortic bodies may exert a greater influence on the cardiovascular system. Increased concentrations of potassium ions in the arterial blood can also stimulate the arterial chemoreceptors.

The response of the arterial chemoreceptors changes *nearly linearly* with the arterial P_{CO_2} over the range of 20 to 60 mm Hg. The exact mechanism by which the chemoreceptors function is uncertain. The carotid body has a very great blood flow (estimated to be as great as 2000 mL/100 g of tissue per minute) and a very small arteriovenous oxygen difference (about 0.5 mL O_2/100 mL blood) even though it has one of the highest metabolic rates in the body. Certain drugs and enzyme poisons that block the cytochrome chain or the formation of adenosine triphosphate (ATP) stimulate the carotid body. For example, both cyanide and dinitrophenol stimulate the carotid body; this may be related to the stimulatory effect of hypoxia on the arterial chemoreceptors. Some studies have shown two different types of cytochrome a_3, with different oxygen affinities, to be present in the carotid body. Ganglionic stimulators such as nicotine also stimulate the carotid body. The mechanism for transducing low arterial P_{O_2}, like that of hypoxic pulmonary vasoconstriction, may involve inhibiting the permeability of the chemosensitive cells to potassium ions. This would decrease the outward flux of potassium ions and lead to depolarization of the chemoreceptors. Heme oxygenase in the cytochromes of mitochondria in the *glomus cells* of the chemoreceptors may also be involved in the transduction process.

Central Chemoreceptors

The central chemoreceptors are exposed to the cerebrospinal fluid and are not in direct contact with the arterial blood. As shown in Figure 9–8, the cerebrospinal fluid is separated from the arterial blood by the blood-brain barrier. Carbon dioxide can easily diffuse through the blood-brain barrier, but hydrogen ions and bicarbonate ions do not. Because of this, alterations in the arterial P_{CO_2} are rapidly transmitted to the cerebrospinal fluid, with a time constant of about 60 seconds. Changes in arterial pH that are not caused by changes in P_{CO_2} take much longer to influence the cerebrospinal fluid; in fact, the cerebrospinal fluid may have changes in hydrogen ion concentration *opposite* to those seen in the blood in certain circumstances, as will be discussed later in this chapter.

The composition of the cerebrospinal fluid is considerably different from that of the blood. It is formed mainly in the choroid plexus of the lateral ventricles. Enzymes, including carbonic anhydrase, play a large role in cerebrospinal fluid formation: The cerebrospinal fluid is not merely an ultrafiltrate of the plasma. The pH of the cerebrospinal fluid is normally about 7.32, compared with the pH of 7.40 of arterial blood. The P_{CO_2} of the cerebrospinal fluid is about 50 mm Hg—about 10 mm Hg higher than the normal arterial P_{CO_2} of 40 mm Hg. The concentration of proteins in the cerebrospinal fluid is only in the range of 15 to 45 mg/100 mL, whereas the concentration of proteins in the *plasma* normally ranges from 6.6 to 8.6 g/100 mL. This does not even include the hemoglobin in the erythrocytes. Bicarbonate is therefore the only buffer of consequence in the cerebrospinal fluid, and the buffer line of the cerebrospinal fluid is lower than and not as steep as that of the blood. Arterial hypercapnia will therefore lead to greater changes in cerebrospinal fluid hydrogen ion concentration than it does in the arterial blood. The brain produces carbon dioxide as an end product of metabolism. Brain carbon dioxide levels are higher than those of the arterial blood, which explains the high P_{CO_2} of the cerebrospinal fluid.

The central chemoreceptors respond to local increases in hydrogen ion concentration or P_{CO_2}, or both. They do not respond to hypoxia.

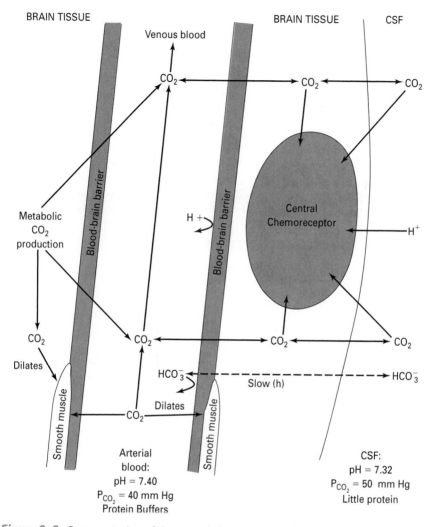

Figure 9–8. Representation of the central chemoreceptor showing its relationship to carbon dioxide (CO_2), hydrogen (H^+), and bicarbonate (HCO_3^-) ions in the arterial blood and cerebrospinal fluid (CSF). CO_2 crosses the blood-brain barrier easily; H^+s and HCO_3^-s do not.

The relative contributions of the peripheral and central chemoreceptors in the ventilatory response to elevated carbon dioxide levels are dependent on the time frame considered. Animals experimentally deprived of the afferent fibers from the arterial chemoreceptors and patients with surgically removed carotid bodies show about 80% to 90% of the normal total *steady-state* response to elevated inspired carbon dioxide concentrations delivered in hyperoxic gas mixtures, indicating that the peripheral chemoreceptors contribute only 10% to 20% of the steady-state response.

Other studies performed on normoxic men indicate that up to one third or one half of the *onset* of the response can come from the arterial chemoreceptors when rapid changes in arterial P_{CO_2} are made. That is, the central chemoreceptors may be mainly responsible for establishing the resting ventilatory level or the long-term response to carbon dioxide inhalation, but the peripheral chemoreceptors may be very important in short-term transient responses to carbon dioxide. Another author proposed that the arterial chemoreceptors monitor alveolar ventilation by detecting arterial P_{CO_2} and pH (and P_{O_2}), whereas the central chemoreceptors monitor the balance of arterial P_{CO_2}, cerebral blood flow, and cerebral metabolism by detecting the interstitial pH of the brain. Many researchers believe that both the arterial and central chemoreceptors respond to hydrogen ion concentration, not P_{CO_2}. Of course they are usually very closely related in the body so it is difficult to distinguish their effects.

Recent investigations have implicated other sensors for carbon dioxide in the body that may influence the control of ventilation. Chemoreceptors within the pulmonary circulation or airways have been proposed but have not as yet been substantiated or localized.

THE RESPONSE TO HYDROGEN IONS

Ventilation increases nearly linearly with changes in hydrogen ion concentration over the range of 20 to 60 nEq/L, as shown in Figure 9–9. As explained in Table 9–3, a metabolic acidosis of nonbrain origin results in hyperpnea coming almost entirely from the peripheral chemoreceptors. Hydrogen ions cross the blood-brain barrier too slowly to affect the central chemoreceptors initially. Acidotic stimulation of the peripheral chemoreceptors increases alveolar ventilation, and the arterial P_{CO_2} falls. Because the cerebrospinal fluid P_{CO_2} is in a sort of dynamic equilibrium with the arterial P_{CO_2}, carbon dioxide diffuses out of

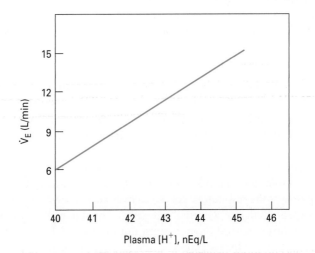

Figure 9–9. The ventilatory response to increased plasma hydrogen ion concentration.

Table 9–3. Effects of Metabolic Acidosis (of Nonbrain Origin) on Arterial and Central Chemoreceptor Ventilatory Drive

	Arterial Blood			Cerebrospinal Fluid		
	pH	P_{CO_2}	Arterial Chemo-receptor Drive	pH	P_{CO_2}	Central Chemo-receptor Drive
Initial acidosis	↓↓	Normal	↑↑	Normal	Normal	Normal
Ventilatory compensation for arterial acidosis	↓	↓↓	↑	Normal	Normal	Normal
"Diffusion" of CO_2 from CSF to blood	↓	↓↓	↑	↑	↓	↓

CSF = cerebrospinal fluid.

the cerebrospinal fluid and the pH of the cerebrospinal fluid *increases,* thus decreasing stimulation of the central chemoreceptor. If the situation lasts a long time (hours to days), the bicarbonate concentration of the cerebrospinal fluid falls slowly, returning the pH of the cerebrospinal fluid toward the normal 7.32. The mechanism by which this occurs is not completely agreed on. It may represent the slow diffusion of bicarbonate ions across the blood-brain barrier, active transport of bicarbonate ions out of the cerebrospinal fluid, or decreased *formation* of bicarbonate ions by carbonic anhydrase as the cerebrospinal fluid is formed.

Similar mechanisms must alter the bicarbonate concentration in the cerebrospinal fluid in the chronic respiratory acidosis of chronic obstructive lung disease because the pH of the cerebrospinal fluid is nearly normal. In this case the cerebrospinal fluid concentration of bicarbonate increases nearly proportionately to its increased concentration of carbon dioxide.

THE RESPONSE TO HYPOXIA

The ventilatory response to hypoxia arises solely from the peripheral chemoreceptors. The carotid bodies are much more important in this response than are the aortic bodies, which are not capable of sustaining the ventilatory response to hypoxia by themselves. In the absence of the peripheral chemoreceptors, the effect of increasing degrees of hypoxia is a progressive direct *depression* of the central respiratory controller. Therefore, when the peripheral chemoreceptors are intact, their excitatory influence on the central respiratory controller must offset the direct depressant effect of hypoxia.

The response of the respiratory system to hypoxia is shown in Figure 9–10. The figure shows that at a normal arterial P_{CO_2} of about 38 to 40 mm Hg, there is very little increase in ventilation until the arterial P_{O_2} falls below about 50 to 60 mm Hg. As expected, the response to hypoxia is potentiated at higher arterial P_{CO_2}s.

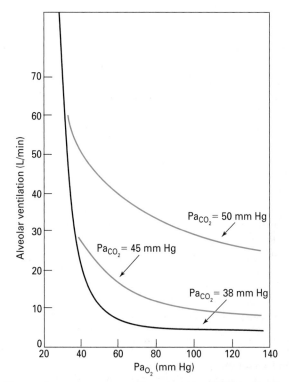

Figure 9–10. The ventilatory responses to hypoxia at three different levels of arterial P_{CO_2}.

Experiments have shown that the respiratory response to hypoxia is related to the change in P_{O_2} rather than the change in *oxygen content.* Therefore, anemia (without acidosis) does not stimulate ventilation because the arterial P_{O_2} is normal and the arterial chemoreceptors are not stimulated.

Hypoxia alone, by stimulating alveolar ventilation, causes a decrease in arterial P_{CO_2}, which may lead to respiratory alkalosis. This will be discussed in the section on altitude in Chapter 11.

THE RESPONSE TO EXERCISE

Exercise increases oxygen consumption and carbon dioxide production; the ventilatory control system must adjust to meet these increased demands. Minute ventilation increases with the level of exercise; it increases linearly with both oxygen consumption and carbon dioxide production up to a level of about 60% of the subject's maximal work capacity. Above that level, minute ventilation increases faster than oxygen consumption but continues to rise proportionally to the increase in carbon dioxide production. This increase in ventilation above oxygen consumption at high work levels is caused by the increased lactic acid production that occurs as a result of anaerobic metabolism. The hydrogen ions liberated in this process can stimulate the arterial chemoreceptors directly; the buffering of hydrogen ions by bicarbonate ions also results in production of carbon dioxide in addition to that derived from aerobic metabolism.

The ventilatory response to constant work-rate exercise consists of three phases. At the beginning of exercise there is an *immediate* increase in ventilation. This is followed by a phase of slowly increasing ventilation, ultimately rising to a final steady-state phase if the exercise is not too severe. The initial immediate increase in ventilation may constitute as much as 50% of the total steady-state response, although it is usually a smaller fraction of the total.

The increase in minute ventilation is usually a result of increases in both tidal volume and breathing frequency. Initially, the tidal volume increases more than the rate, but as metabolic acidosis develops, the increase in breathing frequency predominates.

The mechanisms by which exercise increases minute ventilation remain controversial. They are summarized in Table 9–4. No single factor can fully account for the ventilatory response to exercise, and much of the response is unexplained. The immediate increase in ventilation occurs too quickly to be a response to alterations in metabolism or changes in the blood gases. This "neural component" partly consists

Table 9–4. Ventilatory Response to Exercise

Immediate Response—"neural component"
  Central command
    Learned or conditioned reflex
    Direct connections from motor cortex—collaterals from motor neurons to muscles
    Coordination in hypothalamus
  Proprioceptors or mechanoreceptors in limbs—probably not muscle spindles or Golgi tendon organs
Subsequent Increase
  During moderate exercise
    Arterial chemoreceptors
      P_{O_2}—usually no change in mean
      P_{CO_2}—usually no change in mean
      $[H^+]$—usually no change unless cross anaerobic threshold
      $[K^+]$—minor role
      Oscillations in arterial P_{O_2} and P_{CO_2}
    Metaboreceptors
    Nociceptors—H^+, K^+, bradykinin, arachidonic acid
    Cardiac receptors
    Venous chemoreceptor
    Temperature receptors
  During exercise severe enough to exceed anaerobic threshold
    Lactic acid buffered by HCO_3^- produces CO_2
      Arterial chemoreceptors
        ↑ P_{CO_2}
        ↑ $[H^+]$
      Central chemoreceptors
        ↑ P_{CO_2} → ↑ H^+
      Potentiation of chemoreceptor responses during exercise

of collateral fibers to the respiratory muscles from the motor cortex neurons inner-vating the exercising skeletal muscles and may also be partly accounted for by a con-ditioned reflex, that is, a learned response to exercise. Experiments have also demonstrated that input to the respiratory centers from proprioceptors located in the joints and muscles of the exercising limbs may play a large role in the ventilatory response to exercise. Passive movements of the limbs of anesthetized animals or con-scious human subjects cause an increase in ventilation. The ventilatory and cardio-vascular responses to exercise may be coordinated (and in part initiated) in an "exercise center" in the hypothalamus.

The arterial chemoreceptors do not appear to play a role in the initial immediate ventilatory response to exercise. In mild or moderate exercise (that below the point at which anaerobic metabolism plays a role in energy supply), mean arterial P_{CO_2} and P_{O_2} remain relatively constant, even during the increasing ventilation phase (the "humoral component"), and may actually improve. It is therefore unlikely that hypercapnic or hypoxic stimulation of the arterial chemoreceptors is important in the ventilatory response to exercise in this situation. Nevertheless, patients who have had their carotid bodies surgically removed for medical reasons do show a slower increase in ventilation during the second phase of constant work-rate exercise, even in the absence of lactic acidosis. It is possible that the arterial chemoreceptors are responding to greater *oscillations* in the blood gases during exercise, despite relatively constant mean Pa_{CO_2}s and Pa_{O_2}s. During exercise levels above the "anaerobic thresh-old," these patients do not further increase their ventilation despite metabolic aci-dosis, indicating the importance of the peripheral chemoreceptors in this portion of the response. Another possibility is that elevated arterial potassium concentration causes stimulation of the arterial chemoreceptors. Potassium ions are released into the interstitium during the action potentials of the exercising skeletal muscle, enter the venous blood, and travel through the pulmonary capillaries into the arterial blood, where they can stimulate the arterial chemoreceptors.

Several investigators have suggested that there may be receptors in the pulmonary circulation that could respond to an increased carbon dioxide load in the mixed venous blood or in the heart that could respond to the increased cardiac output or increased cardiac work. Others have proposed that receptors in the exercising muscles that respond to the metabolites released during exercise, some of which can stimulate pain receptors (nociceptors), may send information about the increased muscle metabolism to the respiratory controllers. Thus far, these "mixed venous chemoreceptors" and "metaboreceptors" have not been demonstrated conclusively. The increase in body temperature that occurs during exercise may also contribute to the ventilatory response.

KEY CONCEPTS

*A cycle of inspiration and expiration is **automatically** generated by neurons in the medulla; this cycle can be modified or temporarily suppressed by reflexes or influ-ences from higher brain centers.*

The respiratory control system functions as a **negative-feedback** system; arterial P_{O_2}, P_{CO_2}, and pH and cerebrospinal fluid P_{CO_2} and pH are the regulated variables.

The increases in alveolar ventilation in response to increases in arterial P_{CO_2} and hydrogen ion concentrations are nearly linear within their normal ranges; the increase in alveolar ventilation in response to decreases in arterial P_{O_2} is small near the normal range and very large when the P_{O_2} falls below 50 to 60 mm Hg.

The **arterial chemoreceptors** rapidly respond to changes in arterial P_{O_2}, P_{CO_2}, and pH; the **central chemoreceptors** are on the brain side of the blood-brain barrier and respond to changes in cerebrospinal fluid P_{CO_2} and pH.

CLINICAL PROBLEMS

9–1. Voluntary apnea for 90 seconds will
   a. Increase arterial P_{CO_2}
   b. Decrease arterial P_{O_2}
   c. Stimulate the arterial chemoreceptors
   d. Stimulate the central chemoreceptors
   e. All of the above

9–2. Which of the following conditions would be expected to stimulate the arterial chemoreceptors?
   a. Mild anemia
   b. Severe exercise
   c. Hypoxia due to ascent to high altitude
   d. Acute airway obstruction
   e. Large intrapulmonary shunts

9–3. Stimulation of which of the following receptors should result in decreased ventilation?
   a. Aortic chemoreceptors
   b. Carotid chemoreceptors
   c. Central chemoreceptors
   d. Hering-Breuer inflation (stretch) receptors

9–4. Which of the following would be expected to decrease the ventilatory response to carbon dioxide, shifting the CO_2 response curve to the right?
   a. Barbiturates
   b. Hypoxia
   c. Slow-wave sleep
   d. Metabolic acidosis
   e. Deep anesthesia

SUGGESTED READINGS

Berger AJ. Control of breathing. In: Murray JF, Nadel JA. *Textbook of Respiratory Medicine.* 3rd ed. Philadelphia, Pa: WB Saunders and Company; 2000:179–196.

Berger AJ, Mitchell RA, Severinghaus JW. Regulation of respiration. *N Engl J Med.* 1977;297:92–97, 138–143, 194–201.

Cherniack NS, Coleridge JCG. Pulmonary reflexes: Neural mechanisms of pulmonary defense. *Annu Rev Physiol.* 1994;56:69–91.

Comroe JH Jr. *Physiology of Respiration.* 2nd ed. Chicago, Ill: Year Book; 1974:22–93.

Duffin J. Role of acid-base balance in the chemoreflex control of breathing. *J Appl Physiol.* 2005;99:2255–2265.

Eldridge FL. Central integration of mechanisms in exercise hyperpnea. *Med Sci Sports Exerc.* 1994;26:319–327.

Hannam S, Ingram DM, Rabe-Hesketh S, Milner AD. Characterisation of the Hering-Breuer deflation reflex in the human neonate. *Respir Physiol.* 2000;124:51–64.

Hassan A, Gossage J, Ingram D, Lee S, Milner AD. Volume of activation of the Hering-Breuer inflation reflex in the newborn infant. *J Appl Physiol.* 2001;90:763–769.

Hlastala MP, Berger AJ. *Physiology of Respiration.* 2nd ed. New York, NY: Oxford University Press; 2001:134–147.

Kazemi H, Johnson DC. Regulation of cerebrospinal fluid acid-base balance. *Physiol Rev.* 1986;66:953–1037.

Mahamed S, Ali AF, Ho D, Wang B, Duffin J. The contribution of chemoreflex drives to resting breathing in man. *Exp Physiol.* 2001;86.1:109–116.

Mateika JH, Duffin J. A review of the control of breathing during exercise. *Eur J Appl Physiol.* 1995;71:1–27.

Nattie E. Why do we have both peripheral and central chemoreceptors? *J Appl Physiol.* 2006;100:9–10.

Nunn JF. *Nunn's Applied Respiratory Physiology.* 4th ed. Oxford: Butterworth-Heinemann; 1993:90–116.

Paintal AS. Sensations from J receptors. *News Physiol Sci.* 1995;10:238–243.

Prabhakar NR. Oxygen sensing by the carotid body chemoreceptors. *J Appl Physiol.* 2000;88:2287–2295.

Rabbette PS, Stocks J. Influence of volume dependency and timing of airway occlusions on the Hering-Breuer reflex in infants. *J Appl Physiol.* 1998;85:2033–2039.

Shea SA. Life without ventilatory chemosensitivity. *Respir Physiol.* 1997;110:199–210.

Rekling JC, Feldman JL. Pre Bötzinger complex and pacemaker neurons: Hypothesized site and kernel for respiratory rhythm generation. *Annu Rev Physiol.* 1998;60:385–405.

Schwab RJ, Goldberg AN, Pack AI. Sleep apnea syndromes. In: Fishman AP, ed. *Pulmonary Diseases and Disorders.* 3rd ed. New York, NY: McGraw-Hill; 1998:1617–1637.

Wasserman K. Breathing during exercise. *N Engl J Med.* 1978;298:780–785.

Wasserman K, Casaburi R. Dyspnea: Physiological and pathophysiological mechanisms. *Annu Rev Med.* 1988;39:503–515.

Weir EK, Lopez-Barneo J, Buckler KJ, et al. Acute oxygen-sensing mechanisms. *N Engl J Med.* 2005;353:2042–2055.

Wenninger JM, Pan LG, Klum L, et al. Large lesions in the pre-Boetzinger complex area eliminate eupneic respiratory rhythm in awake goats. *J Appl Physiol.* 2004;97:1629–1636.

Nonrespiratory Functions of the Lung

10

OBJECTIVES

The reader understands the nonrespiratory functions of the components of the respiratory system.

▶ *Lists and describes the mechanisms by which the lung is protected from the contaminants in inspired air.*

▶ *Describes the "air-conditioning" function of the upper airways.*

▶ *Describes the filtration and removal of particles from the inspired air.*

▶ *Describes the removal of biologically active material from the inspired air.*

▶ *Describes the reservoir and filtration functions of the pulmonary circulation.*

▶ *Lists the metabolic functions of the lung, including the handling of vasoactive materials in the blood.*

The main function of the respiratory system in general and of the lung in particular is gas exchange. However, the lung has several other tasks to perform. These nonrespiratory functions of the lung include its own defense against inspired particulate matter, the storage and filtration of blood for the systemic circulation, the handling of vasoactive substances in the blood, and the formation and release of substances used in the alveoli or circulation.

PULMONARY DEFENSE MECHANISMS

 Every day about 10,000 L of air is inspired into the airways and the lungs, bringing it into contact with approximately 50 to 100 m² of what may be the most delicate tissues of the body. This inspired air contains (or may contain) dust, pollen, fungal spores, ash, and other products of combustion;

microorganisms such as bacteria; particles of substances such as asbestos and silica; and hazardous chemicals or toxic gases. As one reviewer (Green) put it, "Each day a surface as large as a tennis court is exposed to a volume of air and contaminants that would fill a swimming pool." In this section, the mechanisms by which the lungs are protected from contaminants in inspired air, as well as from material such as liquids, food particles, and bacteria that may be *aspirated* (accidentally inspired from the oropharynx or nasopharynx) into the airways are discussed.

Air-Conditioning

The temperature and the humidity of the ambient air vary widely, and the alveoli must be protected from the cold and from drying out. The mucosa of the nose, the nasal turbinates, the oropharynx, and the nasopharynx have a rich blood supply and constitute a large surface area. The nasal turbinates alone have a surface area said to be about 160 cm^2. As inspired air passes through these areas and continues through the tracheobronchial tree, it is heated to body temperature and humidified, especially if one is breathing through the nose.

Olfaction

Because the olfactory receptors are located in the posterior nasal cavity rather than in the trachea or alveoli, a person can *sniff* to attempt to detect potentially hazardous gases or dangerous material in the inspired air. This rapid, shallow inspiration brings gases into contact with the olfactory sensors without bringing them into the lung.

Filtration & Removal of Inspired Particles

The respiratory tract has an elaborate system for the filtration of the inspired air and the removal of particulate matter from the airways. The filtration system works better if one is breathing through the nose.

FILTRATION OF INSPIRED AIR

Inhaled particles may be deposited in the respiratory tract as a result of impaction, sedimentation, Brownian motion, and other, less important mechanisms. Air passing through the nose is first filtered by passing through the nasal hairs, or *vibrissae*. This removes most particles larger than 10 to 15 μm in diameter. Most of the particles greater than 10 μm in diameter are removed by impacting in the large surface area of the nasal septum and turbinates (Figure 10–1). The inspired air stream changes direction abruptly at the nasopharynx so that many of these larger particles impact on the posterior wall of the pharynx because of their inertia. The tonsils and adenoids are located near this impaction site, providing immunologic defense against biologically active material filtered at this point. Air entering the trachea contains few particles larger than 10 μm, and most of these will impact mainly at the carina or within the bronchi.

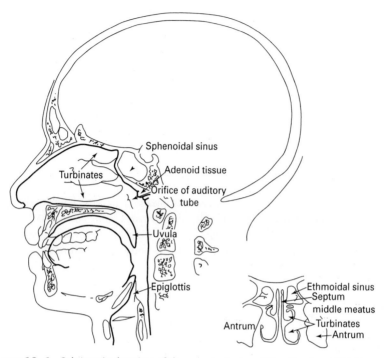

Figure 10–1. Schematic drawing of the upper airways. (After Proctor, 1964. Reproduced with permission.)

Sedimentation of most particles in the size range of 2 to 5 μm occurs by gravity in the smaller airways, where airflow rates are extremely low. Thus, most of the particles between 2 to 10 μm in diameter are removed by impaction or sedimentation and become trapped in the mucus that lines the upper airways, trachea, bronchi, and bronchioles. Smaller particles and all foreign gases reach the alveolar ducts and alveoli. Some smaller particles (0.1 μm and smaller) are deposited as a result of Brownian motion due to their bombardment by gas molecules. The other particles, between 0.1 and 0.5 μm in diameter, mainly stay suspended as aerosols, and about 80% of them are exhaled.

REMOVAL OF FILTERED MATERIAL

Filtered or aspirated material trapped in the mucus that lines the respiratory tract can be removed in several ways.

Reflexes in the Airways—Mechanical or chemical stimulation of receptors in the nose, trachea, larynx, or elsewhere in the respiratory tract may produce bronchoconstriction to prevent deeper penetration of the irritant into the airways and may also produce a cough or a sneeze. A sneeze results from stimulation of receptors in the nose or nasopharynx; a cough results from stimulation of receptors in the trachea. In either case, a deep inspiration, often to near the total lung capacity, is followed by a forced expiration against a closed glottis. Intrapleural pressure may rise to more than 100 mm Hg during this phase of the reflex. The glottis opens suddenly, and pressure in the airways falls rapidly, resulting in compression of the airways and an explosive expiration, with linear airflow velocities said to approach the speed of sound. Such high airflow rates through the narrowed airways are likely to carry the irritant, along with some mucus, out of the respiratory tract. In a sneeze, of course, the expiration is via the nose; in a cough, the expiration is via the mouth. The cough or sneeze reflex is also useful in helping to move the mucous lining of the airways toward the nose or mouth. The term "cough" is not specific to this complete involuntary respiratory reflex. Coughs can be initiated by many causes, including postnasal drip from allergies or viral infections, asthma, gastroesophageal reflux disease, as an adverse effect of the very commonly prescribed angiotensin-converting enzyme inhibitors, mucus production from chronic bronchitis, infections, and bronchiectasis. Voluntary coughs are not usually as pronounced as the violent involuntary reflex described above.

Tracheobronchial Secretions and Mucociliary Transport: The "Mucociliary Escalator"—The entire respiratory tract, from the upper airways down to the terminal bronchioles, is lined by a mucus-covered ciliated epithelium, with an estimated total surface area of 0.5 m^2. The only exceptions are parts of the pharynx and the anterior third of the nasal cavity. A typical portion of the epithelium of the airways (without the layer of mucus that would normally cover it) is shown in Figure 10–2.

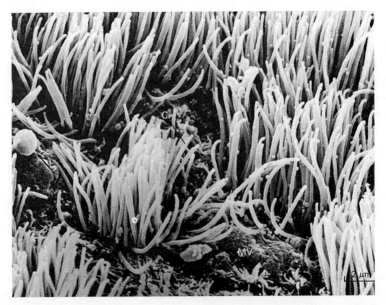

Figure 10–2. Scanning electron micrograph of the surface of bronchiolar epithelium. Ci = cilia; MV = microvilli on surface of unciliated cell. Arrow points to a secretion droplet. (From Weibel, 1998. Reproduced with permission.)

The airway secretions are produced by goblet cells and mucus-secreting glands. The mucus is a complex polymer of mucopolysaccharides. The mucous glands are found mainly in the submucosa near the supporting cartilage of the larger airways. In pathologic states, such as chronic bronchitis, the number of goblet cells may increase and the mucous glands may hypertrophy, resulting in greatly increased mucous gland secretion and increased viscosity of mucus.

The cilia lining the airways beat in such a way that the mucus covering them is always moved up the airway, away from the alveoli and toward the pharynx. Exactly how the ciliary beating is coordinated is unknown—the cilia do not appear to beat synchronously but instead probably produce local waves. The mucous blanket appears to be involved in the mechanical linkage between the cilia. The cilia beat at frequencies between 600 and 900 beats per minute, and the mucus moves progressively faster as it travels from the periphery. In small airways (1 to 2 mm in diameter), linear velocities range from 0.5 to 1 mm/min; in the trachea and bronchi, linear velocities range from 5 to 20 mm/min. Several studies have shown that ciliary function is inhibited or impaired by cigarette smoke.

The "mucociliary escalator" is an especially important mechanism for the removal of inhaled particles that come to rest in the airways. Material trapped in the mucus is continuously moved upward toward the pharynx. This movement can be greatly increased during a cough, as described previously. Mucus that reaches the pharynx is usually swallowed, expectorated, or removed by blowing one's nose. It is important to remember that patients who cannot clear their tracheobronchial secretions (an intubated patient or a patient who cannot cough adequately) continue to produce secretions. If the secretions are not removed from the patient by suction or other means, airway obstruction will develop.

DEFENSE MECHANISMS OF THE TERMINAL RESPIRATORY UNITS

Inspired material that reaches the terminal airways and alveoli may be removed in several ways, including ingestion by alveolar macrophages, nonspecific enzymatic destruction, entrance into the lymphatics, and immunologic reactions.

Alveolar Macrophages—Alveolar macrophages are large mononuclear ameboid cells that inhabit the alveolar surface. Inhaled particles engulfed by alveolar macrophages may be destroyed by their lysosomes. Most bacteria are digested in this manner. Some material ingested by the macrophages, however, such as silica, is not degradable by the macrophages and may even be toxic to them. If the macrophages carrying such material are not removed from the lung, the material will be redeposited on the alveolar surface on the death of the macrophages. The mean life span of alveolar macrophages is believed to be 1 to 5 weeks. The main exit route of macrophages carrying such nondigestible material is migration to the mucociliary escalator via the pores of Kohn and eventual removal through the airways. Particle-containing macrophages may also migrate from the alveolar surface into the septal interstitium, from which they may enter the lymphatic system or the mucociliary escalator. Macrophage function has been shown to be inhibited by cigarette smoke. Alveolar macrophages are also important in the lung's immune and inflammatory responses. They secrete many enzymes, arachidonic acid metabolites,

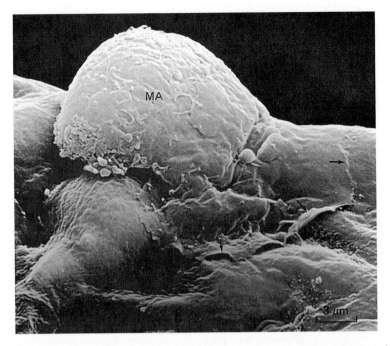

Figure 10–3. Scanning electron micrograph of an alveolar macrophage (MA) on the epithelial surface of a human lung. Arrows point to the advancing edge of the cell. (From Weibel, 1998. Reproduced with permission.)

immune response components, growth factors, cytokines, and other mediators that modulate the function of other cells, such as lymphocytes. A scanning electron micrograph of an alveolar macrophage is shown in Figure 10–3.

Other Methods of Particle Removal or Destruction—Some particles reach the mucociliary escalator because the alveolar fluid lining itself is slowly moving upward toward the respiratory bronchioles. Others penetrate into the interstitial space or enter the blood, where they are phagocytized by interstitial macrophages or blood phagocytes or enter the lymphatics. Particles may be destroyed or detoxified by surface enzymes and factors in the serum and in airway secretions. These include *lysozymes,* found mainly in leukocytes and known to have bactericidal properties; *lactoferrin,* which is synthesized by polymorphonuclear lymphocytes and by glandular mucosal cells and is a potent bacteriostatic agent; *alpha₁ antitrypsin,* which inactivates proteolytic enzymes released from bacteria, dead cells, or cells involved in defense of the lung (e.g., neutrophil elastase); *interferon,* a potent antiviral substance that may be produced by macrophages and lymphocytes; and *complement,* which participates as a cofactor in antigen-antibody reactions and may also participate in other aspects of cellular defense. Finally, many biologically active contaminants of the inspired air may be removed by antibody-mediated or cell-mediated immunologic responses. A diagram summarizing bronchoalveolar pulmonary defense mechanisms is shown in Figure 10–4; respiratory system defense mechanisms are summarized in Table 10–1.

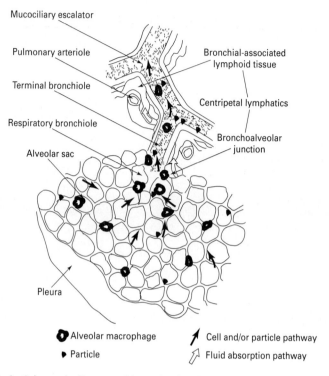

Mucociliary escalator

Pulmonary arteriole

Terminal bronchiole

Respiratory bronchiole

Alveolar sac

Pleura

Bronchial-associated lymphoid tissue

Centripetal lymphatics

Bronchoalveolar junction

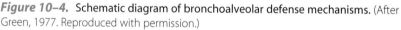

🔴 Alveolar macrophage

▸ Particle

↗ Cell and/or particle pathway

⇗ Fluid absorption pathway

Figure 10–4. Schematic diagram of bronchoalveolar defense mechanisms. (After Green, 1977. Reproduced with permission.)

NONRESPIRATORY FUNCTIONS OF THE PULMONARY CIRCULATION

The pulmonary circulation, strategically located between the systemic veins and arteries, is well suited for several functions not directly related to gas exchange. The entire cardiac output passes over the very large surface area of the pulmonary capillary bed, allowing the lungs to act as a site of blood filtration and storage as well as for the metabolism of vasoactive constituents of the blood.

Reservoir for the Left Ventricle

The pulmonary circulation, because of its high compliance and the negative intrapleural pressure, contains 250 to 300 mL of blood per square meter of body surface area. This would give a typical adult male a pulmonary blood volume of about 500 mL. This large blood volume allows the pulmonary circulation to act as a reservoir for the left ventricle. If left ventricular output is transiently greater than systemic venous return, left ventricular output can be maintained for a few strokes by drawing on blood stored in the pulmonary circulation.

Table 10–1. Integrated System for Defense of the Respiratory Tract

Natural mechanical defenses
  Filtration and impaction remove particles
  Sneeze, cough, and bronchospasm expel particles
  Epithelial barriers and mucus limit particle penetration
  Mucociliary escalator transports particles cephalad
Natural phagocytic defenses
  Effected by airway, interstitial, and alveolar macrophages; polymorphonuclear leukocytes
  Phagocytosis of particulates, organisms, and debris
  Microbicidal and tumoricidal activities
  Degradation of organic particles
Acquired specific immune defenses
  Humoral immunity
    Effected by B lymphocytes
    Biologic activities mediated by specific antibody
    Augments phagocytic and microbicidal defense mechanisms
    Initiates acute inflammatory responses
  Cell-mediated immunity
    Effected by T lymphocytes
    Biologic activities mediated by
      Delayed-type hypersensitivity reaction
      T cell cytotoxicity
    Augments microbicidal and cytotoxic activities of macrophages
    Mediates subacute, chronic, and granulomatous inflammatory responses

Reproduced with permission from Kaltreider, 1994.

The Pulmonary Circulation as a Filter

Because virtually all mixed venous blood must pass through the pulmonary capillaries, the pulmonary circulation acts as a filter, protecting the systemic circulation from materials that enter the blood. The particles filtered, which may enter the circulation as a result of natural processes, trauma, or therapeutic measures, may include small fibrin or blood clots, fat cells, bone marrow, detached cancer cells, gas bubbles, agglutinated erythrocytes (especially in sickle cell disease), masses of platelets or leukocytes, and debris from stored blood or intravenous solutions. If these particles were to enter the arterial side of the systemic circulation, they might occlude vascular beds with no other source of blood flow. This occlusion would be particularly disastrous if it occurred in the blood supply to the central nervous system or the heart.

The lung can perform this very valuable service because there are many more pulmonary capillaries present in the lung than are necessary for gas exchange at rest: Previously unopened capillaries will be recruited. Obviously, no gas exchange can occur distal to a particle embedded in and obstructing a capillary, and so this mechanism is limited by the ability of the lung to remove such filtered material. If particles are experimentally suspended in venous blood and are then trapped in the pulmonary circulation, the diffusing capacity usually decreases for 4 to 5 days and then returns to normal. The mechanisms for removal of material trapped in the pulmonary capillary bed include lytic enzymes in the vascular endothelium, ingestion by macrophages, and penetration to the lymphatic system. Patients on cardiopulmonary bypass do not have the benefit of this pulmonary capillary filtration, and blood administered to these patients must be filtered for them.

Fluid Exchange & Drug Absorption

The colloid osmotic pressure of the plasma proteins normally exceeds the pulmonary capillary hydrostatic pressure. This tends to pull fluid from the alveoli into the pulmonary capillaries and keep the alveolar surface free of liquids other than pulmonary surfactant. Water taken into the lungs is rapidly absorbed into the blood. This protects the gas exchange function of the lungs and opposes transudation of fluid from the capillaries to the alveoli. As noted in Chapter 2, type II alveolar epithelial cells may also actively pump sodium and water from the alveolar surface into the interstitium.

Drugs or chemical substances that readily pass through the alveolar-capillary barrier by diffusion or by other means rapidly enter the systemic circulation. The lungs are frequently used as a route of administration of drugs and for anesthetic gases, such as halothane and nitrous oxide. Aerosol drugs intended for the airways only, such as the bronchodilator isoproterenol, may rapidly pass into the systemic circulation, where they may have large effects. The effects of isoproterenol, for example, could include cardiac stimulation and vasodilation.

METABOLIC FUNCTIONS OF THE LUNG

Until recently, the lung was thought of as an organ with little metabolic activity. The main function of the lung, gas exchange, is accomplished by passive diffusion. Movement of air and blood is accomplished by the muscles of respiration and the right ventricle. Because the lung appeared to do little that required energy and did not appear to produce any substances utilized elsewhere in the body, it was not believed to have any metabolic requirements other than those necessary for the maintenance of its own cells. In the last three decades, however, the metabolic activities of the lung have become an area of intense investigation, and the lung has been shown to be involved in the conversion or uptake of vasoactive substances found in mixed venous blood and the production, storage, and release of substances used locally in the lung or elsewhere in the body.

Metabolism of Vasoactive Substances

Many vasoactive substances are inactivated, altered, or removed from the blood as they pass through the lungs. The site of this metabolic activity is the endothelium of the vessels of the pulmonary circulation, which constitute a tremendous surface area in contact with the mixed venous blood. For example, as shown in Table 10–2, prostaglandins E_1, E_2, and $F_{2\alpha}$ are nearly completely removed in a single pass through the lungs. On the other hand, prostaglandins A_1, A_2, and I_2 (prostacyclin) are not affected by the pulmonary circulation. Similarly, about 30% of the norepinephrine in mixed venous blood is removed by the lung, but epinephrine and isoproterenol are unaffected.

These alterations of vasoactive substances in the lung imply several things. First, some substances released into specific vascular beds for *local* effects are inactivated

Table 10–2. Uptake or Conversion by the Lungs of Chemical Substrates in Mixed Venous Blood

Substance in Mixed Venous Blood	Result of a Single Pass Through the Lung
Prostaglandins E_1, E_2, $F_{2\alpha}$	Almost completely removed
Prostaglandins A_1, A_2, I_2	Not affected
Leukotrienes	Almost completely removed
Serotonin	85% to 95% removed
Acetylcholine	Inactivated by cholinesterases in blood
Histamine	Not affected
Epinephrine	Not affected
Norepinephrine	Approximately 30% removed
Isoproterenol	Not affected
Dopamine	Not affected
Bradykinin	Approximately 80% inactivated
Angiotensin I	Approximately 70% converted to angiotensin II
Angiotensin II	Not affected
Vasopressin	Not affected
Oxytocin	Not affected
Gastrin	Not affected
ATP, AMP	40% to 90% removed

or removed as they pass through the lungs, preventing them from entering the systemic circulation. Other substances, apparently intended for more general effects, are not affected. Second, in the case of those substances that are affected by passing through the lungs, there may be profound differences in the response of a patient receiving an injection or infusion of one of these substances, depending on whether it is administered via an arterial or venous catheter.

Formation & Release of Chemical Substances for Local Use

Several substances that produce effects in the lung have been shown to be synthesized and released by pulmonary cells. The most familiar of these is *pulmonary surfactant,* which is synthesized in type II alveolar epithelial cells and released at the alveolar surface, as shown in Figure 10–5. Surfactant plays an important role in reducing the alveolar elastic recoil due to surface tension and in stabilizing the alveoli, as discussed in Chapter 2. A number of factors may modulate surfactant secretion, including glucocorticoids, epidermal growth factor, cyclic adenosine monophosphate (AMP), and distention of the lung. *Histamine, lysosomal enzymes, prostaglandins, leukotrienes, platelet-activating factor, neutrophil and eosinophil chemotactic factors,* and *serotonin* can be released from mast cells in the lungs in response to conditions such as pulmonary embolism and anaphylaxis. They may cause bronchoconstriction or immune or inflammatory responses, or they may initiate cardiopulmonary reflexes. If there is a *chemical mediator* involved in hypoxic pulmonary vasoconstriction, it is produced in and acts in the lung. As discussed in

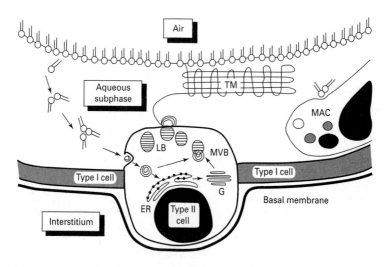

Figure 10–5. Scheme of surfactant metabolism in the alveolus: After synthesis in the endoplasmatic reticulum (ER) and alterations in the Golgi apparatus (G), surfactant is packed in multivesicular bodies (MVB) and stored in the lamellar bodies (LB) of type II alveolar cells. Subsequent to exocytosis, the newly secreted material forms tubular myelin (TM), which appears to act as a reservoir to supply the air-liquid interface with a monomolecular form of surfactant. Material removed from the monolayer may be taken up by the cell again and is either degraded or packed together with newly synthesized surfactant into multivesicular bodies. Macrophages (MAC) also participate in surfactant removal from the alveoli. (Reproduced with permission from Wirtz H, Schmidt M: Ventilation and secretion of pulmonary surfactant. Clin Investig 1992;70:3–13.)

Chapter 4, it is currently believed that hypoxia acts directly on the pulmonary vascular smooth muscle cells by causing decreased permeability to potassium ions, thereby decreasing the efflux of potassium ions and depolarizing the cells. This response, however, may be modulated by mediators released locally. Many substances are also produced by cells of the lung and released into the alveoli and airways, including mucus and other tracheobronchial secretions, the surface enzymes, proteins and other factors, and immunologically active substances discussed earlier in this chapter. These substances are produced by goblet cells, submucosal gland cells, Clara cells, and macrophages.

Formation & Release into the Blood of Substances Produced by Lung Cells

Bradykinin, histamine, serotonin, heparin, prostaglandins E_2 and $F_{2\alpha}$, and the endoperoxides (prostaglandins G_2 and H_2) are all produced and/or stored by cells in the lung and may be released into the general circulation under various circumstances. For example, heparin, histamine, serotonin, and prostaglandins E_2 and $F_{2\alpha}$ are released during anaphylactic shock.

Other Metabolic Functions

The lung must be able to meet its own cellular energy requirements as well as respond to injury. The type II alveolar epithelial cell also plays a major role in the response of the lung to injury. As type I alveolar epithelial cells are injured, type II cells proliferate to reestablish a continuous epithelial surface. Studies in animals have shown that these type II cells can develop into type I cells after injury.

KEY CONCEPTS

Alveolar ventilation brings thousands of liters of air each day into the airways and alveoli, which must be protected from contaminants, microorganisms, low humidity, and cold temperatures.

Metabolic functions of the lung include alterations of many vasoactive substances as they pass through the pulmonary vascular endothelium; formation and release of substances for use in the lungs, such as pulmonary surfactant, or elsewhere in the body; and repair of the alveolar surface in response to injury.

SUGGESTED READINGS

Ali J. Cough. In: Ali J, Summer W, Levitzky M. *Pulmonary Pathophysiology.* 2nd. ed. New York: Lange Medical Books/McGraw-Hill; 2005:21–34.

Banner AS. Cough: Physiology, evaluation, and treatment. *Lung.* 1986;164:79–92.

Green GM, Jakab GJ, Low RB, Davis GS. Defense mechanisms of the respiratory membrane. *Am Rev Respir Dis.* 1977;115:479–514.

Houtmeyers E, Gosselink R, Gayan-Ramirez G, Decramer M. Regulation of mucociliary clearance in health and disease. *Eur Respir J.* 1999;13:1177–1188.

Kaltreider HB. Macrophages, lymphocytes, and antibody- and cell-mediated immunity. In: Murray JF, Nadel JA, eds. *Textbook of Respiratory Medicine.* 2nd ed. Philadelphia, Pa: WB Saunders and Company; 1994:370–401.

Nicod LP. Pulmonary defence mechanisms. *Respiration.* 1999;66:2–11.

Pierce RJ, Worsnop CJ. Upper airway function and dysfunction in respiration. *Clin Exp Pharm Physiol* 1999;26:1–10.

Proctor DF. Physiology of the upper airway. In: Fenn WO, Rahn H, eds. *Handbook of Physiology, sec 3: Respiration.* Washington, DC: American Physiological Society. 1964;1:309–345.

Proctor DF, Andersen I, eds. *The Nose: Upper Airway Physiology and the Atmospheric Environment.* Amsterdam: Elsevier Biomedical; 1982.

Ryan US, Makrides SC. Nonrespiratory functions of the lungs. In: Fishman AP, ed. *Pulmonary Diseases and Disorders.* 3rd ed. New York, NY: McGraw-Hill; 1998:139–148.

Wanner A, Salathé M, O'Riordan TG. Mucociliary clearance in the airways. *Am J Respir Crit Care Med.* 1998;154:1868–1902.

Weibel ER, Taylor CR. Design of the human lung for gas exchange. In: Fishman AP, ed. *Pulmonary Diseases and Disorders.* 3rd ed. New York, NY: McGraw-Hill; 1998:21–61.

Wirtz H, Schmidt M. Ventilation and secretion of pulmonary surfactant. *Clin Investig.* 1992;70:3–13.

The Respiratory System Under Stress

OBJECTIVES

The reader uses the knowledge he or she gained from the preceding chapters to predict the response of the respiratory system to three physiologic stresses: exercise, ascent to altitude, and diving.

▶ *Identifies the physiologic stresses involved in exercise.*

▶ *Predicts the responses of the respiratory system to acute exercise.*

▶ *Describes the effects of long-term exercise programs (training) on the respiratory system.*

▶ *Identifies the physiologic stresses involved in the ascent to altitude.*

▶ *Predicts the initial responses of the respiratory system to the ascent to altitude.*

▶ *Describes the acclimatization of the cardiovascular and respiratory systems to residence at high altitudes.*

▶ *Identifies the physiologic stresses involved in diving.*

▶ *Predicts the responses of the respiratory system to various types of diving.*

This chapter is mainly intended to be a review of the preceding chapters of the book. The responses of the respiratory system to three physiologic stresses are examined as they relate to the material already covered; the discussions of the responses to each stress will therefore be brief and rather superficial. For a more complete discussion of each stress, consult the Suggested Readings at the end of this chapter.

EXERCISE & THE RESPIRATORY SYSTEM

 Exercise increases the metabolism of the working muscles. It stresses the respiratory system by increasing the demand for oxygen and increasing the production of carbon dioxide. Moderate to severe levels of exercise also cause increased lactic acid production. The respiratory and cardiovascular systems must increase the volume of oxygen supplied to the exercising tissues and increase the removal of carbon dioxide and hydrogen ions from the body.

Acute Effects

The effects of exercise in an untrained person are mainly a function of an increase in the cardiac output coupled with an increase in alveolar ventilation.

CONTROL OF BREATHING

As discussed at the end of Chapter 9, both the tidal volume and the breathing frequency are increased during exercise. The causes of the increased alveolar ventilation during exercise were discussed in that section.

MECHANICS OF BREATHING

The work of breathing is increased during exercise. Larger tidal volumes result in increased work necessary to overcome the elastic recoil of the lungs and chest wall during inspiration because the lungs are less compliant at higher lung volumes and because the elastic recoil of the chest wall is inward at high thoracic volumes. Of course, the greater elastic recoil tends to make expiration easier, but this is offset by other factors. The high airflow rates generated during exercise result in a much greater airways resistance component of the work of breathing. Greater turbulence and dynamic compression of airways secondary to active expiration combine to greatly increase the work of breathing. (Recall that during turbulent airflow $\Delta P = \dot{V}^2 R$.) Increasing airflow rates especially increases the resistive work of breathing through the nose: Minute ventilations above about 40 L/min are normally accomplished by breathing through the mouth.

ALVEOLAR VENTILATION

In normal adults, the resting minute ventilation ($\dot{V}E$) of 5 to 6 L/min can be increased to as much as 150 L/min during short periods of maximal exercise. Maximal increases in cardiac output during exercise are only in the range of four to six times the resting level in healthy adults compared with this 25-fold potential increase in minute ventilation. Therefore, it is the cardiovascular system rather than the respiratory system that is the limiting factor in exercise by healthy people.

As discussed in Chapter 9, at less strenuous levels of exercise, the increase in ventilation is accomplished mainly by increasing the tidal volume. During strenuous exercise, the tidal volume usually increases to a maximum of about 50% to 60% of the vital capacity of a normal subject, or about 2.5 to 3.0 L in an average-sized man. This increase in tidal volume appears to occur mainly at the expense of the inspiratory reserve volume, with the expiratory reserve volume somewhat less affected. An increase in the central blood volume (caused by increased venous return) may decrease the total lung capacity slightly. The residual volume and functional residual capacity may be unchanged or slightly elevated. The vital capacity may be slightly decreased or unchanged. The breathing frequency may increase to 40 to 50 breaths per minute in healthy adults (and as high as 70 breaths per minute in children) with strenuous exercise.

The anatomic dead space may increase slightly in inspiration during exercise because of airway distention at high lung volumes; any alveolar dead space present at rest normally decreases as cardiac output increases. As a result, there is little change in physiologic dead space during exercise. Because the tidal volume does increase, however, the ratio of physiologic dead space to tidal volume (V_D/V_T) decreases.

The arterial P_{O_2} stays relatively constant during even strenuous exercise. Arterial P_{CO_2} also stays relatively constant until anaerobic metabolism results in appreciable lactic acid generation. The hydrogen ions liberated directly stimulate alveolar ventilation and may cause arterial P_{CO_2} to fall a few millimeters of mercury below the resting arterial P_{CO_2}.

The regional differences in alveolar ventilation seen in upright lungs (which were discussed in Chapter 3) are probably slightly attenuated during exercise. The larger tidal volumes, occurring at the expense of both the inspiratory and expiratory reserve volumes, indicate that alveoli in more dependent regions of the lung are more fully inflated. However, these alveoli may also suffer airway collapse during active expirations. Similarly, alveoli in upper portions of the lung (with respect to gravity) should deflate more fully during expiration, resulting in greater ventilation of upper parts of the lung.

PULMONARY BLOOD FLOW

As already mentioned, the cardiac output increases linearly with oxygen consumption during exercise. This normally occurs more as a result of an autonomically mediated increase in heart rate than from an increase in stroke volume. An increased venous return, due to deeper inspiratory efforts (in addition to extravascular compression by the exercising muscles and by a decrease in venous capacitance), also contributes to the increase in cardiac output. Mean pulmonary artery and mean left atrial pressures increase, but the increase is not as great as the increase in pulmonary blood flow. This indicates a decrease in pulmonary vascular resistance. As discussed in Chapter 4, this decrease occurs passively by recruitment and distention of pulmonary vessels. Much of the recruitment of pulmonary blood vessels occurs in upper regions of the lung, thus tending to decrease the regional inhomogeneity of pulmonary blood flow discussed in Chapter 4. The expected effect of the deeper tidal volumes and active expirations that occur during exercise is to increase pulmonary vascular resistance. During active expiration the extraalveolar vessels should be compressed; during inspiration the alveolar vessels should be stretched. Mean pulmonary vascular resistance decreases, so the effects of recruitment and distention must be greater than the effects of extravascular compression.

VENTILATION-PERFUSION RELATIONSHIPS

The more uniform regional perfusion that occurs during exercise results in a much more uniform matching of ventilation and perfusion throughout the lung. Studies done on normal subjects engaged in exercise in the upright position have demonstrated a greatly increased perfusion of upper regions of the lung, resulting in improved matching of ventilation and perfusion. Because in moderate to severe exercise ventilation increases more than perfusion, the whole lung ventilation-perfusion ratio ($\dot{V}_A/\dot{Q}c$) increases to a range of 2.0 to 4.0, as seen in Figure 11–1, where the $\dot{V}_A/\dot{Q}c$ for the whole lung is approximately 2.5. A comparison of these findings with the ventilation-perfusion ratios seen at rest in the figure and in Figure 5–7

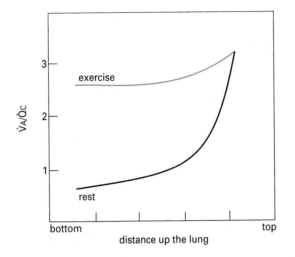

Figure 11–1. Representation of regional differences in the ventilation-perfusion ratio of an upright lung during rest and exercise. Compare with Figure 5–7.

demonstrates the reduced "scatter" of ventilation-perfusion ratios during exercise. Thus, the *location* of the perfusion is better matched to the *location* of the ventilation during exercise, but the ventilation-perfusion ratios increase in most alveolar-capillary units. The increased ventilation-perfusion ratios may enhance the alveolar-capillary diffusion gradients for oxygen and carbon dioxide in many units. On the other hand, several investigations have demonstrated *increased* $\dot{V}_A/\dot{Q}_C$ inequality for the whole lung during exercise. The mechanism for this is unclear, but it may involve increased perfusion of poorly ventilated alveoli. This may occur as increased pulmonary artery pressure interferes with hypoxic pulmonary vasoconstriction. Increased perfusion of poorly ventilated alveoli would act as an intrapulmonary shunt (or a "shunt-like" area). This is one explanation for the *decrease* in arterial P_{O_2} and increased alveolar-arterial P_{O_2} difference (the $(A-a)D_{O_2}$) seen in normal people as exercise levels increase. The $(A-a)D_{O_2}$, which is normally 5 to 15 mm Hg at rest in a young person, usually increases to 20 to 30 mm Hg in normal healthy untrained people at maximal exercise and may be even greater in athletes. Another explanation for the decreased arterial P_{O_2} and the increased $(A-a)D_{O_2}$ during severe exercise is that intrapulmonary arteriovenous shunts may open as exercise levels increase. These intrapulmonary arteriovenous shunts, which appear to anatomically bypass pulmonary capillaries, may open to help keep pulmonary vascular pressures low to prevent pulmonary edema caused by either high pulmonary capillary hydrostatic pressure or vessel failure caused by mechanical stress ("stress failure"). Furthermore, as exercise levels increase, mixed venous P_{O_2} decreases (see below), which would also increase the effect on the $(A-a)D_{O_2}$. Finally, the development of diffusion limitation of oxygen transfer (see the next section) from the alveolus to the pulmonary capillary may contribute to the increased $(A-a)D_{O_2}$ in severe exercise.

DIFFUSION THROUGH THE ALVEOLAR CAPILLARY BARRIER

The diffusing capacities for oxygen and carbon dioxide normally increase substantially during exercise. Some studies have shown a nearly linear increase in diffusing capacity as oxygen uptake increases, although the diffusing capacity may reach a maximum level before the $\dot{V}_{O_2}$ does. The increase in diffusing capacity during exercise is largely a result of the increase in pulmonary blood flow. Recruitment of capillaries, especially in upper regions of the lungs, increases the surface area available for diffusion. Increased linear velocity of blood flow through pulmonary capillaries reduces the time that red blood cells spend in contact with the alveolar air to less than the 0.75 seconds normally seen at rest, decreasing the perfusion limitation of gas transfer. As noted in Chapter 6, the P_{O_2} and P_{CO_2} of the plasma in the pulmonary capillaries normally equilibrate with the alveolar P_{O_2} and P_{CO_2} within about the first 0.25 seconds of the time blood spends in the pulmonary capillaries. After this equilibration, no further gas diffusion between the equilibrated blood and the alveoli takes place because the partial pressure gradient ($P_1 - P_2$ in Fick's law) is equal to zero. Increased velocity of blood flow through the lung therefore increases the diffusing capacity by bringing unequilibrated blood into the lung faster, thus maintaining the partial pressure gradient for diffusion. On the other hand, very great blood flow velocities may increase the possibility of diffusion limitation of gas transfer, even in a healthy person. Diffusion limitation is likely to develop in a person who has some diffusion impairment, as can be seen in Figure 6–2.

Another related factor, less dependent on the increased cardiac output, that helps increase diffusion during exercise is that the mixed venous P_{O_2} may be lower and the mixed venous P_{CO_2} may be higher than those seen at rest. These factors may also help increase and maintain the partial pressure gradients for diffusion.

The total effect on diffusion through the alveolar-capillary barrier of the increased surface area and the better maintenance of the alveolar-capillary partial pressure gradients may be seen by reviewing Fick's law for diffusion:

$$\dot{V}_{gas} \propto \frac{A \times D \times (P_1 - P_2)}{T}$$

The thickness of the alveolar-capillary barrier may also be affected during exercise, but the net effect may be either an increase or a decrease. At high lung volumes, the alveolar vessels are stretched and the thickness of the barrier may decrease. On the other hand, high cardiac outputs may be associated with vascular congestion, increasing the thickness of the barrier.

The alveolar-arterial oxygen difference increases during exercise. This is probably because of a number of factors, including $\dot{V}_A/\dot{Q}_C$ mismatch, diffusion limitation of gas transfer, a decreased mixed venous P_{O_2}, an increased alveolar P_{O_2}, and alterations in the oxyhemoglobin dissociation curve.

OXYGEN AND CARBON DIOXIDE TRANSPORT BY THE BLOOD

The loading of carbon dioxide into the blood and the unloading of oxygen from the blood are enhanced in exercising muscles. Oxygen unloading is improved because the P_{O_2} in the exercising muscle is decreased, causing a larger percentage of deoxyhemoglobin. Oxygen unloading is also enhanced by the rightward shift of the oxyhemoglobin dissociation curve caused by the elevated P_{CO_2}s (the Bohr effect), hydrogen ion concentrations, and temperatures (and possible 2,3-bisphosphoglycerate [2,3-BPG]) found in exercising muscle. Low capillary P_{O_2}s should also lead to improved carbon dioxide loading because lower oxyhemoglobin levels shift the carbon dioxide dissociation curve to the left (the Haldane effect).

ACID-BASE BALANCE

Exercise severe enough to cause a significant degree of anaerobic metabolism results in metabolic acidosis secondary to the increased lactic acid production. As discussed previously, the hydrogen ions generated by this process stimulate the arterial chemoreceptors (especially the carotid bodies) and cause a further compensatory increase in alveolar ventilation, maintaining arterial pH near the normal level.

The responses of the normal respiratory system to acute exercise are summarized in Table 11–1.

Table 11–1. Response of the Respiratory System to Acute Moderate or Severe Exercise

Variable	Moderate Exercise	Severe Exercise
Mechanics of breathing		
Elastic work of breathing	↑	↑↑
Resistance work of breathing	↑	↑↑
Alveolar ventilation		
Tidal volume	↑↑	↑↑
Frequency	↑	↑↑
Anatomic dead space	↑	↑
Alveolar dead space (if present)	↓	↓
V_D/V_T	↓	↓↓
Pulmonary blood flow	↑	↑↑
Perfusion of upper lung	↑	↑↑
Pulmonary vascular resistance	↓	↓↓
Linear velocity of blood flow	↑	↑↑
Ventilation-perfusion relationships		
Ventilation-perfusion matching	↑	↑
Ventilation-perfusion ratio	↑	↑↑
Diffusion through the alveolar-capillary barrier		
Surface area	↑	↑↑
Perfusion limitation	↓	↓↓
Partial pressure gradients	↑	↑↑
Oxygen unloading at the tissues	↑	↑↑
Carbon dioxide loading at the tissues	↑	↑↑
$P_{A_{O_2}}$	↔	↑
Pa_{O_2}	↔	↑, ↔, or ↓
Pa_{CO_2}	↔	↓
pHa	↔	↓
Arteriovenous O_2 difference	↑	↑↑

Training Effects

The ability to perform physical exercise increases with training. Most of the changes that occur as a result of physical training, however, are a function of alterations in the cardiovascular system and in muscle metabolism rather than changes in the respiratory system. The maximal oxygen uptake increases with physical training. This increase appears to be mainly a result of an increased maximal cardiac output. As was stated earlier in this chapter, the maximal cardiac output is probably a limiting factor in exercise. Physical training lowers the resting heart rate and increases the resting stroke volume. The maximal heart rate does not appear to be affected by physical training, but the heart rate of a trained person is lower than that of an untrained person at any level of physical activity. Stroke volume is increased. The arterial hemoglobin concentration and the hematocrit do not appear to change with physical training at sea level, but the arteriovenous oxygen content difference does appear to increase with physical training. This is probably a function of the increased effects of local pH, P_{CO_2}, and temperature in the exercising muscles, as well as an increased ability of the muscles to use oxygen. Blood volume is usually increased by training.

Physical training increases the oxidative capacity of skeletal muscle by inducing mitochondrial proliferation and increasing the concentration of oxidative enzymes and the synthesis of glycogen and triglyceride. These alterations result in lower concentrations of blood lactate in trained subjects than those found in untrained people, reflecting increased aerobic energy production. Nevertheless, blood lactate levels during maximal exercise may be higher in trained athletes than in untrained people.

Maximal ventilation and resting ventilation do not appear to be affected by physical training, but ventilation at submaximal loads is decreased, probably because of the lower lactic acid levels of the trained person during submaximal exercise. The strength and endurance of the respiratory muscles appear to improve with training. Total lung capacity is not affected by training; vital capacity may be normal or elevated. Pulmonary diffusing capacity is often elevated in athletes, probably as a result of their increased blood volumes and maximal cardiac outputs.

ALTITUDE & ACCLIMATIZATION

As one ascends to greater altitudes, the total barometric pressure decreases because the total barometric pressure at any altitude is proportional to the weight of the air above it. Air is attracted to the earth's surface by gravity. Because air is compressible, the change in barometric pressure per change in vertical distance is not constant. There is a greater change in barometric pressure per change in altitude closer to the earth's surface than there is at very great altitudes.

The fractional concentration of oxygen in the atmosphere does not change appreciably with altitude. Oxygen constitutes about 21% of the total pressure of dry ambient air, and so the P_{O_2} of dry air at any altitude is about 0.21 times total barometric pressure at that altitude. Water vapor pressure, however, must also be considered in calculations of the P_{O_2}. The water vapor pressure depends on the temperature and humidity of the air. As the inspired air passes through the airways, it is warmed to body temperature and completely humidified. Therefore, the partial pressure exerted by the water vapor in the air entering the alveoli is fixed at 47 mm Hg.

The alveolar P_{O_2} can therefore be calculated by using the alveolar air equation discussed in Chapter 3:

$$P_{A_{O_2}} = P_{I_{O_2}} - \frac{P_{A_{CO_2}}}{R} + [F]$$

The inspired P_{O_2} is equal to 0.21 times the total barometric pressure (if ambient air is breathed) after the subtraction of the water vapor pressure of 47 mm Hg:

$$P_{I_{O_2}} = 0.21 \times (P_B - 47 \text{ mm Hg})$$

The alveolar P_{CO_2} falls at greater altitudes because hypoxic stimulation of the arterial chemoreceptors increases alveolar ventilation. For example, at an altitude of 15,000 ft, the total barometric pressure is about 429 mm Hg. The inspired P_{O_2} is therefore $0.21 \times (429 - 47)$ mm Hg, or 80.2 mm Hg. The alveolar P_{CO_2} is likely to be decreased to about 32 mm Hg, resulting in a $P_{A_{O_2}}$ of about 45 mm Hg. At 18,000 ft, the total barometric pressure is about 380 mm Hg; at 20,000 ft, it is 349 mm Hg. At 50,000 ft, the total barometric pressure is only 87 mm Hg. Even if 100% oxygen is breathed, the $P_{A_{O_2}}$ plus the $P_{A_{CO_2}}$ divided by R can only *total* 40 mm Hg after water vapor pressure is subtracted. At 63,000 ft, the total barometric pressure is 47 mm Hg and the fluid in blood "boils."

Acute Effects

An unacclimatized person suffers a deterioration of nervous system function when ascending rapidly to great heights. Similar dysfunctions occur if cabin pressure is lost in an airplane. The symptoms are mainly due to hypoxia and may include sleepiness, laziness, a false sense of well-being, impaired judgment, blunted pain perception, increasing errors on simple tasks, decreased visual acuity, clumsiness, and tremors. Severe hypoxia, of course, may result in a loss of consciousness or even death.

If an unacclimatized person ascends to a moderate altitude, he or she may suffer from a group of symptoms known collectively as *acute mountain sickness.* The symptoms include headache, dizziness, breathlessness at rest, weakness, malaise, nausea, anorexia, sweating, palpitations, dimness of vision, partial deafness, sleeplessness, fluid retention, and dyspnea on exertion. These symptoms are a result of hypoxia and hypocapnia, and alkalosis or cerebral edema, or both.

CONTROL OF BREATHING

The decreased alveolar and arterial P_{O_2}s that occur at altitude result in stimulation of the arterial chemoreceptors and an increase in alveolar ventilation; the central chemoreceptors are not responsive to hypoxia. At an arterial P_{O_2} of 45 mm Hg, minute ventilation is approximately doubled. Because carbon dioxide production is initially normal (it does increase with the elevated work of breathing caused by greater alveolar ventilation), alveolar and arterial P_{CO_2} fall, causing respiratory alkalosis. Arterial hypocapnia also results in "diffusion" of carbon dioxide out of the cerebrospinal fluid, causing an increase in the pH of the cerebrospinal fluid. The central chemoreceptors are therefore not only unresponsive to the hypoxia of altitude; their activity is depressed by the secondary hypocapnia and alkalosis of the cerebrospinal fluid.

MECHANICS OF BREATHING

The increased rate and depth of breathing increase the work of breathing. Greater transpulmonary pressures are necessary to generate greater tidal volumes and also to overcome the possible effects of vascular engorgement and increased interstitial fluid volume of the lung, which may also decrease the vital capacity during the first 24 hours at altitude. High ventilatory rates may be accompanied by active expiration, resulting in dynamic compression of airways. This airway compression, coupled with a reflex parasympathetic bronchoconstriction in response to the arterial hypoxemia, results in elevated resistance work of breathing. More turbulent airflow, which is likely to be encountered at elevated ventilatory rates, may also contribute to elevated resistance work. Maximum airflow rates may increase because of decreased gas density.

ALVEOLAR VENTILATION

The anatomic dead space may decrease slightly at altitude because of the reflex bronchoconstriction or increase slightly because of the opposing effect of increased tidal volumes. In any event the ratio of dead space to tidal volume falls with greater tidal volumes. A more uniform regional distribution of alveolar ventilation is also expected at altitude because of deeper inspirations and fuller expirations. Previously collapsed or poorly ventilated alveoli will be better ventilated.

PULMONARY BLOOD FLOW

There is an increase in cardiac output, heart rate, and systemic blood pressure at altitude. These effects are probably a result of increased sympathetic stimulation of the cardiovascular system secondary to arterial chemoreceptor stimulation and increased lung inflation. There may also be a direct stimulatory effect of hypoxia on the myocardium. Alveolar hypoxia results in pulmonary vasoconstriction—hypoxic pulmonary vasoconstriction. The increased cardiac output, along with hypoxic pulmonary vasoconstriction and sympathetic stimulation of larger pulmonary vessels, results in an increase in mean pulmonary artery pressure and tends to abolish any preexisting zone 1 by recruiting previously unperfused capillaries. Undesirable consequences of these effects include vascular distention and engorgement of the lung secondary to the pulmonary hypertension, which may lead to "high-altitude pulmonary edema" and a greatly increased right ventricular workload. Some climbers seem particularly susceptible to high-altitude pulmonary edema; it is possible that they do not have as extensive or responsive intrapulmonary arteriovenous shunts (described in the exercise section earlier) as those climbers less susceptible to high-altitude pulmonary edema. People who are more susceptible to high-altitude pulmonary edema also seem to have greater hypoxic pulmonary vasoconstriction responses than less susceptible individuals. Furthermore, their pulmonary blood flow appears to be more heterogeneous during hypoxia, which may be a result of uneven hypoxic pulmonary vasoconstriction. Analysis of the fluid from high-altitude pulmonary edema shows that it contains large molecular weight proteins, which indicates that the edema is caused by increased capillary permeability as well as increased capillary hydrostatic pressure. The increased capillary permeability may result from capillary stress failure caused by high pulmonary artery pressure and blood flow and by altered release of cytokines or other mediators.

VENTILATION-PERFUSION RELATIONSHIPS

The increase in pulmonary blood flow seen acutely at high altitude, coupled with the more uniform alveolar ventilation, would be expected to make regional $\dot{V}A/\dot{Q}c$ more uniform. Surprisingly, studies have not shown striking differences in $\dot{V}A/\dot{Q}c$ relationships at high altitude, although they do appear to improve.

DIFFUSION THROUGH THE ALVEOLAR-CAPILLARY BARRIER

At high altitude, the partial pressure gradient for oxygen diffusion is decreased because the alveolar P_{O_2} is decreased more than the mixed venous P_{O_2} (see Figure 6–2B). This decrease in the partial pressure gradient is partly offset by effects of the increase in cardiac output and increased pulmonary artery pressure, which increase the surface area available for diffusion and decrease the time erythrocytes spend in pulmonary capillaries. The thickness of the barrier may be slightly decreased at higher lung volumes or increased because of pulmonary vascular distention.

OXYGEN AND CARBON DIOXIDE TRANSPORT BY THE BLOOD

Oxygen loading in the lung may be compromised at alveolar P_{O_2}s low enough to be below the flat part of the oxyhemoglobin dissociation curve, causing a low arterial oxygen content. Hypocapnia may aid somewhat in oxygen loading in the lung but will interfere with oxygen unloading at the tissues. The main short-term compensatory mechanism for maintenance of oxygen *delivery* is the increased cardiac output. The hemoglobin concentration may increase slightly within the first 2 days. This is a result of hemoconcentration secondary to fluid shifting into the extravascular space, not an increase in erythrocyte production.

CEREBRAL CIRCULATION

The cerebral circulation is an area of special difficulty at high altitude. Hypocapnia is a strong cerebral vasoconstrictor. The brain therefore receives not only blood with a low oxygen content but could also receive reduced blood flow. On the other hand, hypoxia causes cerebral vasodilation and can cause hyperperfusion and distention of cerebral vessels.

Hypoxic stimulation of the arterial chemoreceptors causes hypocapnia and respiratory alkalosis, as already discussed. Cerebral arterial hypocapnia not only could cause constriction of the cerebral blood vessels, it would also cause alkalosis of the cerebrospinal fluid (as discussed under Control of Breathing above; see also Figure 9–8). Most of the central nervous system symptoms of acute mountain sickness could be attributed to cerebral hypoperfusion, alkalosis, or both. However, it now appears that in most cases the symptoms of acute mountain sickness result from *cerebral hyperperfusion and edema.* This hyperperfusion is mainly a result of vasodilation, which is the direct effect of hypoxia on the cerebral blood vessels. As the cerebral arterioles dilate, the hydrostatic pressure in the cerebral capillaries increases, increasing the tendency of fluid to leave the cerebral capillaries and cause cerebral edema. The hyperperfusion and cerebral edema elevate intracranial pressure, compressing and distorting intracranial structures. This may lead to a general increase in sympathetic activity in the body, increasing the possibility of pulmonary edema and promoting renal salt and water retention.

Acid-Base Balance

As already mentioned, the increased alveolar ventilation at altitude results in hypocapnia and respiratory alkalosis.

Prevention of Acute Mountain Sickness

Acetazolamide, a carbonic anhydrase inhibitor, taken for a few days before ascending to altitude can prevent the symptoms of acute mountain sickness in many people. The mechanism by which it does this is unclear because acetazolamide has several actions that may help prevent acute mountain sickness. It decreases reabsorption of bicarbonate by the proximal tubule of the kidney. This may lead to a moderate metabolic acidosis that may partly offset the respiratory alkalosis and therefore also help stimulate ventilation. Acetazolamide is also a diuretic, so it may help prevent fluid retention and edema. Similarly, a recent study demonstrated that subjects less prone to acute mountain sickness have decreased levels of antidiuretic hormone at simulated altitudes, whereas subjects prone to acute mountain sickness have increased levels of antidiuretic hormone at simulated altitudes and therefore more fluid retention. Therefore acetazolamide may act to prevent acute mountain sickness by preventing fluid retention. It is likely that both proposed mechanisms are involved. Acetazolamide may also inhibit hypoxic pulmonary vasoconstriction.

Acclimatization

Longer-term compensations to the ascent to high altitude begin to occur after several hours and continue for days or even weeks. The immediate responses to the ascent and the early and late adaptive responses are summarized in Table 11–2.

Renal compensation for respiratory alkalosis begins within a day: Renal excretion of base is increased, and hydrogen ions are conserved. A second major compensatory mechanism is erythropoiesis. Within 3 to 5 days, new red blood cells are produced, increasing the hematocrit and the oxygen-carrying capacity. Thus, although the arterial P_{O_2} is not increased, the arterial oxygen content increases because of the increased blood hemoglobin concentration. This is at the cost of increased blood viscosity and ventricular workload. Increased concentrations of 2,3-BPG may help release oxygen at the tissues.

Hypoxic stimulation of the arterial chemoreceptors persists indefinitely, although it may be somewhat diminished after prolonged periods at high altitude. A more immediate finding is that the ventilatory response curve to carbon dioxide shifts to the left. That is, for any given alveolar or arterial P_{CO_2}, the ventilatory response is greater after several days at high altitude. This increased response probably reflects alterations in central acid-base balance. It occurs at about the same time as

Table 11–2. Physiologic Responses to High Altitude Relative to Sea Level Control Values*

	Immediate	Early Adaptive (72h)	Late Adaptive (2 to 6 weeks)
Spontaneous ventilation			
Minute ventilation	↑	↑	↑
Respiratory rate	Variable	Variable	Variable
Tidal volume	↑	↓	↑
Arterial P_{O_2}	↓	↓	↓
Arterial P_{CO_2}	↓	↓	↓
Arterial pH	↑	↑ ↔	↑ ↔
Arterial HCO_3^-	↔	↓	↓
Evaluation of lung function			
Vital capacity	↔ ↓	↔	↔
Maximum airflow rates	↑	↑	↑
Functional residual capacity	↔	↔	↔
Ventilatory response to inhaled CO_2	↔	↑	↑
Ventilatory response to hypoxia	↔	↔	↔
Pulmonary vascular resistance	↑	↑	↑
Oxygen transport			
Hemoglobin	↔	↑	↑
Erythropoietin	↑	↔	↔
P_{50}	↓	↑	↑
2, 3-BPG	↔	↑	↑
Cardiac output	↑	↔	↔ ↓
Central nervous system			
Headaches, nausea, insomnia	↑	↔	↔
Perception, judgment	↓	↔	↔
Spinal fluid pH	↑	↔	↔
Spinal fluid HCO_3^-	↔	↓	↓
Cerebral edema	↑	↔	↔

*These values apply to native sea-level inhabitants.
Adapted with permission from Guenter, 1977.

the alleviation of central nervous system symptoms and a return of the cerebrospinal fluid pH toward normal because of a reduction of the bicarbonate concentration of the cerebrospinal fluid. Although it was initially believed that this bicarbonate reduction reflected active transport of the bicarbonate out of the cerebrospinal fluid, that belief is now somewhat controversial. Bicarbonate may instead simply diffuse out of the cerebrospinal fluid, or the reduced cerebrospinal fluid levels of bicarbonate may reflect decreased production of bicarbonate in the cerebrospinal fluid.

Resolution of the cerebral edema and increased intracranial pressure probably also occurs at about the same time as the alleviation of central nervous system symptoms. This probably occurs because of increased reabsorption of cerebrospinal fluid, autoregulation of cerebral blood flow, and a sympathetically mediated vasoconstriction that for some reason takes several days to develop. It is also possible that the cerebral vessels produce less nitric oxide, which probably mediates the cerebral vasodilation in response to hypoxia.

The elevated cardiac output, heart rate, and systemic blood pressure return to normal levels after a few days at high altitude. This probably reflects a decrease in sympathetic activity or changes in sympathetic receptors. Nevertheless, hypoxic pulmonary vasoconstriction and pulmonary hypertension persist (along with increased blood viscosity), leading to right ventricular hypertrophy and frequently chronic cor pulmonale (right ventricular failure secondary to pulmonary hypertension).

Many of the predicted responses of the respiratory system to chronic and acute altitude may be seen in the data obtained from one of two medical scientist climbers who made it to the top of Mount Everest without supplemental oxygen in 1981. They were members of the American Medical Research Expedition and had undergone lengthy periods of acclimatization at somewhat less severe high altitudes. Total barometric pressure on top of Mount Everest was 253 mm Hg. This was about 17 mm Hg greater than expected and was explained by local weather conditions and because barometric pressure is higher at lower latitudes. The alveolar P_{CO_2} of the scientist who reached the summit and was able to take samples was an incredibly low 7.5 mm Hg, with a calculated arterial pH of 7.76. This extreme hyperventilation allowed an alveolar P_{O_2} of 35 mm Hg, resulting in a calculated arterial P_{O_2} of 28 mm Hg.

The scientist's arterial hemoglobin concentration was elevated to 18.4 g/100 mL of blood, and his extremely high levels of 2,3-BPG should have shifted his oxyhemoglobin dissociation curve to the right, with a P_{50} of 29.6 at a pH of 7.40. However, his respiratory alkalosis actually shifted the curve to the left, resulting in a P_{50} of 19.4. This leftward shift allowed sufficient loading at the summit to saturate 75% of his hemoglobin with oxygen.

Similar results were obtained under the more controlled conditions of a simulated 40-day "ascent" (in a decompression chamber) to a maximum altitude of 29,028 ft. Arterial blood samples taken from five subjects at the simulated summit had a mean P_{O_2} of 30 mm Hg, a mean P_{CO_2} of 12 mm Hg, and a mean pH of 7.56.

DIVING & THE RESPIRATORY SYSTEM

The major physiologic stresses involved in diving include elevated ambient pressure, decreased effects of gravity, altered respiration, hypothermia, and sensory impairment. The severity of the stress involved depends on the depth attained, the length of the dive, and whether the breath is held or a breathing apparatus is used. The first three physiologic stresses are the focus of this discussion.

Physical Principles

The pressure at the bottom of a column of liquid is proportional to the height of the column, the density of the liquid, and the acceleration of gravity. For example, for each 33 ft of seawater (or 34 ft of fresh water) ambient pressure increases by

1 atmosphere (atm). Thus, at a depth of 33 ft of seawater, total ambient pressure is equal to 1520 mm Hg.

The tissues of the body are composed mainly of water and are therefore nearly incompressible, but gases are compressible and follow Boyle's law. Thus, in a breath-hold dive the *volume* of gas in the lungs is inversely proportional to the depth attained. At 33 ft of depth (2 atm) lung volume is cut in half; at 66 ft (3 atm) it is one third the original lung volume. As gases are compressed, their *densities* increase.

As the total pressure increases, the *partial pressures* of the constituent gases also increase, according to Dalton's law. The biologic effects of gases are generally dependent on their partial pressures rather than on their fractional concentrations. Also, as the partial pressures of gases increase, the amounts *dissolved* in the tissues of the body increase, according to Henry's law.

Effects of Immersion up to the Neck

Merely immersing oneself up to the neck in water causes profound alterations in the cardiovascular and pulmonary systems. These effects are mainly a result of an increase in pressure outside the thorax, abdomen, and limbs.

MECHANICS OF BREATHING

The pressure outside the chest wall of a person standing or seated in neck-deep water is greater than atmospheric, averaging about 20 cm H_2O. This positive pressure outside the chest opposes the normal outward elastic recoil of the chest wall and decreases the functional residual capacity by about 50%. This occurs at the expense of the expiratory reserve volume, which may be decreased by as much as 70%. The intrapleural pressure is less negative at the functional residual capacity because of decreased outward elastic recoil of the chest wall. The work that must be done to bring air into the lungs is greatly increased because extra inspiratory work is necessary to overcome the positive pressure outside the chest. Nonetheless, the vital capacity and total lung capacity are only slightly decreased. As was already pointed out, the expiratory reserve volume is decreased by neck-deep immersion, and the inspiratory reserve volume is therefore increased. The residual volume is slightly decreased because of an increase in pulmonary blood volume. Immersion up to the neck in water results in an increase in the work of breathing of about 60%.

The hydrostatic pressure effects of water outside the chest prevent a submerged person who is trying to breathe through a tube that is communicating with the air above the surface of the water from descending more than about 3 ft. This is true even if the increased airways resistance offered by the tube were negligible and if the person avoided increasing the effective dead space by occluding the mouth end of the tube and exhaling directly into the water (or by using a one-way valve). The reason is that the maximal inspiratory pressure that normal individuals can generate with their inspiratory muscles is about 80 to 100 cm H_2O (that is, intrapleural pressures of -80 to -100 cm H_2O). Because 100 cm is 1 m, or 39.37 in, the maximum depth a person can attain while breathing through a tube in this manner is a little more than 3 ft.

PULMONARY BLOOD FLOW

During neck-deep immersion, increased pressure outside the limbs and abdomen results in less pooling of systemic venous blood in gravity-dependent regions of the body. If the water temperature is below body temperature, a sympathetically mediated venoconstriction occurs, also augmenting venous return. The increased venous return increases the central blood volume by approximately 500 mL. Right atrial pressure increases from about −2 to +16 mm Hg. As a result, the cardiac output and stroke volume increase by about 30%. The increases in pulmonary blood flow and pulmonary blood volume probably result in elevated mean pulmonary artery pressure, capillary recruitment, an increase in the diffusing capacity, and a somewhat improved matching of ventilation and perfusion.

An additional effect of neck-deep immersion is "immersion diuresis." Within a few minutes of immersion, urine flow increases 4- to 5-fold. Osmolal clearance increases only slightly. These findings are consistent with stimulation of stretch receptors in the left atrium and elsewhere in thoracic vessels by the increased thoracic blood volume. This, in turn, is believed either to decrease the secretion of antidiuretic hormone (ADH) by the posterior pituitary gland or to cause the release of a natriuretic hormone from the atria.

Breath-Hold Diving

During a breath-hold dive, the total pressure of gases within the lungs is approximately equal to ambient pressure. Therefore, the *volume* within the thorax must decrease proportionately and partial pressures of gases increase.

THE DIVING REFLEX

Many subjects demonstrate a profound bradycardia (decreased heart rate) and increased systemic vascular resistance with face immersion (especially into cold water) as well as apnea. This "diving reflex" is initiated by as yet unknown sensors in the face or nose. A similar (but greater) response is seen when aquatic mammals such as whales and seals dive. The reflex decreases the workload of the heart and severely limits perfusion to all systemic vascular beds except for the strongest autoregulators—namely, the heart and brain. The cardiovascular effects of the diving reflex are similar to those produced by stimulation of the arterial chemoreceptors when no increase in ventilation can occur, except that the diving reflex also appears to cause the spleen to slowly contract, which releases erythrocytes stored in the spleen into the venous blood. This increases the oxygen-carrying capacity of the blood and therefore the oxygen content of the blood at the same arterial P_{O_2}. The bradycardic component of the diving reflex is demonstrated in Figure 11–2.

GAS EXCHANGE IN THE LUNGS

Breath-hold divers usually hyperventilate before a dive so that typical alveolar P_{O_2}s and P_{CO_2}s might be 120 and 30 mm Hg, respectively. Indeed, breath-hold divers must take care not to hyperventilate so much that their P_{CO_2} gets so low that they do not reach their "breakpoint" (mainly determined by Pa_{CO_2}) until after they lose consciousness from arterial hypoxemia. During a breath-hold dive to a depth of 33 ft,

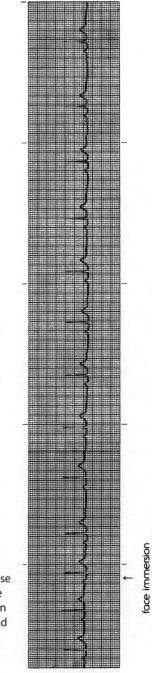

Figure 11–2. The author's electrocardiographic response to face immersion in ice water. The experiment was done with the author in the prone position, and face immersion was performed without changing the position of the head to avoid the effects of changes in baroreceptor activity. Note that heart rate decreased from about 75 to about 43 beats per minute.

lung volume decreases and gases are compressed. Total gas pressure approximately doubles: Thus after 20 seconds at 33 ft the alveolar P_{O_2} may be 160 to 180 mm Hg; even after 1 minute at 33 ft the alveolar P_{O_2} is well above 100 mm Hg. The alveolar P_{CO_2} (which would be less than 40 mm Hg at the surface because of hyperventilation before the dive) also increases during descent to above 40 mm Hg, reversing the gradient for CO_2 transfer. Carbon dioxide therefore diffuses from the alveoli into the pulmonary capillary blood. The alveolar P_{CO_2} therefore does not increase as much as would be predicted by the compression of gases caused by the increased pressure as CO_2 diffuses into the blood. This is believed to result from the much greater solubility of CO_2 than O_2 in the blood. Thus, the transfer of oxygen from alveolus to blood is undisturbed until ascent; however, the normal transfer of carbon dioxide from blood to alveolus is reversed during descent and results in significant retention of carbon dioxide in the blood.

During ascent, the ambient pressure falls rapidly, lung volume increases, and alveolar gas partial pressures decrease accordingly. Alveolar P_{CO_2} falls, allowing CO_2 to diffuse from pulmonary capillary blood into the alveoli. However, the rapid decrease in alveolar P_{O_2} during ascent may result in a decrease in arterial P_{O_2} sufficient to cause the breath-hold diver to lose consciousness. This loss of consciousness can occur rapidly and without warning and usually occurs as divers ascend to a depth of approximately 15 ft or less. It is therefore known as *"shallow water blackout."*

The Use of Underwater Breathing Apparatus

Self-contained underwater breathing apparatus, or scuba gear, mainly consists of a tank full of compressed gas that can be delivered by a demand regulator to the diver when the diver's mouth pressure decreases (during inspiration) to slightly less than the ambient pressure. Expired gas is simply released into the water as bubbles. Therefore, during a dive with scuba gear, gas pressure within the lungs remains close to the ambient pressure at any particular depth. The physiologic stresses on the respiratory system during scuba diving are therefore mainly a consequence of elevated gas densities and partial pressures.

MECHANICS OF BREATHING

During scuba diving, the inspiratory work of breathing is not a great problem at moderate depths because gas is delivered at ambient pressures. At very great depths, however, increased gas *density* becomes a problem because it elevates the airways resistance work of breathing during turbulent flow. For example, in long-term experiments done with subjects *simulating* dives of over 2000 ft inside hyperbaric chambers, all subjects reported that they could breathe only through their mouths: The work of breathing through the nose was too great. This is one reason for replacing nitrogen with helium for deep dives. Helium is only about one seventh as dense as nitrogen.

CONTROL OF BREATHING

The respiratory system's sensitivity to carbon dioxide is decreased at great depths because of increased gas densities and high arterial P_{O_2}s and because divers learn to suppress carbon dioxide drive to conserve compressed gas.

OTHER HAZARDS AT DEPTH

Other hazards that may be encountered in diving to great depths include barotrauma, decompression illness, nitrogen narcosis, oxygen toxicity, and high-pressure nervous syndrome.

Barotrauma—Barotrauma occurs when ambient pressure increases or decreases but the pressure in a closed unventilated area of the body that cannot equilibrate with ambient pressure does not. The barotrauma of descent is called "squeeze." It can affect the middle ear, if the eustachian tube is clogged or edematous, so that a person cannot equilibrate pressure in the middle ear; the sinuses; the lungs, resulting in pulmonary congestion, edema, or hemorrhage; and even cavities in the teeth. The barotrauma of ascent can occur if gases are trapped in areas of the body and begin to expand as the diver ascends. If a diver does not exhale while ascending, expanding pulmonary gas may overdistend and rupture the lung ("burst lung"). This may result in hemorrhage, pneumothorax, or air embolism. Gases trapped in the gastrointestinal tract may cause abdominal discomfort and eructation or flatus as they expand. Barotrauma of the ears, sinuses, and teeth may also occur on rapid ascent from great depths.

Decompression Illness—Decompression illness occurs when gas bubbles form in the blood and body tissues as the ambient pressure decreases. The term "decompression illness" encompasses two different problems, both of which involve gas bubbles. *Arterial gas embolism* is gas bubbles in the arterial blood. Because bubbles do not seem to form in the arterial blood itself, arterial gas embolism usually occurs when airway obstruction prevents expanding gas from being exhaled. As expanding alveoli rupture, gas bubbles may enter pulmonary capillaries and be carried into the arterial blood. Arterial gas embolism is a likely consequence of an ascending diver neglecting to exhale upon rapid ascent. Bubbles resulting from arterial gas embolism are often carried to cerebral blood vessels. The second component of decompression illness, *decompression sickness,* occurs when bubbles form in tissues of the body. During a dive, the increasing ambient pressure causes an elevation of the partial pressure of nitrogen in the body. The high partial pressure of nitrogen causes this normally poorly soluble gas to dissolve in the body tissues and fluids according to Henry's law. This is especially the case in body fat, which has a relatively high nitrogen solubility. At great depths, body tissues become supersaturated with nitrogen.

During a fast ascent, ambient pressure falls rapidly and nitrogen comes out of solution, forming bubbles in body tissues and fluids. The effect is the same as opening a bottle of a carbonated beverage. During the production of a carbonated beverage it is exposed to higher than atmospheric pressures of gases, mainly carbon dioxide, and then capped. The total pressure in the gas layer above the liquid remains greater than atmospheric pressure. The partial pressures of gases dissolved in the liquid phase are in equilibrium with the partial pressures in the gas phase. Gases dissolve in the liquid phase according to Henry's law. When the bottle is uncapped, the pressure in the gas phase drops suddenly and the gas dissolved in the liquid phase comes out of solution, forming bubbles.

The bubbles formed in decompression sickness may enter the venous blood or affect the joints of the extremities. Bubbles that enter the venous blood are usually trapped in the pulmonary circulation and rarely cause symptoms. The symptoms that do occasionally occur, which are known as "the chokes" by divers, include substernal chest pain, dyspnea, and cough and may be accompanied by pulmonary hypertension, pulmonary edema, and hypoxemia. These symptoms are obviously an extremely dangerous form of decompression illness. Even more dangerous, of course, are bubbles in the circulation of the central nervous system, which may result in brain damage and paralysis. They may result from alveolar rupture and arterial gas embolism, as discussed previously, or be carried from the venous blood to the arterial side through a patent foramen ovale or an intrapulmonary shunt. Bubbles that form in the joints of the limbs cause pain ("the bends"). Osteonecrosis of joints may also be caused by inadequate decompression.

The treatment for decompression illness is immediate recompression in a hyperbaric chamber, followed by slow decompression. Decompression illness may be prevented by slow ascents from great depths (according to empirically derived decompression tables) and by substituting helium for nitrogen in inspired gas mixtures. Helium is only about half as soluble as nitrogen in body tissues.

Gas bubbles, although they are sterile, are perceived by the body as foreign. They elicit inflammatory and other responses, including platelet activation, blood clotting, the release of cytokines and other mediators, leukocyte aggregation, free radical production, and endothelial damage. These responses are not reversed by recompression and may continue unless additional treatment is initiated.

Divers who ascend from submersion with no immediate effects of decompression may subsequently suffer decompression illness if they ride in an airplane within a few hours of the dive. Commercial airplanes normally maintain cabin pressures well below 760 mm Hg, with cabin pressures similar to those at altitudes 5000 to 8000 ft above sea level.

Nitrogen Narcosis—Very high partial pressures of nitrogen directly affect the central nervous system, causing euphoria, loss of memory, clumsiness, and irrational behavior. This "rapture of the deep" occurs at depths of 100 ft or more and at greater depths may result in numbness of the limbs, disorientation, motor impairment, and ultimately unconsciousness. The mechanism of nitrogen narcosis is unknown.

Oxygen Toxicity—Inhalation of 100% oxygen at 760 mm Hg or of lower oxygen concentrations at higher ambient pressures can cause central nervous system, visual system, and alveolar damage, although pulmonary manifestations are rare among divers. The mechanism of oxygen toxicity is controversial but probably involves the formation of superoxide anions or other free radicals.

High-Pressure Nervous Syndrome—Exposure to very high ambient pressures, such as those encountered at very great depths (greater than 250 ft), is associated with tremors, decreased mental ability, nausea, vomiting, dizziness, and decreased manual dexterity. This high-pressure nervous syndrome (HPNS) usually occurs when nitrogen has been replaced by helium to decrease gas density, prevent nitrogen narcosis, and help avoid decompression sickness. Small amounts of nitrogen added to the inspired gas mixture help counteract the problem. One hypothesis explaining HPNS is that the syndrome may result from alterations in cerebral neurotransmission.

KEY CONCEPTS

1. The main physiologic stresses of **exercise** on the respiratory system are increased oxygen demand and increased removal of carbon dioxide and hydrogen ions; in a healthy young person, exercise is limited by the cardiovascular system, not the respiratory system.

2. The main physiologic stresses of **altitude** are hypoxia and secondary hypocapnia and respiratory alkalosis; **acclimatization** occurs mainly by renal compensation for the respiratory alkalosis, erythropoiesis, elevated 2,3-BPG concentrations, and resolution of cerebral edema.

3. The main physiologic stresses of **diving** are caused by increased ambient pressures causing gas compression, leading to increased partial pressures and densities and viscosities of gases.

CLINICAL PROBLEMS

11–1. Which of the following would be expected to occur as an untrained person begins to exercise?

   a. Decreased pulmonary vascular resistance

   b. Increased cardiac output

   c. More homogeneous ventilation-perfusion ratios throughout the lung

   d. Increased diffusing capacity

   e. All of the above

11–2. Which of the following responses would be expected in a normal person after 6 days of residence at an altitude of 15,000 ft?

   a. Elevated mean pulmonary artery pressure

   b. Alveolar ventilation greater than at sea level

   c. Increased hematocrit

   d. Decreased plasma bicarbonate

   e. Normal arterial P_{CO_2}

11–3. Which of the following are expected consequences of neck-deep immersion in water?

   a. Increased work of breathing

   b. Decreased functional residual capacity

   c. Increased expiratory reserve volume

   d. Decreased inspiratory reserve volume

SUGGESTED READINGS

Exercise

Eldridge MW, Dempsey JA, Haverkamp HC, Lovering AT, Hokanson JS. Exercise-induced intrapulmonary arteriovenous shunting in healthy humans. *J Appl Physiol.* 2004;797–805.

Hammond MD, Gale GE, Kapitan KS, Ries A, Wagner PD. Pulmonary gas exchange in humans during exercise at sea level. *J Appl Physiol.* 1986;60:1590–1598.

Harf A, Pratt T, Hughes JMB. Regional distribution of $\dot{V}A/\dot{Q}$ in man at rest and with exercise measured with Krypton-81 m. *J Appl Physiol.* 1978;44:115–123.

Wasserman K, Whipp BJ. Exercise physiology in health and disease. *Am Rev Respir Dis.* 1975;112:219–249.

Whipp BJ. Breathing during exercise. In: Fishman AP, ed. *Pulmonary Diseases and Disorders.* 3rd ed. New York, NY: McGraw-Hill; 1998:229–241.

Altitude

Bartsch P, Mairbaurl H, Maggiorini M, Swenson ER. Physiological aspects of high-altitude pulmonary edema. *J Appl Physiol.* 2005;98:1101–1110.

Guenter CA, Welch MH, Hogg JC. *Clinical Aspects of Respiratory Physiology.* Philadelphia, Pa: Lippincott; 1977:3–37.

Hackett PH, Roach RC. High altitude illness. *N Engl J Med.* 2001;345:107–114.

Hohne C, Krebs MO, Seiferheld M, Boemke W, Kaczmarczyk G, Swenson ER. Acetazolamide prevents hypoxic pulmonary vasoconstriction in conscious dogs. *J Appl Physiol.* 2004;97:515–521.

Hopkins SR, Garg J, Bolar DS, Balouch J, Levin DL. Pulmonary blood flow heterogeneity during hypoxia and high-altitude pulmonary edema. *Am J Respir Crit Care Med* 2005;171:83–87.

Houston CS. Mountain sickness. *Sci Am.* 1992;267:58–66.

Houston CS, Sutton JR, Cymerman A, Reeves JT. Operation Everest II: Man at extreme altitude. *J Appl Physiol.* 1987;63:877–882.

Lahiri S, Milledge JS. Pulmonary adaptation and clinical disorders related to high altitude. In: Fishman AP, ed. *Pulmonary Diseases and Disorders.* 3rd ed. New York, NY: McGraw-Hill; 1998:965–977.

Loeppky JA, Icenogle MV, Maes D, Riboni K, Hinghofer-Szalkay H, Roach RC. Early fluid retention and severe mountain sickness. *J Appl Physiol.* 2005;98:591–597.

Richalet J-P, Rivera M, Bouchet P, Chirinos E, Onnen I, Petitjean O, Bienvenu A, Lasne F, Moutereau S, Leon-Velarde F. Acetazolamide: A treatment for chronic mountain sickness. *Am J Respir Crit Care Med.* 2005;172:1427–1433.

Schoene RB, Hackett PH, Hornbein TF. High altitude. In: Murray JF, Nadel JA, eds. *Textbook of Respiratory Medicine.* 3rd ed. Philadelphia, Pa: WB Saunders and Company; 2000:1915–1950.

West JB. *Everest: The Testing Place.* New York, McGraw-Hill, 1985.

West JB, Hackett PH, Maret KH, et al. Pulmonary gas exchange on the summit of Mount Everest. *J Appl Physiol.* 1983;55:678–687.

Winslow RM, Samaja M, West JB. Red cell function at extreme altitude on Mount Everest. *J Appl Physiol.* 1984;56:109–116.

Diving

Clark JM. Diving injuries and air embolism. In: Fishman AP, ed. *Pulmonary Diseases and Disorders.* 3rd ed. New York, NY: McGraw-Hill; 1998:980–987.

Espersen K, Frandsen H, Lorentzen T, Kanstrup I-L, Christensen NJ. The human spleen as an erythrocyte reservoir in diving-related interventions. *J Appl Physiol.* 2002;92:2071–2079.

Hong SK, Ceretelli P, Cruz JC, Rahn H. Mechanics of respiration during submersion in water. *J Appl Physiol.* 1969;27:535–538.

Liner MH. Cardiovascular and pulmonary responses to breath-hold diving in humans. *Acta Physiol Scand.* 1994;151(suppl 620):1–32.

Moon RE, Vann RD, Bennett PB. The physiology of decompression illness. *Sci Am.* 1995;273:70–77.

Muth CM, Radermacher P, Pittner A, Steinacker J, Schabana R, Hamich S, Paulat K, Calzia E. Arterial blood gases during diving in elite apnea divers. *Int J Sports Med.* 2003;24:104–107.

Neuman TS. Arterial gas embolism and decompression sickness. *News Physiol Sci.* 2002;17:77–81.

Pollock NW, Natoli MJ, Gerth WA, Thalman ED, Vann RD. Risk of decompression sickness during exposure to high cabin altitude after diving. *Aviat Space Environ Med.* 2003;74:1163–1168.

Strauss RH (ed). *Diving Medicine.* New York, NY: Grune & Stratton; 1976.

Strauss RH. Diving medicine. *Am Rev Respir Dis.* 1979;19:1001–1023.

Clinical Problem Answers

CHAPTER 2

2–1. The correct answer is:

$$\text{Compliance} = \frac{\Delta V}{\Delta P}$$

Remember to use *transmural* pressure differences in calculations of compliance:

Transmural pressure = pressure inside − pressure outside

Compliance of lungs is

$$C_L = \frac{\Delta V}{\underset{\text{end inspiration}}{(P_A - P_{ip})} - \underset{\text{preinspiration}}{(P_A - P_{ip})}}$$

where P_A = alveolar pressure
P_{ip} = intrapleural pressure

$$C_L = \frac{0.500 \text{ L}}{[0 - (-10) \text{ cm H}_2\text{O}] - [0 - (-5) \text{ cm H}_2\text{O}]}$$

$$C_L = 0.10 \text{ L/cm H}_2\text{O}$$

2–2. The correct answer is:

a. $$C_L = \frac{0.500 \text{ L}}{(20 - 10 \text{ cm H}_2\text{O}) - [0 - (-3) \text{ cm H}_2\text{O}]}$$

$$C_L = 0.07 \text{ L/cm H}_2\text{O}$$

b. $$C_T = \frac{\Delta V}{\underset{\text{end inspiration}}{(P_A - P_B)} - \underset{\text{preinspiration}}{(P_A - P_B)}}$$

$$C_T = \frac{0.500 \text{ L}}{(20 - 0) \text{ cm H}_2\text{O} - (0 - 0) \text{ cm H}_2\text{O}}$$

250

$$C_T = \frac{0.500 \text{ L}}{20 \text{ cm H}_2\text{O}}$$

$$C_T = 0.025 \text{ L/cm H}_2\text{O}$$

where P_B = pressure outside the chest wall. It is considered to be 0 cm H_2O in this calculation.

c. $\dfrac{1}{C_T} = \dfrac{1}{C_L} + \dfrac{1}{C_W}$

$$\frac{1}{C_W} = \frac{1}{C_T} - \frac{1}{C_L}$$

$$\frac{1}{C_W} = \frac{1}{0.025 \text{ L/cm H}_2\text{O}} - \frac{1}{0.07 \text{ L/cm H}_2\text{O}}$$

$$\frac{1}{C_W} = (40 - 14.3)/\text{L/cm H}_2\text{O}$$

$$\frac{1}{C_W} = 25.7/\text{L/cm H}_2\text{O}$$

$$C_W = 0.039 \text{ L/cm H}_2\text{O}$$

2–3. The correct answer is **e.**
All of the conditions lead to decreased compliance. Surgical removal of one lobe would decrease pulmonary compliance because the lobes of the lung are in parallel and compliances in parallel add directly.

2–4. The correct answer is **e.**

2–5. The correct answer is **e.**

2–6. The correct answer is **e.**

2–7. The correct answer is **d.**
Alveolar elastic recoil is greater at high lung volumes, which helps oppose dynamic compression and decrease airways resistance by traction on small airways. During a forced expiration, as soon as dynamic compression occurs the effective driving pressure for airflow becomes alveolar pressure minus intrapleural pressure (instead of alveolar pressure minus atmospheric pressure). However, alveolar pressure minus intrapleural pressure equals the alveolar elastic recoil pressure.

CHAPTER 3

3–1. The correct answer is **f.**
Fibrosis increases lung elastic recoil, but emphysema decreases elastic recoil of the lungs. In the supine position, the outward recoil of the chest wall is decreased, as it is in obesity and pregnancy.

3–2. As a person stands up, the effects of gravity alter the mechanics of breathing (and also decrease venous return). The contents of the abdomen are pulled away from the diaphragm, thus increasing the outward elastic recoil of the chest wall. The inward recoil of the lungs is not affected, and so the *functional residual capacity* (FRC) is increased. The *residual volume* (RV) is relatively unaffected. The *expiratory reserve volume* (ERV) increases because the FRC is increased and the RV is relatively unchanged. The total lung capacity (TLC) may increase slightly because of the slightly decreased inward elastic recoil of the chest wall at high lung volumes and because the abdominal contents are pulled away from the diaphragm. The tidal volume (VT) is probably unchanged. The higher FRC and similar TLC and VT lead to a decrease in the *inspiratory reserve volume* (IRV) and a decrease in the *inspiratory capacity* (IC). The *vital capacity* (VC) is also relatively unchanged, although it may be slightly increased because of the slight increase in TLC and the decreased intrathoracic blood volume.

3–3. Assuming general good health and normal weight, the main changes seen with age are a *loss of pulmonary elastic recoil* and a slight *increase* of the elastic recoil of the chest wall, especially at higher volumes. The loss of pulmonary elastic recoil has the secondary effect of *increasing airway closure* in dependent areas of the lung at the lower lung volumes. For these reasons, the *FRC* will be increased and the *RV* may be greatly increased, with the *TLC* slightly decreased. The *VT* should be unchanged or may be either slightly increased or decreased, depending on whether the increased lung compliance, increased airways resistance, or decreased chest wall compliance predominates. The *ERV* will decrease because the increase in *RV* due to airway closure is greater than the increase in FRC. *IRV* and *IC* are decreased, as is the *VC*. The *closing volume* is also increased.

3–4. The correct answer is:

$$V_2 = V_1 \times \text{temperature correction} \times \text{pressure correction}$$

$$\text{Temperature correction} = \frac{V_2}{V_1} = \frac{T_2}{T_1}$$

$$\text{Therefore, } V_2 = V_1 \times \frac{T_2}{T_1}$$

$$\text{Pressure correction} = P_1 V_1 = P_2 V_2$$

$$\text{Therefore, } V_2 = V_1 \times \frac{P_1}{P_2}$$

Combining the two, we get

$$V_2 = V_1 \times \frac{T_2}{T_1} \times \frac{P_1}{P_2}$$

Note that temperatures must be expressed in degrees Kelvin (K) when these corrections are made.

a. The V_{STPD} is

$$V_{STPD} = V_{ATPS} \times \frac{T_{STPD}}{T_{ATPS}} \times \frac{P_{ATPS}}{P_{STPD}}$$

$$V_{STPD} = 1\ L \times \frac{273\ K}{(273 + 23)\ K} \times \frac{(770 - 21)\ mm\ Hg}{760\ mm\ Hg}$$

$$V_{STPD} = 0.91\ L$$

b. The V_{BTPS} is

$$V_{BTPS} = V_{ATPS} \times \frac{T_{BTPS}}{T_{ATPS}} \times \frac{P_{ATPS}}{P_{BTPS}}$$

$$V_{BTPS} = 1\ L \times \frac{(273 + 37)\ K}{(273 + 23)\ K} \times \frac{(770 - 21)\ mm\ Hg}{(770 - 47)\ mm\ Hg}$$

$$V_{BTPS} = 1.1\ L$$

3–5. The volume of N_2 in the spirometer is 0.056×36 L, or 2.0 L. This is the volume of N_2 in the subject's lungs when the test began (at her FRC). Since N_2 constituted 80% of her FRC, her FRC is equal to $100 \div 80 \times 2.0$ L, or 1.25×2.0 L, which is equal to 2.5 L.

3–6. Because helium is not absorbed or given off by the lung, the initial amount of helium in the system must equal the final amount of helium in the system. The amount is equal to the fractional concentration times the volume:

$$F_{HE_i} \times V_{sp_i} = F_{HE_f}(V_{sp_f} + V_{L_f})$$

where F = fractional concentration
$\quad\quad\ V$ = volume
$\quad\quad sp$ = spirometer
$\quad\quad\ \ L$ = lungs
$\quad\quad\ \ i$ = initial
$\quad\quad\ \ f$ = final (after equilibration)

Because the test was ended at the end of a normal expiration, V_{L_f} equals the subject's FRC.

$$0.15 \times 10\ L = 0.11\ (10.64\ L + FRC)$$
$$1.5\ L = 1.17\ L + 0.11 \times FRC$$
$$0.11 \times FRC = 1.5\ L - 1.17\ L$$
$$FRC = \frac{0.33\ L}{0.11}$$
$$FRC = 3.0\ L$$

3–7. The correct answer is:

$$P_{M_i} \times V_{L_i} = P_{M_f} \times (V_{L_i} + \Delta V)$$

where P = pressure
  V = volume
  M = mouth
  L = lung
  i = initial
  f = final

Because the valve was closed at the end of a normal expiration, V_{L_i} equals the subject's FRC.

$$760 \text{ mm Hg} \times FRC = 750 \text{ mm Hg (FRC} + 50 \text{ mL)}$$
$$10 \text{ FRC} = 37{,}500 \text{ mL}$$
$$FRC = 3.75 \text{ L}$$

3–8. Assuming that the two tests have been done correctly, this patient has approximately 750 mL of *trapped gas* at her FRC.

3–9. The correct answer is:

a. $\dot{V}_E$ is

$$\dot{V}_E = n \times V_T = \frac{10 \text{ breaths}}{\text{min}} \times \frac{500 \text{ mL}}{\text{breath}} = \frac{5000 \text{ mL}}{\text{min}}$$

b. $\dot{V}_A$ is

$$V_T = V_A + V_D$$

Multiply by rate

$$\dot{V}_E = \dot{V}_A + \dot{V}_D$$

$$\dot{V}_A = \dot{V}_E - \dot{V}_D = \frac{10 \text{ breaths}}{\text{min}} \left(\frac{500 \text{ mL}}{\text{breath}} - \frac{150 \text{ mL}}{\text{breath}} \right)$$

$$\dot{V}_A = \frac{3500 \text{ mL}}{\text{min}}$$

c. The new $\dot{V}_E$ and $\dot{V}_A$ are

$$\dot{V}_E = \frac{15 \text{ breaths}}{\text{min}} \times \frac{500 \text{ mL}}{\text{breath}} = \frac{7500 \text{ mL}}{\text{min}}$$

$$\dot{V}_A = \frac{15 \text{ breaths}}{\text{min}} \left(\frac{500 \text{ mL}}{\text{breath}} - \frac{150 \text{ mL}}{\text{breath}} \right) = \frac{5250 \text{ mL}}{\text{min}}$$

d. The new $\dot{V}_E$ and $\dot{V}_A$ are

$$\dot{V}_E = \frac{10 \text{ breaths}}{\text{min}} \times \frac{750 \text{ mL}}{\text{breath}} = \frac{7500 \text{ mL}}{\text{min}}$$

$$\dot{V}_A = \frac{10 \text{ breaths}}{\text{min}} \left(\frac{750 \text{ mL}}{\text{breath}} - \frac{150 \text{ mL}}{\text{breath}} \right) = \frac{6000 \text{ mL}}{\text{min}}$$

3–10. The correct answer is:

$$\frac{V_{D_{CO_2}}}{V_T} = \frac{Pa_{CO_2} - P\bar{E}_{CO_2}}{Pa_{CO_2}}$$

$$P\bar{E}_{CO_2} = 0.04\ (747\ mm\ Hg - 47\ mm\ Hg)$$
$$P\bar{E}_{CO_2} = 28\ mm\ Hg$$

$$\frac{V_{D_{CO_2}}}{V_T} = \frac{40\ mm\ Hg - 28\ mm\ Hg}{40\ mm\ Hg}$$

$$\frac{V_{D_{CO_2}}}{V_T} = 0.3$$

Since $V_T = \dfrac{\dot{V}_E}{n}$

$$V_T = \frac{6000\ mL/min}{12\ breaths/min}$$
$$V_T = 500\ mL$$
$$V_{D_{CO_2}} = 0.3 \times 500\ mL$$
$$V_{D_{CO_2}} = 150\ mL$$

Since $V_{D_{CO_2}}$ = anatomic dead space + alveolar dead space, the alveolar dead space = 50 mL. The presence of alveolar dead space results in an arterial end-tidal P_{CO_2} difference, so arterial P_{CO_2} should exceed end-tidal.

3–11. The correct answer is:

$$PA_{CO_2} \propto \frac{\dot{V}_{CO_2}}{\dot{V}_A}$$

If alveolar ventilation doubles, alveolar P_{CO_2} is cut in half:

$$PA_{CO_2} = 20\ mm\ Hg$$

$$PA_{O_2} = PI_{O_2} - \frac{PA_{CO_2}}{R} + F$$

$$PI_{O_2} = 0.2093 \times (760 - 47)\ mm\ Hg$$
$$PI_{O_2} = 149\ mm\ Hg$$

$$PA_{O_2} = 149\ mm\ Hg - \frac{20\ mm\ Hg}{0.8}$$

$$PA_{O_2} = 149\ mm\ Hg - 25\ mm\ Hg = 124\ mm\ Hg$$

3–12. The correct answer is **b.**

At the residual volume, airways in gravity-dependent portions of the lungs are likely to be collapsed. Alveoli in upper regions of the lung are on the steep portion of their pressure-volume curves (i.e., they are more compliant than they are at higher lung volumes), and so most of the labeled gas will enter the alveoli in the upper portions of the lung.

CHAPTER 4

4–1. The correct answer is:

$$\Delta P = \dot{Q} \times R$$

$$R = \frac{\Delta P}{\dot{Q}}$$

Pulmonary vascular resistance (PVR):

$$PVR = \frac{MPAP - MLAP}{\dot{Q}t}$$

where MPAP = mean pulmonary artery pressure
MLAP = mean left atrial pressure
$\dot{Q}t$ = cardiac output

$$PVR = \frac{(15 - 5)\ mm\ Hg}{5\ L/min}$$

$$PVR = 2\ mm\ Hg/L/min$$

Systemic vascular resistance (SVR):

$$SVR = \frac{MABP - RAP}{\dot{Q}t}$$

where MABP = mean arterial blood pressure
RAP = right atrial pressure
$\dot{Q}t$ = cardiac output

$$SVR = \frac{(100 - 2)\ mm\ Hg}{5\ L/min}$$

$$SVR = 19.6\ mm\ Hg/L/min$$

4–2. The correct answer is **d.**
Only moderate exercise would be expected to cause a decrease in pulmonary vascular resistance (PVR). Exercise increases the cardiac output and raises pulmonary artery pressure, which cause recruitment of pulmonary vessels, distention of pulmonary vessels, or both.

At 15,000 ft above sea level, barometric pressure is only about 429 mm Hg. Breathing ambient air, the inspired P_{O_2} is about 80 mm Hg and alveolar P_{O_2} is about 50 mm Hg. This degree of alveolar hypoxia elicits hypoxic pulmonary vasoconstriction and increases PVR.

PVR is high at both high and low lung volumes, as shown in Figure 4–4.

Blood loss leads to decreased venous return and a decrease in cardiac output and mean pulmonary artery pressure. This causes a derecruitment of pulmonary vessels and decreases their distention, increasing PVR.

4–3. The correct answers are **b** and **d.**

Zone 1 is defined as an area of the lung in which no blood flow occurs because alveolar pressure is greater than pulmonary artery pressure. Blood loss secondary to trauma lowers venous return and cardiac output. As a result, pulmonary artery pressure is likely to fall, increasing the likelihood of zone 1 conditions in the lung. Positive-pressure ventilation with PEEP (positive airway pressure during *expiration,* often used on patients at risk for spontaneous atelectasis, causes positive alveolar and pleural pressures throughout the respiratory cycle) would also increase the likelihood of zone 1 conditions in the lung.

Ascent to 15,000 ft (see Chapter 11) increases pulmonary artery pressure by activating hypoxic pulmonary vasoconstriction and increasing cardiac output; moderate exercise increases mean pulmonary artery pressure by increasing venous return and cardiac output. Both of these would decrease the tendency toward zone 1 conditions. Lying down lowers the hydrostatic pressure gradient that must be overcome to perfuse nondependent portions of the lung. It also increases, at least transiently, venous return and cardiac output by decreasing the amount of blood held in the systemic veins by gravity.

4–4. The correct answer is **f.**

Each of the above conditions could contribute to the formation of pulmonary edema. Left ventricular failure and overtransfusion with saline both increase pulmonary capillary hydrostatic pressure, which increases the tendency toward pulmonary edema, as given by the Starling equation. Low plasma protein concentration, caused by a protein-poor diet or renal problems or by *dilution* in overtransfusion with saline, is another predisposing factor that may lead to pulmonary edema because it lowers the plasma colloid osmotic pressure. Destruction of portions of the pulmonary capillary endothelium or occlusion of the lymphatic drainage of portions of the lung may also be causative factors in pulmonary edema.

CHAPTER 5

5–1. The correct answer is **e.**

With a partial obstruction of its airway the right lung will have a ventilation-perfusion ratio lower than that of the left lung; therefore, it will have a lower alveolar P_{O_2} and a higher alveolar P_{CO_2}. With more alveolar-capillary units overperfused, the calculated shunt will increase. The overperfusion may be somewhat attenuated if *hypoxic pulmonary vasoconstriction* diverts some blood flow away from hypoxic and hypercapnic alveoli to the better-ventilated left lung, but this response never functions perfectly. As a result, the arterial P_{O_2} will fall.

5–2. The correct answers are **a, b,** and **c.**

The right lung, which is more gravity-dependent, will have a greater blood flow per unit volume than will the left lung because hydrostatic forces increase the intravascular pressures, causing more distention, recruitment, or both. The pleural surface pressure is less negative in the more gravity-dependent region, and so the alveolar-distending pressure is lower in the right lung and the alveoli are smaller. Because of this, the alveoli of the right lung are on a steeper portion of their pressure-volume curves and are therefore better ventilated. The difference in blood flow between the two lungs, however, is greater than is the difference in ventilation, so the right lung has a lower $\dot{V}A/\dot{Q}c$ than does the left. This leads to a lower $P_{A_{O_2}}$ and a higher $P_{A_{CO_2}}$ in the right lung.

CHAPTER 6

6–1. Explanations of how each condition or circumstance affects the diffusing capacity of lungs follow:

a. Changing from the supine to the upright position slightly decreases the diffusing capacity by decreasing the venous return because of pooling of blood in the extremities and abdomen. The decreased venous return decreases the central blood volume and may slightly decrease the right ventricular output, resulting in derecruitment of pulmonary capillaries and decreased surface area for diffusion.

b. Exercise increases the diffusing capacity by increasing the cardiac output. This recruits previously unperfused capillaries, increasing the surface area available for diffusion. Oxygen transfer across the alveolar-capillary barrier will also increase because at high cardiac outputs the linear velocity of the blood moving through the pulmonary capillaries increases and there is less perfusion limitation of oxygen transfer.

c. A Valsalva maneuver (an expiratory effort against a closed glottis) greatly decreases the pulmonary capillary blood volume and therefore decreases the diffusing capacity.

d. Anemia decreases the diffusing capacity by decreasing the hemoglobin available to chemically combine with oxygen. The partial pressure of oxygen in the plasma in the pulmonary capillaries therefore equilibrates more rapidly with the alveolar P_{O_2}, leading to increased perfusion limitation of oxygen transfer.

e. A low cardiac output because of blood loss decreases the diffusing capacity by decreasing the venous return and the central blood volume. Pulmonary capillary blood volume decreases, resulting in derecruitment and decreased surface area for diffusion.

f. Diffuse interstitial fibrosis of the lungs thickens the alveolar-capillary barrier (as does interstitial edema), resulting in decreased diffusion of gases across the alveolar-capillary barrier, in accordance with Fick's law.

g. Emphysema destroys the alveolar interstitium and blood vessels, decreasing the surface area for diffusion.

6–2. The correct answer is **a.**

If the pulmonary capillary partial pressure equals the alveolar partial pressure before the blood leaves the capillary, its transfer is perfusion limited, not diffusion limited. Increasing the cardiac output will increase the diffusion of the gas both by increasing the velocity of blood flow through the capillary and by recruiting more capillaries. Recruiting more capillaries increases the surface area for gas exchange; increasing the alveolar partial pressure will increase the partial pressure gradient. Surface area and partial pressure gradient are both in the numerator of Fick's law.

CHAPTER 7

7–1. The correct answers are **b** and **d.**
The blood oxygen-carrying *capacity* (excluding physically dissolved O_2) will decrease from 20.1 to 16.08 mL O_2/100 mL of blood. The arterial P_{O_2} is not affected by the decreased hemoglobin concentration, and so the oxygen saturation of the hemoglobin that is present is also unaffected. If alveolar P_{O_2} is approximately 104 mm Hg, then the arterial P_{O_2} is about 100 and hemoglobin is about 97.4% saturated. The arterial oxygen content (excluding physically dissolved O_2) is therefore reduced from 19.58 to 15.66 mL O_2/100 mL of blood.

7–2. The correct answer is:
Physically dissolved:

$$\frac{0.003 \text{ mL } O_2/100 \text{ mL blood}}{\text{mm Hg } P_{O_2}} \times 100 \text{ mm Hg} = \frac{0.3 \text{ mL } O_2}{100 \text{ mL blood}}$$

Bound to hemoglobin:

$$\frac{1.34 \text{ mL } O_2}{\text{g Hb}} \times \frac{10 \text{ g Hb}}{100 \text{ mL blood}} \times 0.974 = \frac{13.05 \text{ mL } O_2}{100 \text{ mL blood}}$$

Total: 13.35 mL O_2/100 mL of blood

7–3. The correct answer is:
Oxygen-carry *capacity:*

$$\frac{1.34 \text{ mL } O_2}{\text{g Hb}} \times \frac{10 \text{ g Hb}}{100 \text{ mL blood}} = \frac{13.4 \text{ mL } O_2}{100 \text{ mL blood}}$$

$$\text{Saturation} = \frac{\text{content}}{\text{capacity}} = \frac{10}{13.4} = 0.75 \times 100\%$$

Saturation = 75%

7–4. The correct answer is **e.**
Hypercapnia, acidosis, increased blood levels of 2, 3-BPG, and increased body temperature all shift the oxyhemoglobin dissociation curve to the right and should therefore increase the P_{50}.

CHAPTER 8

8–1. The correct answer is **d.**
The pH is low, the Pa_{CO_2} is high, and the plasma bicarbonate concentration is slightly elevated. The Pa_{O_2} is low and the anion gap is normal. This appears to be uncompensated respiratory acidosis secondary to hypoventilation caused, for example, by acute respiratory depression, acute airway obstruction, or hypoventilation of a patient on a mechanical ventilator.

8–2. The correct answer is **a.**
The pHa and Pa_{CO_2} are both elevated and the Pa_{O_2} and anion gap are within normal limits. Bicarbonate is elevated. This appears to be partly compensated metabolic alkalosis, as might be seen 10 minutes after vomiting.

8–3. The correct answer is **e.**
The pHa is very high and the Pa_{CO_2} is very low. The Pa_{O_2} is abnormally *high*. The plasma bicarbonate concentration is slightly depressed, but it falls on the normal buffer line for a pH of 7.60. This is uncompensated respiratory alkalosis secondary to hyperventilation. Since the Pa_{O_2} is *high,* it is not caused by hypoxic stimulation of alveolar ventilation (see Chapters 9 and 11) but is probably of voluntary or psychological origin, caused by drugs that stimulate ventilation or by overadministration of mechanical ventilation.

8–4. The correct answer is **f.**
The arterial pH is low but close to the normal range. The arterial P_{CO_2} is high and the Pa_{O_2} is low. The plasma bicarbonate concentration is above the normal buffer line. This is chronic respiratory acidosis (caused by hypoventilation) with renal compensation. This is a familiar pattern in patients with chronic obstructive pulmonary disease.

8–5. The correct answer is **c.**
The arterial pH is low, indicating acidosis, but the arterial P_{CO_2} is also low. The arterial P_{O_2} is normal or even slightly elevated, and the plasma bicarbonate is low. This appears to be metabolic acidosis with respiratory compensation, as indicated by the low Pa_{CO_2} and somewhat elevated Pa_{O_2}. The anion gap is within the normal range, as would be seen with diarrhea.

8–6. The correct answer is **b.**
The data are identical to those in problem 8–5, except for the high anion gap. This is consistent with metabolic acidosis with respiratory compensation caused by lactic acidosis, diabetic ketoacidosis, renal retention of anions, or ingestion of organic anions such as salicylate, ethylene glycol, ethanol, or methanol.

8–7. The correct answer is **b.**
The patient clearly has obstructive disease. His FEV_1/FVC, FEV_3/FVC, PEF, and $FEF_{25-75\%}$ are all very low. His high TLC, high FRC, and very high RV, combined with his low FEV_1/FVC, rule out restrictive disease. Inspiratory flow data are not provided, and so we must assume that the patient's problem is primarily expiratory.

8–8. The correct answer is **c.**
The patient's problem probably is not asthma because there was no improvement in his dynamic lung volumes after he received a bronchodilator. Sarcoidosis and alveolar fibrosis, both restrictive diseases, have already been ruled out, leaving the choice of emphysema or chronic bronchitis. (Remember that patients often have both.) The patient only sometimes produces sputum, does not appear to be cyanotic, and has a low diffusing capacity for carbon monoxide. His disease is therefore more likely to be emphysema than chronic bronchitis.

8–9. The correct answer is **a.**
The patient does not appear to have an obstructive disease. His FEV_1/FVC is greater than predicted. He does appear to have a restrictive disease—his lung volumes and capacities are all approximately two thirds of the predicted values.

8–10. The correct answer is **c.**
Emphysema and chronic bronchitis are obstructive diseases and have therefore been ruled out. Interstitial alveolar fibrosis is the most likely of the remaining three choices because of the patient's very low diffusing capacity.

CHAPTER 9

9–1. The correct answer is **e.**
Voluntary apnea (breath holding) for 90 seconds causes alveolar P_{O_2} to decrease and alveolar P_{CO_2} to increase (about 15 mm Hg). These alterations are reflected in the arterial P_{O_2} and P_{CO_2}. The decrease in arterial P_{O_2} and the increase in arterial P_{CO_2} (and the increase in hydrogen ion concentration) stimulate the arterial chemoreceptors. Ninety seconds is a sufficient period for the carbon dioxide to begin to diffuse into the cerebrospinal fluid and stimulate the central chemoreceptors. The hypoxia and acidosis should have little effect on the central chemoreceptors: The central chemoreceptors are not responsive to hypoxia, and few hydrogen ions would be expected to get across the blood-brain barrier in 90 seconds.

9–2. The correct answers are **b, c, d,** and **e.**
Mild anemia without metabolic acidosis does not stimulate the arterial chemoreceptors because the arterial chemoreceptors are stimulated by low arterial P_{O_2} rather than by a low arterial oxygen content. Severe exercise may cause a lactic acidosis that stimulates the arterial chemoreceptors. Intrapulmonary shunts and hypoxia stimulate the arterial chemoreceptors, as does acute airway obstruction, which leads to hypoxia and hypercapnia.

9–3. The correct answer is **d.**

9–4. The correct answers are **a, c,** and **e.**

CHAPTER 11

11–1. The correct answer is **e.**

As cardiac output increases in response to exercise, previously unperfused capillaries are recruited. This recruitment, which occurs primarily in upper regions of the lung, results in a decreased pulmonary vascular resistance, more homogeneous ventilation-perfusion ratios, and a greater surface area for diffusion. The increased cardiac output also results in increased linear velocity of blood flow through the lung, which helps increase the diffusing capacity.

11–2. The correct answers are **a, b, c,** and **d.**

Mean pulmonary artery pressure is elevated because of the continued presence of hypoxic pulmonary vasoconstriction. Alveolar ventilation continues to be elevated because of hypoxic drive of the arterial chemoreceptors. This results in hypocapnia. The respiratory alkalosis caused by the hypocapnia, however, is partially compensated for by renal excretion of base, resulting in a decreased plasma bicarbonate concentration. Hematocrit is increased secondary to increased erythropoiesis as mediated by erythropoietin.

11–3. The correct answers are **a** and **b.**

The outward elastic recoil of the chest wall is decreased by the hydrostatic pressure of neck-deep water. This increases the work that must be done to bring air into the lungs and decreases the FRC. The decrease in FRC occurs mainly at the expense of the ERV, which decreases. Because the VC decreases only slightly, the IRV is increased.

Appendix

I. SYMBOLS USED IN RESPIRATORY PHYSIOLOGY

P   Partial pressure of a gas (mm Hg)

V   Volume of a gas (mL)

$\dot{V}$ Flow of gas (mL/min, L/s)

Q   Volume of blood (mL)

$\dot{Q}$ Blood flow (mL/min)

F   Fractional concentration of a gas

C   Content or concentration of a substance in the blood (milliliters per 100 mL of blood)

S   Saturation in the blood (%)

I   Inspired

E   Expired

$\bar{\text{E}}$ Mixed expired

A   Alveolar

T   Tidal

D   Dead space

a   Arterial

v   Venous

$\bar{\text{v}}$ Mixed venous

c   Capillary

c′   End capillary

II. THE LAWS GOVERNING THE BEHAVIOR OF GASES

1. **Avogadro's hypothesis** Equal volumes of different gases at equal temperatures contain the same number of molecules. Similarly, equal numbers of molecules in identical volumes and at the same temperature will exert the same pressure. (One mole of any gas will contain 6.02×10^{23} molecules and will occupy a volume of 22.4 L at a temperature of 0°C and a pressure of 760 mm Hg.)

2. **Dalton's law** In a gas mixture the pressure exerted by each individual gas in a space is independent of the pressures of other gases in the mixture, e.g.,

$$P_A = P_{H_2O} + P_{O_2} + P_{CO_2} + P_{N_2}$$
$$P_{gas,\, x} = F_{gas\, x} \times P_{tot}$$

3. **Boyle's law**

$$P_1V_1 = P_2V_2 \text{ (at constant temperature)}$$

4. **Charles' law or Gay Lussac's law**

$$\frac{V_1}{V_2} = \frac{T_1}{T_2} \text{ (at constant pressure, with T the absolute temperature in K)}$$

5. **Ideal gas law**

$$PV = nRT$$

6. **Henry's law** The weight of a gas absorbed by a liquid with which it does not combine chemically is directly proportional to the pressure of the gas to which the liquid is exposed (and its solubility in the liquid).

7. **Graham's law** The rate of diffusion of a gas (in the gas phase) is inversely proportional to the square root of its molecular weight.

8. **Fick's law of diffusion**

$$\dot{V}_{gas} = \frac{A \times D \times (P_1 - P_2)}{T}$$

$$D \propto \frac{solubility}{\sqrt{molecular\ weight}}$$

III. FREQUENTLY USED EQUATIONS

1. The alveolar air equation:

$$P_{A_{O_2}} = P_{I_{O_2}} - \frac{P_{A_{CO_2}}}{R} + F$$

2. The Bohr equation:

$$\frac{V_{D_{CO_2}}}{V_T} = \frac{Pa_{CO_2} - P\bar{E}_{CO_2}}{Pa_{CO_2}}$$

3. Components of alveolar pressure:

$$P_A = P_{ip} + P_{elas}$$

4. The diffusing capacity equation:

$$D_{L_x} = \frac{\dot{V}_x}{P_{x_1} - P_{x_2}}$$

5. The Fick equation:

$$\dot{V}_x = \frac{A \times D \times P_{x_1} - P_{x_2}}{T}$$

6. The Henderson-Hasselbalch equation:

$$pH = pK' + \log \frac{[HCO_3^-]}{.03 \times P_{CO_2}}$$

7. Oxygen-carrying capacity of hemoglobin:

$$1.34 \text{ mL } O_2/\text{g Hb}$$

8. The shunt equation:

$$\frac{\dot{Q}s}{\dot{Q}T} = \frac{Cc'_{O_2} - Ca_{O_2}}{Cc'_{O_2} - C\bar{v}_{O_2}}$$

9. Solubility of oxygen in plasma:

$$0.003 \text{ mL } O_2/100 \text{ mL blood/mm Hg } P_{O_2}$$

IV. PULMONARY FUNCTION TEST DECISION TREE

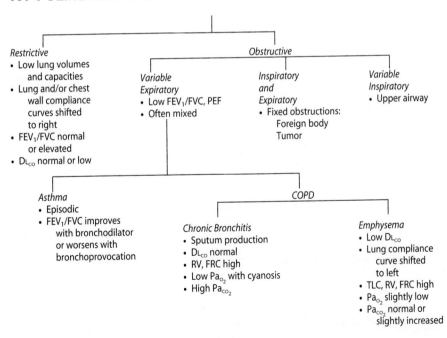

Restrictive
- Low lung volumes and capacities
- Lung and/or chest wall compliance curves shifted to right
- FEV_1/FVC normal or elevated
- DL_{CO} normal or low

Obstructive

Variable Expiratory
- Low FEV_1/FVC, PEF
- Often mixed

Inspiratory and Expiratory
- Fixed obstructions: Foreign body Tumor

Variable Inspiratory
- Upper airway

Asthma
- Episodic
- FEV_1/FVC improves with bronchodilator or worsens with bronchoprovocation

COPD

Chronic Bronchitis
- Sputum production
- DL_{CO} normal
- RV, FRC high
- Low Pa_{O_2} with cyanosis
- High Pa_{CO_2}

Emphysema
- Low DL_{CO}
- Lung compliance curve shifted to left
- TLC, RV, FRC high
- Pa_{O_2} slightly low
- Pa_{CO_2} normal or slightly increased

V. TABLE OF NORMAL RESPIRATORY AND CIRCULATORY VALUES

	Term Newborn	1 Year	8 Years	Adult
Breaths/min	40	25	18	12
Tidal volume (mL/kg)	7	8	7	7
Dead space (mL/kg)	2	2	2.8	2
Alveolar ventilation (mL/kg)	130	120	80	60
Vital capacity (mL/kg)	40	45	60	60
Functional residual capacity (mL/kg)	28	25	40	35
Heart rate/min	133 ± 18	120 ± 2	85 ± 10	75 ± 5
Cardiac index (L/min/m^2)	2.5 ± 0.6	2.5 ± 0.6	4.0 ± 1.0	3.7 ± 0.3
Systolic blood pressure (mm Hg)*	73 ± 8	96 ± 30	100 ± 15	122 ± 30
Diastolic blood pressure (mm Hg)	50 ± 8	66 ± 25	56 ± 9	75 ± 20
Oxygen consumption (mL/kg/min)	6.0 ± 1.0	5.2 ± 1.0	4.9 ± 0.9	3.4 ± 0.6

*The lower limit for normal systolic blood pressure can be approximated by the formula 70 + (2 × age in years) for pediatric patients; the lower limit for normal systolic blood pressure for term newborns is 60 mm Hg. (Reproduced with permission from Levitzky MG, Hall SM, McDonough KH. *Cardiopulmonary Physiology in Anesthesiology.* New York: McGraw-Hill; 1997.)

VI. GENERAL SUGGESTED READINGS

Fishman AP, Elias JA, Fishman JA, Grippi MA, Kaiser LR, Senior RM, eds. *Fishman's Pulmonary Diseases and Disorders.* 3rd ed. New York, NY: McGraw-Hill; 1998.

Fishman AP, ed. *Handbook of Physiology, section 3: The Respiratory System,* Bethesda, Md: American Physiological Society.

Fishman AP, Fisher AB, eds. *Volume I: Circulation and Nonrespiratory Functions.* Bethesda, Md: American Physiological Society; 1985.

Cherniack NS, Widdicombe JG, eds. *Volume II: Control of Breathing, Parts 1 and 2.* Bethesda, Md: American Physiological Society; 1986.

Macklem PT, Mead J, eds. *Volume III: Mechanics of Breathing, Parts 1 and 2.* Bethesda, Md: American Physiological Society; 1986.

Farhi LE, Tenney SM, eds. *Volume IV: Gas Exchange.* Bethesda, Md: American Physiological Society; 1987.

Murray JF, Nadel JA, Mason RJ, Boushey HA, eds. *Textbook of Respiratory Medicine.* 3rd ed. Philadelphia, Pa: WB Saunders and Company; 2000.

Nunn JF. *Nunn's Applied Respiratory Physiology.* 4th ed. Oxford: Butterworth-Heinemann; 1993.

Index